THE ECOLOGY OF MALNUTRITION IN THE CARIBBEAN

The Bahamas, Cuba, Jamaica, Hispaniola (Haiti and the Dominican Republic), Puerto Rico, The Lesser Antilles, and Trinidad and Tobago

THE NUTRITIONAL NICHE

LAND AND WATER ENVIRONMENT= PHYSICAL GEOGRAPHY

FOOD PRODUCTION AND RESOURCES= ECONOMIC GEOGRAPHY

TRADITION AND CULTURE= HUMAN GEOGRAPHY

DIETS AND NUTRITIONAL DISEASES= MEDICAL GEOGRAPHY

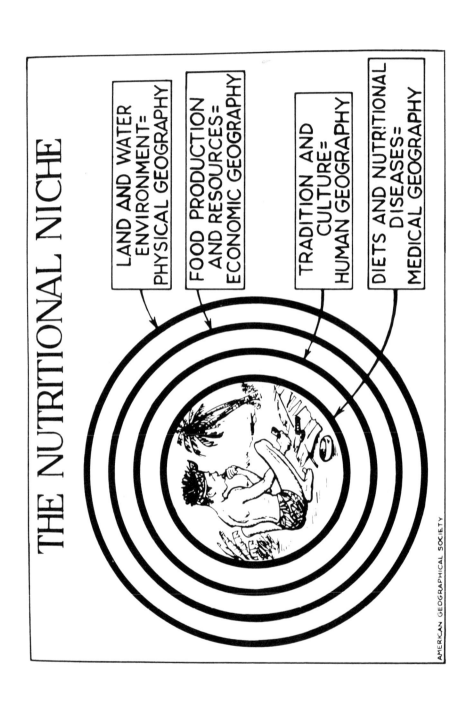

AMERICAN GEOGRAPHICAL SOCIETY

THE ECOLOGY OF MALNUTRITION IN THE CARIBBEAN

The Bahamas, Cuba, Jamaica, Hispaniola (Haiti and the Dominican Republic), Puerto Rico, The Lesser Antilles, and Trinidad and Tobago

by
Jacques M. May, M.D.
and
Donna L. McLellan

Studies in Medical Geography, Volume 12

HAFNER PRESS
NEW YORK
1973

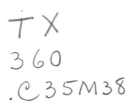

First Edition 1973

Printed and Published by

HAFNER PRESS
A Division of Macmillan Publishing Co., Inc.
866 Third Avenue
New York, N.Y. 10022

Library of Congress Catalog Number: 73-76140

ISBN: 02-848920-X

This study was sponsored by the Office, Chief of Research and Development, United States Army, under Contract No. DAAG17-71-C-0042 and was monitored by the Earth Sciences Division, Geographic Sciences Laboratory, United States Army Engineer Topographical Laboratories, Fort Belvoir, Virginia. The findings and interpretations contained herein are not to be regarded as reflecting official Department of the Army policy.

Printed in U.S.A. by
NOBLE OFFSET PRINTERS, INC.
New York, N.Y. 10003

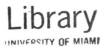

TABLE OF CONTENTS

Page

ACKNOWLEDGMENTS

The authors would like to thank Dr. Kendall King, Dr. Ivan Beghin and Dr. William Fougère for permission to reproduce tables from their very useful volume on Haiti entitled *L'Alimentation et la Nutrition en Haiti* (Paris, Presses Universitaires de France, 1970). Thanks also go to Dr. Henry Sebrell, Dr. Kendall King and their collaborators for sharing the valuable information compiled in their survey of the Dominican Republic. The authors are also indebted to Dr. Derrick B. Jelliffe, former Director of the Caribbean Food and Nutrition Institute, for making available the nutrition surveys carried out by the Institute. The chapter on diets in Puerto Rico relied heavily on the excellent series of surveys carried out by Dr. Nelson Fernández, Dr. Conrado Asenjo and their colleagues at the University of Puerto Rico. Miss Carmen Rosaly, Librarian at the Office of the Commonwealth of Puerto Rico in Washington, D.C., was very helpful in providing general information on Puerto Rico. Special thanks go to Dr. Jaime Suchlicki, Associate Director of Inter-American Studies at the University of Miami, and to Mr. Frank Soler of the *Miami Herald* for providing valuable documentation as well as personal communications on the situation in Cuba.

Dr. William Robison, Dr. Jack Planalp and Miss Pauline Riordan of the Earth Sciences Division, Geographic Sciences Laboratory at Fort Belvoir, carefully and critically reviewed the manuscript in draft. The authors are grateful for their constructive comments and observations. Thanks go to Mr. Tibor Toth for drawing the maps which enhance this volume. Finally, the book could not have been prepared without the very able assistance of our irreplacable secretary, Mrs. Rhoda Durkan, who typed the successive drafts of the manuscript.

INTRODUCTION

The Caribbean island group dealt with in this volume has a visage all its own. Located at the gateway to the great American continents, it bears the scars left by the various conquerors who fought for domination of the great land masses that lay beyond. For 300 years, Spain, France and Great Britain struggled for possession of the Caribbean islands and continued to fight well after the question of which culture would rule which parts of the continents had been settled. Some of the islands changed hands as many as 14 times, but somehow the economic, political and military forces at play eventually neutralized each other and a compromise resulted which is the frame for the ecological study we are presenting to our readers. Not that this pattern has any permanence. A newcomer—the Soviet Union—has now claimed an important foothold in the area and, like its predecessors, is challenging the whole structure of the lands well beyond the gate.

The modern history of the Caribbean can be viewed in three periods. The first was the period of the Spanish Conquest. The Spaniards initially landed by accident and, not knowing very well what to do, sought their Caribbean vocation in gold mining, cattle-raising, farming and propagation of the faith. It was during this period that the aboriginal Indian population practically disappeared as a result of the harsh treatment and diseases introduced by their conquerors.

The second period was the multinational sugar era. Before Napoleon discovered by necessity the sweet virtues of the beet root, the countries of Europe and North America were in need of cane sugar and there was a heavy demand for its byproduct, rum. This was the period when Great Britain was ready to exchange Canada for Guadeloupe, but the French would not let themselves be duped and preferred to keep their lucrative sugar island. This was also the period when Africans were imported en masse to work the canefields, eventually becoming the most significant population group of the islands. The third period could be called the tourist era. While sugar is still important, the hope of most of these islands is to replace the bounty that flowed from cane syrup with the income which flows from currency exchange counters. The dream of the canecutter is now to become a waiter in a tourist hotel. It is during this period that a new power never yet seen in these waters has taken a firm grip on one major island and, following the Caribbean tradition, has made sugar still more important to the Cuban economy than it ever was and foreign dominance still more compelling.

Whatever the period considered, the diets of the islanders have been poor. Preemption of land for sugar at the expense of food crops, reliance on imported foods which cost more than the common people can afford, lack of education about food values, all have played a role in creating malnutrition. Moreover, European or American continental wars have often cut off supplies, reinforcing dependence upon local resources that were not adequately husbanded. The traditional diet of imported cod, local beans, rice and a rich variety of fruits could have provided adequately balanced intakes, however monotonous and dreary. Why it did not and why (as in the rest of the developing world) the populations of the Caribbean islands have continuously suffered from malnutrition are questions which will be analyzed in the following pages.

CONVERSION TABLES

Weights and Measures

Metric Unit	Abbreviation	Approximate U.S. Equivalent
kilometer	km	0.62 miles
meter	m	39.37 inches — 1.09 yards
millimeter	mm	0.04 inches
square kilometer	sq km	0.3861 square miles
hectare	ha	2.47 acres
hectoliter	hl	26.4 gallons
liter	l	2.11 pints
milliliter	ml	0.06 cubic inches
metric ton	t	1.1 tons
quintal	q	220.46 pounds
kilogram	kg	2.2046 pounds
gram	g	0.035 ounces
milligram	mg	0.015 grains

Temperatures

Degrees Centigrade	Approximate Degrees Fahrenheit
0	32
5	41
10	50
15	59
20	68
25	77
30	86
35	95
40	104

Currencies

All local currencies have been converted into U.S. dollars.

THE COMMONWEALTH OF
THE BAHAMA ISLANDS

TABLE OF CONTENTS

THE COMMONWEALTH OF THE BAHAMA ISLANDS

I. BACKGROUND INFORMATION

A. PHYSICAL SETTING [3] [2] [4] [1] [17] [11]

The Bahama Islands are an archipelago of about 700 coralline islands or islets and more than 2,000 reefs stretching over 800 kilometers from the southeastern coast of Florida to the southern tip of Cuba. The total land area of the Bahamas is over 13,934 square kilometers but only about 30 islands are inhabited. The largest is Andros (4,144 square kilometers) while the most important one is relatively small (150 square kilometers) New Providence where the capital city of Nassau is located. Other important islands are Great and Little Abaco (2,010 square kilometers), Inagua (1,455 square kilometers), Grand Bahama (1,114 square kilometers) and Eleuthera (425 square kilometers).

The Bahamas are mainly flat or gently rolling. The highest point is on Cat Island (65.5 meters above sea level). Because the islands rise from two broad submarine banks, the offshore waters are generally shallow and dangerous for ocean-going vessels. Two indentations in the banks, however (Exuma Sound and Tongue of the Ocean), provide deepwater channels giving access to the various ports. Coral reefs abound on the eastern (windward) side of the islands, the longest being the 32-kilometer barrier reef off Andros Island.

The soils are shallow, comprising a thin layer over a coralline and oölitic limestone base. On higher, better drained land the soil tends to be reddish clay and in low-lying areas black, humus-rich loam and white sandy types. In general, fertility is low, water retention potentials are poor and the tendency toward erosion is high. Added to the general mediocre quality of the soil is the stony nature of the terrain, making cultivation difficult. In some places, farmers sow in potholes (called banana holes) which have filled with soil over time and can usually accommodate no more than one plant each.

3

Only the island of Andros has any real rivers and most water bodies found scattered over the islands are brackish salt-water reservoirs connected to the sea by underground natural crypts. Traditionally, rainwater has been collected for drinking purposes, and to meet the growing demands of the tourist industry, a desalination plant has been established on New Providence Island.

Considerable forests are found on Abaco, Grand Bahama, Andros and some smaller islands, with Caribbean pine dominating and providing a valuable source of income. Low scrub covers extensive areas of the islands and mangrove swamps are found in sheltered coastal regions. Edible grasses capable of supporting dairy herds are present on New Providence and Eleuthera.

B. CLIMATE   [2] [3] [4] [1] [17] [11]

The Bahamas lie in the path of the warm Gulf Stream which contributes to the prevalence of a subtropical climate. Winter temperatures average $21°C$ and the summer range is between $26°$ and $32°C$. Rainfall averages 1,143 millimeters annually and occurs mainly in May, June, September and October. The archipelago lies within the North American hurricane belt, but tropical storms seldom cause serious damage.

C. POPULATION [2] [4] [1] [13] [17] [12]

The 1970 population was estimated at 177,000 (see Table No. 1). Many of the islands are uninhabited, others are only sparsely settled. The greatest concentration of people is on New Providence where more than half of the total population lives. About 85 percent of the inhabitants are of African extraction, descendants of slaves brought to the islands during the American Revolution by the many Loyalists who migrated to the Bahamas. As in the other Caribbean islands, the black slaves were used as plantation labor, but following emancipation in 1834 they began farming small subsistence plots on the edges of the plantations. The remaining 15 percent of the present population is primarily Caucasian, although there are a few Asians. There are no survivors of the original Arawak Indian population, which was depleted between 1492 and 1550 when Spanish raiders carried off almost all the Indians to work in the mines of Cuba and Hispaniola and on the sugar plantations of the West Indies.

The rate of natural population increase is estimated to be around 2.3 percent per annum. In addition, there is some immigration of workers from Haiti and Jamaica. The infant mortality rate is about 45.8 per 1,000 live births. Education is free and compulsory between the ages of 5 and 14. The literacy rate is deemed to be fairly high.

D. HISTORY AND GOVERNMENT [12] [2]

The Bahamas were discovered by Columbus in 1492 when he made his first landfall in the New World at San Salvador (Watlings) Island. The Spaniards prospected the islands for silver and gold but found none and hence had no interest in colonizing. The native Indian inhabitants were sent off to work in other Spanish colonies. The islands remained unoccupied until 1629 when England claimed the Bahamas for herself. Only a few people came to the islands until the 1640's when a group of fortune seekers known as the "Eleutherian Adventurers" migrated from Bermuda to the Bahamas. Many were Independent Puritans seeking freedom from religious persecution. They named the island on which they settled Eleutheria (from the Greek *eleuthros* meaning "freedom") which was later contracted to Eleuthera.

The colonists found farming to be difficult on the hard limestone soil and soon preferred to try their luck at commerce, exporting tropical woods, turtles, seals, fish and ambergris. One of their main occupations, however, came to be salvaging ships which had run aground off the islands. Among the later settlers there was even a certain degree of deliberate shipwrecking. There were some attempts at establishing cotton plantations but production was never widespread and collapsed entirely with the abolition of slavery. The islands have never had a reliable agricultural export, although various crops, such as sisal and pineapples, have been tried. Sponge fishing was remunerative until the 1930's when disease and competition from synthetic substitutes killed the industry. Since the 1920's the Bahamas have been increasingly reliant upon tourism for income and the islands' present prosperity is due almost entirely to the tourist trade. Manufacturing began to develop in the 1960's due to favorable tax rates established at Freeport and Nassau.

The 1964 Constitution as amended in 1968 gives the Commonwealth of the Bahamas full internal self-government. Great Britain retains responsibility for defense and internal security through a Governor wh ɔ is the Queen's representative. The head of government is the Prime Minist.r who is the leader of the majority party in the bicameral legislature. There is a 16-seat Senate, nine of whose members are appointed by the Governor on advice of the Premier, four on the advice of the Leader of the Opposition and three at the Governor's own discretion. The 38 members of the General Assembly are elected by universal suffrage. Justice is administered by an independent judiciary.

E. AGRICULTURAL POLICIES [1] [16]

Agriculture is of only secondary importance to the economy of the Bahamas as a result of the emphasis placed on tourism. About three-fourths of the islands' food supply is purchased from abroad annually, but incomes are well above the average for the Caribbean and unemployment is relatively low so the inhabitants appear to be able to afford the expensive imported foods. Although agriculture is impeded by the thinness and poor quality of the soils, the rockiness of the terrain, the forests in areas where fertile land is located, the scarcity of water and the unreliability of interisland transportation, the Government has adopted a policy of improving and diversifying the production of food crops, and of increasing the output of cattle and pigs. A land resources survey was recently undertaken to determine the optimum utilization of all land and water resources.

F. FOREIGN AID

Due to the relative affluence of the Bahamas as a result of tourism, the island Commonwealth receives no external assistance.

II. FOOD RESOURCES

A. GENERAL [3] [2] [1] [17]

The total land area of the Bahamas does not exceed 14,000 square kilometers. The area under forests covers 316,000 hectares or just about 23.1 percent of the total. By contrast, only 14,170 hectares (or 1 percent of the total land area) are cultivated. Hence, it is obvious that the vast majority of the food consumed on the islands has to be imported or fished out of the sea. This is not surprising, given the history of the islands. As already pointed out, there is no extensive tradition of agriculture. Farming has never been a major occupation, although many of the inhabitants have at all times produced some food on a subsistence basis. Now, because of the tourist explosion, more interest than before seems to be focused on food production. However, agriculture is still practiced in very primitive ways, using the traditional pattern of crop rotation and shifting cultivation. Moreover, the soils are very poor and the farmers have to make do with a layer of topsoil less than 3 centimeters thick which limits the use of mechanical equipment. As in Africa, the stick and the hoe are the best tools for the circumstances. In some parts of the islands, ancient potholes filled with loam can be used for individual banana bulbs. When many of these holes are located in the same field, a banana grove can be established. In other places, the farmer creates cultivable craters by blasting a few holes in the limestone crust.

According to Bounds, the first year's planting consists of cabbages, tomatoes, corn, manioc, yams, pigeon peas, and beans. This is the year of plenty, but the next year only manioc and legumes will grow. The third year the yield drops substantially and the farmer moves elsewhere to initiate a new 3-year cycle. Successful application of such a system requires an extensive supply of cropland, which does not exist in the Bahamas. In any case, the yearly diminution of output on a single plot implies considerable inadequacy of subsistence crops. The small farmer also grows a few cash crops, including bananas, pineapples and all kinds of vegetables, for the hotel and tourist trade. Most of this garden production occurs on Cat Island where the soil is better than that of the other islands. Larger estates on Eleuthera, Great Abaco and Andros also engage in commercial cropping. It is estimated that while agricultural production and fishing now provide only about 33 percent of the total food requirements, in the future this percentage will increase as a result of the introduction of modern techniques.

B. MEANS OF PRODUCTION

1. Agricultural Labor Force [3] [1] [16]

Estimates of the agricultural labor force vary from 10 to 15 percent of the total work force. This would represent approximately 7,000-8,000 people based on a total force of about 55,000 people (1963 census: 51,948). A similar number of people work in construction, while in 1963 about 25 percent were engaged in personal services (hotels and tourism). By now there must be some 14,000 people working in this last occupation. There is virtually no unemployment on the islands. The demand for labor in the timber industry has to be met by attracting immigrants from other islands. There used to be a seasonal migration of workers from the Bahamas to the United States but this was canceled by the U.S. Government after 1965. There is no minimum wage.

Thirty-eight percent of the farmhands are females. Young men view agricultural work as demeaning and conducive to poverty because of the poor results obtained on unfertile soil. This attitude may change when returns from agriculture increase in value and quantity as a result of the influx of tourists, and when the use of mechanical equipment wherever soil conditions permit makes farming more prestigious.

2. Farms [1] [2] [17]

Only 2,849 square kilometers of the islands' total land are privately-owned. The rest, which is mostly rocky, barren or swampy, is owned by the Crown. Crown land includes many islets or cays which can be rented on a lease basis for 2-5 years during which time the tenant is required to make some permanent improvements. Most of the privately-owned land is on New Providence where the capital city of Nassau is located.

Food is produced on small- and medium-sized farms, some consisting of tiny separate plots, some of one integrated piece of land. However, the trend is toward larger estates which can be exploited economically. Much land has now been cleared on Great Abaco, Andros, Eleuthera and Cat islands. The largest of these commercial farms, catering to the United States market as well as to the tourist trade, have been established at Marsh Harbor on Great Abaco and at Mastic Point and Fresh Creek on Andros. The climate works to their advantage, permitting the winter sale of crops in the U.S. when prices are high.

3. Fertilizers and Mechanical Equipment [5] [2]

There is no information on the amount of fertilizer used in the Bahamas. Bounds reports that an American earthmoving company has devised a limestone crusher which can change any rocky field into an acceptable soil which needs only to be adequately fertilized and mineralized to provide crops. The extent to which this is done has not been reported but obviously such an operation is undoubtedly too costly for the small farmer. There are no recent and reliable statistics on the mechanical equipment used in the Bahamas. It must be very limited and available only to the few large estates now in the process of expansion.

C. PRODUCTION [1]

Agricultural production in the Bahamas is estimated to total $8 million annually by value. Adding fishing and forestry, the total rises to make a $14.4 million contribution to the gross national product.

1. Food Crops [2] [1] [5]

Local production provides about 33 percent of the islands' food needs. Fruits and vegetables, grown mostly on small farms, include mangoes, avocados, papayas, pineapples, citrus fruit, melons, tomatoes, onions, cucumbers, cabbage, legumes of many kinds, potatoes, eggplants and pumpkins. While cucumbers and tomatoes were at one time important exports to Florida, cultivation of these crops is said to be diminishing as more land is devoted to the expansion of the sugar industry. Tomatoes occupy 500 hectares.

2. Cash Crops [2] [1] [5]

Many Bahamian food crops are also cash crops. As stated earlier, pineapples, tomatoes, yams and other foodstuffs originate on Cat Island and are sold on the Bahamian market. Bananas from northern Eleuthera feed the local and tourist markets for 9 months of the year. Dwarf Cavendish and Sugar are the most popular of the banana varieties. Citrus fruits are grown in all the inhabited islands but commercial production of Valencia, seedless and navel oranges, limes, lemons, tangerines, and grapefruit is concentrated mostly in Nassau nurseries. Tomatoes have lost ground on the export market since 1961 when Florida production began to increase, but the local market absorbs great quantitities during the winter months. Dried onions (Texas Grand) are produced on Eleuthera and Exuma. Fresh and dried pigeon peas are still harvested, but commerical production is limited because of the high cost of labor. Sisal, mostly grown on Cat Island, provides the raw material for the handicrafts sold to tourists at Nassau's famous straw market. There, baskets, mats, handbags and hats of every description are sold, bringing an income of $1.5 million a year, some of which goes into the farmers' pockets. A sugarcane plantation has recently been established in the central and northern area of Great Abaco Island covering 6,680 hectares. This plantation supplies the rum distillery of the Bahamas and exports some sugar to the United States. The establishment of this estate may explain the drop in sugar imports in recent years (see *Trade*).

3. Animal Husbandry [2] [1] [5]

a. *Livestock and Poultry*

The climate of the Bahamas facilitates animal husbandry. A herd of 4,000 cattle, located mostly at Rock Sound in southern Eleuthera, provides milk and high quality meat on the local market. The herd is composed mostly of Charolais stock, reputed for the quality of their meat. Cows, mainly Holstein and a few Jerseys imported from the U.S. and Canada, supply milk for local consumption. Yearling bulls are exported in small numbers. Pig-raising is high on the list of expansion plans. The number of these animals has risen from a yearly average of 8,000 in 1952 to 11,000 in 1968. The mild climate without extremes favors the development of sheep, which number 24,000. Goats, whose meat is a favorite of the local population, number 14,000 and the size of the herd has remained static for the last 20 years. There are an estimated 650,000 chickens in the islands.

b. *Meat, Milk and Eggs*

Meat is provided by beef cattle, pigs and poultry. In 1969 the poultry industry was considered to be self-supporting and capable of meeting all local demands. There are two large dairy herds, one on New Providence, the other at Hatchet Bay on Eleuthera. The value of the meat obtained from cattle, sheep, goats and pigs was estimated at $300,000 in 1969. Fresh and reconstituted milk are also produced at Hatchet Bay—2,000 tons of cow's milk and 3,000 tons of goat's milk. Milk is always in short supply. Fresh and frozen chicken is another output of Hatchet Bay. The value of the eggs, broilers and milk produced in the islands in 1968 was estimated at $5.5 million.

4. Fisheries [1]

Fishing takes place almost everywhere, but the most important grounds are on the Great and Little Bahama boats. The variety of fish is considerable. Crayfish, or spiny lobster, is the most important export of the fishing industry. All boats and equipment are owned by individuals. Exporters and buyers operate under licenses issued by the Ministry of Agriculture and Fisheries. The season for crayfish begins on September 1st and ends on March 15th. Licensed buyers export whole crayfish to Miami and West Palm Beach, Florida.

The next important exportable sea product is really not a fish but a reptile: the turtle. Loggerhead, hawksbill and green species all live in the waters of the Commonwealth. In 1968 the landings at Nassau amounted to 1,260 bundles of turtle meat weighing 34,000 kilos. An equal amount was brought in on the out islands.* Conch is a traditional element of the Bahamian diet and the export of both meat and shell is prohibited due to the increasing scarcity of the species. Over 1 million conch worth $217,000 are landed at Nassau each year. Fishing is done by about 3,500 men, all individual boat owners. They sell their landings at the Nassau wharfs directly to the consumers or to exporters.

D. FOOD INDUSTRIES [2] [1]

While manufacturing is not extensively developed, there are a few modern prosperous food industries. Frozen lobster tails, tomatoes and pineapples are all processed for export. A rum distillery located at New Providence exports some of its output to the United Kingdom. The plant can also process 50,000 tons of sugar annually. A brewery and a mineral water plant also operate at New Providence. Salt is an important resource and two large companies, one at Great Inagua, the other at Long Island, export their salt all over the world. Canning of tomatoes is done at Eleuthera.

According to Bounds, at the beginning of 1969 there were 82 industrial enterprises in the Bahamas, not all of them directly concerned with food. Thirty-one were located in Nassau, 47 in Freeport and four in some of the out islands. Table No. 2 summarizes the main agricultural and industrial activities of the 10 most important islands.

E. TRADE [1] [2] [6]

The economy of the Bahamas is really based on the growing tourist trade from North America. The number of visitors reached 1 million in 1968 and is still increasing. This influx creates a demand for food, stimulates agriculture and creates jobs. The income derived offsets the trade deficit incurred as a result of having to import about three-fourths of the food needed in the islands. In 1967, for instance, the trade deficit amounted to $133,539,636 but was amply balanced by the $145 million spent in the islands by a million visitors.

Table No. 3 shows the kinds and quantities of imported food items needed to support the Commonwealth's 177,000 inhabitants and its over 1 million visitors. The most important single food import item, in terms of both quantity and cost, is meat, followed by a variety of cereals (wheat, rice and corn) in terms of

---

*Bahamians consider New Providence to be the center of their world and all the other islands are consequently referred to as "the out islands."

quantity, and beverages (mainly alcoholic drinks) in terms of value. Only a fraction of the alcoholic beverages are purchased by local inhabitants, who probably consume their own rum. Most of the wheat imported is consumed in the form of bread. The importation of sugar has diminished drastically since 1963, reflecting the increase in domestic production which followed the establishment of local sugar refineries.

Agricultural exports still remain significant and consist mainly of tomatoes, cucumbers (either fresh or pickled), peppers, squash, papayas, pineapples, eggplant and salt. Nonedible exports include pulpwood. Forest products, together with cement, which is probably the largest single item of export, are also the largest cash earners. The following tables indicate the most important domestic exports and the Commonwealth's major trading partners.

Principal Domestic Exports – Bahamas, 1966 and 1967
(in million tons)

Item	1966	1967
Pulpwood	3.5	3.7
Salt	1.9	1.2
Crayfish	.5	.7
Cucumbers	.05	.04
Rum	3.0	4.6
Cement	4.8	6.2

Source: Barclays Bank D.C.O. *The Bahamas.*

Main Recipients of Bahama Exports, 1966 and 1967
(in percent)

Country	1966	1967
United States	82.0	75.0
United Kingdom	7.1	9.4
Canada	.4	6.5
Others	10.5	9.1

Source: Barclays Bank D.C.O. *The Bahamas.*

These tables illustrate the small role agriculture plays in the export trade of the Bahamas and the growing importance of pulpwood, rum and cement. The expansion of the British and Canadian markets at the expense of the United States is also worth considering.

F. FOOD SUPPLY

1. Storage [1] [2] [3] [17]

There is no published information on the food supply of the Bahama Islands at the household or national warehouse levels. Only very general conclusions can be drawn from other facts elicited by this research: mainly that there are no food shortages and none are likely to occur because of the tradition of fishing. The nearness of the sea cancels out to a large extent the problems of cold storage. Moreover, the wharves, warehouses and storage rooms which are sufficient to keep the reserves needed for 1 million visitors a year must be sufficient to keep the food needed by the 177,000 permanent inhabitants, half of whom live in Nassau near the storage space. The problem of supplying food to little islands with few inhabitants does not appear to present any major difficulty because of the abundance of small farms whose output should be sufficient for both subsistence and commercial needs, and because of the possibility of improvising interisland transportation by sea and air as needed.

While there seems to be no problem in bringing food to the Bahamas, there is a problem of water supply. There are no natural sources of fresh water except at Andros where two small rivers exist. All other ponds and bodies of water are brackish because of their underground communication with the sea. Rainwater is collected in cisterns from roofs and slopes and a seawater desalination plant operates in New Providence. This plant provided 3 million gallons a day until 1970 when the capacity was raised to 4.5 million gallons daily. The cost of 1,000 gallons to the consumer is $1.40.

2. Transportation [3] [2]

New Providence has 306 kilometers, Eleuthera 161 kilometers and Grand Bahama 105 kilometers of motorable roads maintained by the Government. Good roads exist or are being built on Great Abaco, Cat, San Salvador, Long Island, Great and Little Exuma, Andros (which already had 40 kilometers), Crooked Island, Mayaguana and Great Inagua. Many roads owned and maintained by private enterprises also exist. There are large airports at Nassau on New Providence and Freeport and West End on Grand Bahama. There are also 41 smaller airports and airstrips for interisland communications. Where no landing strips exist, seaplanes are used. The main seaports are Nassau, Freeport and Matthew Town (on Inagua).

III. DIETS

A. GENERAL [6] [1] [2]

One of the most important facts concerning the diets of Bahamians is that the small amount of arable land makes it impossible for the territory to support its permanent population on indigenous agricultural resources. The history of Bahamian diets has been a succession of periods of plentiful imports separated by long periods of belt-tightening depressions. These were usually correlated with the great wars of history which temporarily brought navigation in the area to a halt. The American Revolutionary War, the Napoleonic wars, the American Civil War and finally the First World War were such periods. The American Prohibition Era, by contrast, was a period of prosperity for the islands, where bootlegging flourished. The tourist boom, which began in the early 20th century and gained momentum with the commercialization of air travel, finally brought consistently good diets to the Bahamians.

B. NATIVE DIETS

Native diets have been based on fish or other seafood, especially conch which is consumed mostly as a chowder but is also prepared in the form of fritters eaten with rice and chilies. Green turtle soup, peas and rice fried with onions, salt pork and herbs, baked crabs and roast chicken are all popular native dishes. Snacking is becoming increasingly popular. Although snacks were always part of the African way of life, eaten when the occasion presented itself, they used to consist of berries, fruit and small animals or fish caught on the spot. Even very young children knew how to make the most of these opportunities, and adolescents as well as adults were not slow in picking up mangoes in season or roasting a small rodent on an improvised wooden fire. Now, however, it appears that with increased Westernization, traditional feeding habits have changed. It has been estimated that 80 percent of the people live according to Western standards practically all the time while the rest are still living and eating according to a mixed pattern of ancient and new. An older Bahamian housewife is quoted as saying that she does not prepare meals any more because her whole family snacks outside continuously; but a typical snack nowadays consists of saltines and a bowl of conch soup washed down with Coca-Cola. The caloric value of such a mixture cannot be measured without knowing how many crackers, how much soup, how many bottles of Coke.

Turning to the food import list, it appears that about 12,355 tons of meat are imported per year for the 177,000 inhabitants and over 1 million tourists. An average stay of 5 days per tourist and 365 days per permanent resident would give 5 million man days for visitors and 64 million man days for the inhabitants, or a total of 69 million man days of food consumption. This would yield an approximate availability of 175 grams of imported meat per capita per day, a more than satisfactory intake. Cereals, most of which are eaten by the local population, would come to about 2 kilos per capita per day by applying the same speculative computation. If the average tourist stay in the Bahamas were 10 days per person instead of 5, then the meat and cereal availabilities would drop to 166 grams and 1.8 kilograms, respectively, which is still more than acceptable, even after animal feed and other preemptions have been deducted. As a result of this quick review, it would seem that malnutrition does not exist in the Bahamas, at least not on the basis of food availability. Consumption is another matter, and there is the possibility that the distribution of resources is less equitable than appears. Tourists can and do waste as much food as they consume. But then—in compensation—we have not introduced into our computation the local resources in meat, fish, dairy products, fruits and vegetables.

IV. ADEQUACY OF FOOD RESOURCES

According to the figures available, while only 33 percent of the total consumption of foodstuffs is derived from local resources, the island is nearing self-sufficiency in milk, eggs and dairy products, as well as in some kinds of meats. Given also the abundant resources in seafood, it can be safely concluded that the food resources of the Bahamas are adequate to feed the permanent population and the considerable surplus of temporary visitors represented by tourists. Only a combination of blockade and hurricanes could conceivably create a problem of food supply, but in such an instance, tourists would stay away, thus substantially reducing the number of consumers. How the 177,000 inhabitants would fare under these circumstances is impossible to guess but undoubtedly a very serious situation would be created since they would have to survive on very limited domestic resources.

V. NUTRITIONAL DISEASE PATTERNS [3]

No nutrition survey has been conducted in the Bahamas, hence a description of the patterns of nutritional diseases is impossible. However, it is stated that the main diseases observed in the islands are: "chest ailments" (which probably means tuberculosis of the respiratory system), diseases of early infancy, and "social diseases" resulting from poor housing and lack of sanitation in certain areas. Principal causes of death are listed as gastroenteritis, pneumonia, cancer, anemia, tetanus and cirrhosis of the liver. This list strongly suggests the existence of malnutrition in the children dying of gastroenteritis. Moreover, the likelihood that the anemias are of nutritional origin is high in an area where no malaria is reported and the incidence of hookworm must be extremely light due to the stoniness of the soil. The possibility that the tetanus cases observed originated in contamination through the umbilical cord is also high, as wound contamination would be accidental and not listed as a health problem. A picture of very low levels of public health and nutrition among certain isolated population groups thus comes to mind. While the numbers must be small, there seems to be little doubt that cases of deficiency diseases are probably found among those who are not participating in the prosperity brought about by the tourist trade.

VI. CONCLUSIONS

The emergence of a country like the Commonwealth of the Bahamas is a new phenomenon, representative of the mid-20th century. Tourists who used to be the frosting on the economic cake have become the cake itself. Examples are few, indeed, of nations that can afford $165 million of foreign purchases while earning only $32 million from exports and still maintain a balance of payments surplus. A tourist industry providing 87.8 percent of the cost of imports is a rare experience. It makes it difficult to assess what is the carrying capacity of the land—the "ecological ratio" of population to habitat resources. Yet, such a ratio is important to know since the tourist trade could conceivably fail, leaving the Commonwealth to its own devices. As long as the tourist boom lasts, however, the growth and development of the Bahama Islands seems secure.

BIBLIOGRAPHY

1. Barclays Bank D.C.O. *The Bahamas.* Economic Survey. London, Barclays Bank, 1969.

2. Bounds, J.H. "The Bahamas." *Focus,* 1969, XIX (9), 1-7.

3. British Information Services. "The Bahamas." *Fact Sheets on the Commonwealth.* New York, BIS, 1968.

4. *Encyclopedia Britannica.* Chicago, William Benton Publisher, 1970.

5. Food and Agriculture Organization of the United Nations. *Production Yearbook 1969.* Volume 23. Rome, FAO, 1970.

6. _____ . *Trade Yearbook 1969.* Volume 23. Rome, FAO, 1970.

7. Inter-American Development Bank. *Eleventh Annual Report.* Washington, D.C., IDB, 1970.

8. _____ . *Socio-Economic Progress in Latin America.* Social Progress Trust Fund. Tenth Annual Report. Washington, D.C., IDB, 1970.

9. International Bank for Reconstruction and Development. *Statement of Loans.* Washington, D.C., IBRD, 1971.

10. International Development Association. *Statement of Development Credits.* Washington, D.C., IDA, 1971.

11. James, P.E. *Latin America*. Fourth Edition. New York, The Odyssey Press, 1969.

12. Paxton, J. Ed. *The Statesman's Yearbook 1970-1971*. New York, St. Martin's Press, 1970.

13. United Nations (Department of Economic and Social Affairs). *Demographic Yearbook 1969*. New York, UN, 1970.

14. United Nations Children's Fund. *Digest of Projects Aided by UNICEF in the Americas*. New York, UNICEF, 1969.

15. United Nations Development Program. *Projects in the Special Fund Component as of January 31, 1971*. DP/SF/Reports Series B, No. 11. New York, UNDP, 1971.

16. U.S. Department of Agriculture (Economic Research Service). *Agriculture and Trade of the Caribbean Region*. ERS-Foreign 309. Washington, D.C., U.S. Government Printing Office, 1971.

17. West R.C. and Augelli, J.P. *Middle America: Its Lands and Peoples*. Englewood Cliffs, Prentice Hall, 1966.

LIST OF TABLES

LIST OF MAPS

TABLE NO. 1

Population by Islands – Bahama Islands, 1963-1970

Island	1963 Census	1970 Estimate
Abacos	6,527	8,802
Acklins	1,235	1,655
Andros	7,560	10,185
Berry Islands	266	336
Bimini	1,704	2,299
Cat Island	3,145	4,230
Cay Labos	6	8
Crooked Island	794	1,039
Eleuthera	7,283	9,803
Exuma	3,445	4,635
Grand Bahama	8,490	11,430
Harbour Island	1,005	1,355
Inagua	1,252	1,672
Long Cay	34	45
Long Island	4,177	5,612
Mayaguana	708	953
New Providence	81,592	110,117
Ragged Island	389	484
Rum Cay	81	101
San Salvador	971	1,286
Spanish Wells	861	1,141
	131,525	177,188

Source: After Barclays Bank D.C.O. *The Bahamas.*

TABLE NO. 2

Agricultural and Industrial Activity – Bahamas, 1970

Island	Agriculture	Industry
New Providence	Nurseries for a variety of citrus fruits.	Tourism, brewery, mineral water plant, rum distillery, sugar refinery, processing of turtle meat, freezing of lobster tails.
Great Abaco	Commercial farm at Marsh Harbor, sugarcane plantation of 6,680 hectares, pineapples.	Pulpwood, crayfish processing, conch processing.
Bimini	Cucumbers, tomatoes, sugarcane.	Marine laboratory, Bahamas Agricultural Industries, Ltd. treating sugarcane.
Freeport		Bahamas Cement Co., Syntex Corporation, Bahamas Oil Refinery.
Eleuthera	Dairy farm at Hatchet Bay in central Eleuthera, poultry for the Bahamas market, food crops, truck gardening, pineapples, citrus fruit, bananas, onions in northern Eleuthera, tomatoes, cattle ranch at Rock Sound in southern Eleuthera.	Tomato canning, freezing of chicken, milk processing at Hatchet Bay.
Exuma	Palm trees, onions.	Tourism, preparation of palm straws, drying of onions.
Andros	Commercial farm at Mastic Point, year-round garden agriculture (cucumbers, squashes, peppers, tomatoes), underwater farming of lobster, crab, conch turtles.	Pulpwood cutting by the Bahama Agricultural Industries, Ltd.
Great Inagua		Salt processing (Diamond Co., Morton Co.).
Long Island		Salt processing.
Cat Island	Sisal, pineapples, tomatoes, yams.	Sisal processing.

Sources: Barclays Bank D.C.O. *The Bahamas.*
          J.H. Bounds, "The Bahamas."

TABLE NO. 3

Food Imports – Bahama Islands, 1963-1967

Food Item	Quantity (tons)		Value ($1,000)	
	1963	1968	1963	1968
Bovine cattle	3,170	5,320	357	671
Poultry ⎰ fresh, chilled	496	876	492	761
Other meats ⎱ and frozen	6	55	12	112
Meat preserves (dried, salted)	1,856	2,630	1,535	2,625
Bacon and other preserved pig meat	910	1,258	818	1,440
Other offals	945	1,372	717	1,185
Other preserves	521	844	439	715
	7,904	12,355	4,370	7,509
Milk and cream (evaporated, condensed, dry, fresh)	NA	NA	1,196	1,702
Butter	667	693	397	659
Cheese and curd	240	365	247	426
Eggs in shell	40	59	28	40
Cereals (wheat, rice, corn)	11,800	14,600	1,570	2,320
Lemons and limes	17	68	9	36
Apples	460	1,100	124	254
Potatoes	2,510	3,480	257	368
Legumes	240	320	84	143
Onions	785	1,047	106	165
Sugar (raw basis)	3,700	1,900	790	470
Coffee	80	120	120	190
Tea	21	44	73	125
Margarine	1,552	1,796	576	771
Beverages	NA	NA	5,400	6,900
Animal fats	130	190	69	115
Total other food imports	22,242	25,782	11,046	14,684
Total all food imports	30,146	38,137	15,416	22,193

Source: Food and Agriculture Organization of the United Nations. *Trade Yearbook 1969.*

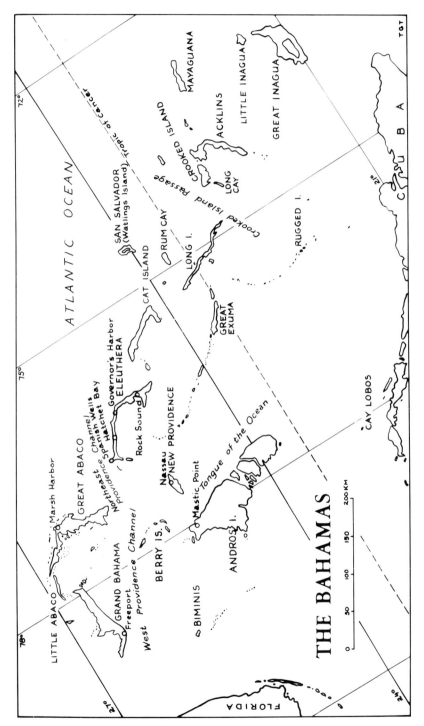

MAP NO. I.

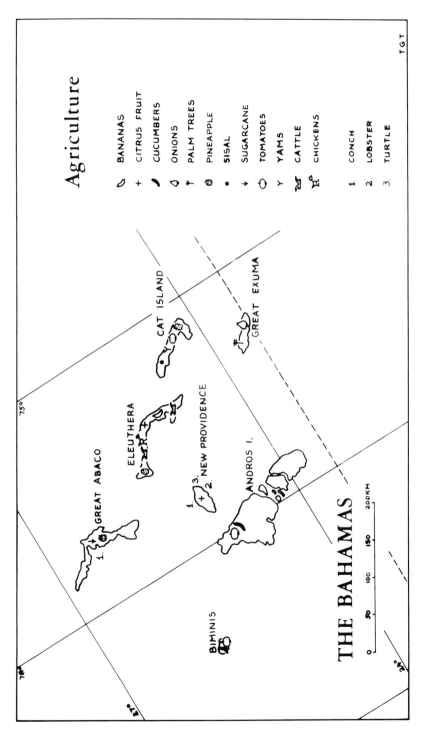

Agriculture

∂ BANANAS
+ CITRUS FRUIT
⊃ CUCUMBERS
∂ ONIONS
🌴 PALM TREES
🍍 PINEAPPLE
• SISAL
→ SUGARCANE
○ TOMATOES
Y YAMS
CATTLE
CHICKENS

1. CONCH
2. LOBSTER
3. TURTLE

GREAT ABACO

ELEUTHERA

CAT ISLAND

NEW PROVIDENCE

GREAT EXUMA

ANDROS I.

BIMINIS

THE BAHAMAS

0   50   100   150   200KM

TGT

MAP NO. 2.

THE REPUBLIC OF CUBA

TABLE OF CONTENTS

INTRODUCTION

A discussion of Cuban diets in 1972 is made difficult by the absence of incontrovertible sources on the subject of nutrition as well as data pertaining to the infrastructure of Cuban diets. Information sources on Cuba fall into three categories:

1. Those tainted with an overwhelming favorable bias;
2. Those tainted with an overwhelming unfavorable bias; and
3. Those which are favorable to the revolution but deplore the way it has been conducted.

To those of the first category there are hardly any dark sides to the changes that have occurred in Cuba since 1959 and the few negative aspects they see are blamed on the United States. To the second group, nothing has been accomplished which would justify the events of the last decade. To the last group, most of the faults identified in Cuba since the revolution should be charged to the incompetence and prideful ignorance of the leaders and to the lack of skilled personnel.

The present authors have tried their best to present and analyze the facts impartially.

THE REPUBLIC OF CUBA

I. BACKGROUND INFORMATION

A. PHYSICAL SETTING [38] [24] [65] [5] [4] [6]

The island of Cuba lies 90 nautical miles from Key West, Florida, at the entrance to the Gulf of Mexico, between parallels 19°49' and 23°15' north and meridians 74°8' and 84°57' west. The island extends for 1,256 kilometers in an east-west direction and the width varies from 40 to 192 kilometers. Cuba is the largest of the Antilles: the total area of the island is 114,524 square kilometers, including the Isle of Pines (3,061 square kilometers) and some adjacent islets. The island enjoys a coastline of about 3,500 kilometers with an unusually large number of good harbors. There are many swampy areas along the shoreline covered by mangrove forests, especially along the southern coast. Cuba is the least mountainous of the Greater Antilles, with an average elevation of about 100 meters above sea level. Gently sloping land and plains characterize three-fourths of the countryside, thus making cultivation and transportation relatively easy. Over 200 rivers drain Cuba, most of them originating along the island's axis and running in a northerly or southerly direction. In general they are short; the longest and most important river is the Cauto which extends 249 kilometers in western Oriente Providence and waters the Central Valley (see Map No. 1).

There are three mountain complexes on the island: the eastern, the central and the western. The eastern system, which covers most of Oriente Province and extends into Camagüey, is composed primarily of the Sierra Maestra running parallel to the southern coast, and a northern coastal range which includes the Sierra de Nipe and the Cuchillas de Toar. The highest elevation in Cuba occurs in the Sierra Maestra at Pico-Turquino (1,973 meters). Between the southern and northern ranges of the eastern system lies the Central Valley. The central mountain complex is smaller in area and lower in elevation than the eastern. The most important ranges of this system are the Trinidad and Sancti Spíritus

27

mountains. The western mountain system consists mainly of the Sierra de los Organos and the Sierra del Rosario. Here the basic rock is limestone, honeycombed with caves due to progressive erosion by water. There are also tall columns of erosion-resistant rocks resembling organ pipes which have given the Sierra de los Organos its name. Below the strange limestone formations of this region lie flat valleys of irregular shape.

Limestone is the basic ingredient of Cuban soils, which generally have a high clay content. The red clay soils of Matanzas, southern La Habana and western Camagüey provinces are among the best on the island. These soils are deep and have excellent permeability, supporting such crops as sugarcane, rice and vegetables. Another zone of fertile soil is found in the plain north of Cienfuegos Bay and the plain running from the Sancti Spíritus mountains to the Caribbean coast. Alluvial soils, when they occur, are fertile; however, they are found only in the narrow flood plains bordering rivers and streams. The soils of the Central Valley and Guantánamo Basin in eastern Cuba are compatible with sugarcane production. Fairly large areas of sandy soils are found in southern Pinar del Río, western Las Villas and part of Camagüey Province. These soils are characterized by an inability to retain much moisture, and hence support only sparse vegetation, such as palm trees, shrubs and grass suitable for pasturage. The plains of Camagüey have good soils capable of sustaining sugarcane cultivation.

Ecologically, Cuba can be divided into four regions: western, central, east-central and eastern.

The Western Region

The western region encompasses the provinces of Pinar del Río, La Habana and Matanzas. It extends to the savannas of western Las Villas Province and covers about 26 percent of the island's surface. About 40 percent of the country's population inhabits this sector. In the extreme west is the lowland area of Cape San Antonio where the soils range from medium to poor and there is little agriculture except for a small area of rice cultivation. To the northeast of the Cape is the Sierra de los Organos, interspersed with a number of fertile valleys where tobacco farming is the primary activity. To the east of the Sierra de los Organos is the Sierra del Rosario where coffee is cultivated in the high valleys. The southern plain of Pinar del Río is used primarily for pastures due to the poor quality of the soil. In places where fertilizers have been used, however, tobacco is raised (*Vuelta Abajo* region) and in certain areas irrigation has stimulated rice production. The so-called red plains of La Habana and Matanzas provinces are the sites of sugarcane, rice, pineapple, plantain, vegetable and other crop production. Much of the non-cane agricultural produce is marketed in the city of Habana and its suburbs. The peninsula of Zapata is covered with mangrove swamps and hence is relatively unpopulated. Its few inhabitants earn their livelihood primarily by making charcoal.

Central Region

The central region covers most of Las Villas Province, with the exception of the Zapata Peninsula, and a small portion of western Camagüey Province. It includes about 20 percent of Cuba's territory and an equal percentage of its population. In the western part of Las Villas the Trinidad Mountains dominate, and east of the Ayabama River the highlands continue as the Sancti Spíritus Mountains. In those valleys where agriculture can be practiced, coffee, sugarcane and tobacco are the main crops. North of the Trinidad Mountains are the rolling Santa Clara Hills where cattle are grazed and tobacco is cultivated. Still farther north, in the valleys of the Sagua la Grande and Sagua la Chica rivers and along the coastal plain, the soils are very productive, supporting sugarcane and tobacco cultivation. To the west of the Trinidad-Sancti Spiritus mountains is the plain of Cienfuegos, which is very fertile and hence intensively cultivated in sugar. Population density in this area is very high. To the east of the Sancti Spíritus mountains another plain extends to the coast and it, too, is a very productive zone with sugarcane, tobacco, dairy products and some rice as the primary commodities.

East-Central Region

The east-central region extends from western Camagüey Province to Nipe Bay in northwestern Oriente Province, giving a home to about 25 percent of the Cuban population. The western part of Camagüey Province consists mainly of La Trocha Plain, which runs the width of the island and which encompasses some of the country's most fertile soils. Sugarcane, pineapples, oranges, potatoes, rice and other crops are grown. The Central Plain, which runs from the city of Camagüey southeastward to Holguín in Oriente Province is covered with savanna and represents Cuba's major livestock area. About 20 percent of the island's cattle population grazes on the pastures of the Central Plain where the soil is too sandy and gravelly to support crop cultivation. Legumes and other staple food crops are cultivated around Holguín where heavier soils permit agriculture. To the north and south of the central lowland, where other plains slope gently to the Atlantic and Caribbean coasts, sugarcane is produced, and in parts of the southern plain livestock is raised.

The Eastern Region

The eastern region covers most of Oriente Province, from Holguín eastward. It encompasses around 20 percent of the island's territory and the same proportion of the population. A broad plain drained by the Río Cauto extends from around Nipe Bay to the Gulf of Guacanayabo but is not heavily populated. The Guacanayabo coastal area is marshy but inland, around Bayamo, livestock-raising is an important activity. Sugarcane is produced wherever possible, but extensive flooding during the rainy season prohibits agriculture in many places. The eastern region includes the Sierra Maestra which represents the most rugged terrain on the island. The southern slopes of the Sierra are practically uninhabited and are covered with dense forests, but coffee is cultivated in the valleys of the northern slopes. The eastern and northeastern parts of Oriente Province are covered by the Highlands of Baracoa, large parts of which still remain to be penetrated. Bananas, coffee and cocoa are cultivated around the coastal city of Baracoa. To the west of the Baracoa Highlands are the Nipe Mountains which create a broad plateau covered with pine trees. The soils there are too poor for cultivation but they are rich in deposits of iron, aluminum, manganese and other minerals which are being mined for export. Between the Sierra Maestra to the south and the Sierra de Nipe and Sierra de Toar to the northeast, lie the fertile Central Valley and Guantánamo Basin. Sugarcane is the major crop in both lowland areas and coffee is grown on the mountain slopes.

B. CLIMATE [24] [38] [67]

Although it lies within the torrid zone, the island of Cuba enjoys a maritime subtropical climate due to the tempering effect of trade winds. Seasonal temperature averages for the island range from 21.1°C in January and February to 27.2°C in July and August. As could be expected, temperatures decrease with elevation. Freezing temperatures are frequently recorded in the mountains but minimum readings below 10°C are rare elsewhere, as are maximums above 32.2°C.

Since temperatures throughout the year vary only slightly, the change of seasons is marked by rainfall rather than temperature. The rainy season lasts from May through October and the dry season from November through April. In 1968 the average precipitation for the whole island was 1,437 millimeters with 75 percent of the rainfall occurring during the summer months. The mountains of Pinar del Río receive the heaviest precipitation (over 1,700 millimeters) and the Guantánamo Basin receives the least (under 1,270 millimeters), but no area is deficient in rainfall. Cuba lies within the hurricane zone and is frequently ravaged by tropical storms.

C. POPULATION [67] [61] [58] [55]

In 1970 the estimated population of Cuba was 8.66 million and the overall density was about 75 persons per square kilometer. The area of greatest population concentration is La Habana Province (about 250 inhabitants per square kilometer) and the most sparsely populated is Camagüey Province (approximately 30 per square kilometer). Table No. 1 shows the population distribution by province as estimated in 1967. Rural inhabitants represent 41.6 percent of the total. The overall rate of population increase is about 2.3 percent per year and the rate of urbanization is about 2.45 percent per annum. The infant mortality rate is reported to be 37.6 per 1,000 live births, an increase from 33 per 1,000 in 1958. Almost half of all Cubans are under 15 years of age.

Like the other islands of the Caribbean, Cuba has a racially mixed population. About 73 percent of the inhabitants are Caucasian (mainly of Spanish descent), about 12 percent are Negro (descendants of African slaves and immigrants from other West Indian islands) and about 15 percent are of mixed heritage, primarily Caucasian and Negro. There is a small Oriental community (numbering about 20,000) composed mostly of Chinese who are descendants of indentured laborers brought to the island in the middle of the 19th century.

The original inhabitants of Cuba were Ciboney and Taino Indians, but none seem to have survived the Spanish occupation. The cultural heritage of the Indians, however, is evidenced in the *bohío* (thatch-roofed wooden dwelling typical of the rural countryside) and the cultivation and use of such native plants as tobacco and manioc.

The Spaniards began colonizing Cuba in 1511, but immigration was slow until the late 18th century when the financial rewards to be reaped from sugar plantations attracted an influx of settlers. The heaviest flow of Spanish immigrants, however, occurred in the first three decades of the 20th century. Other Caucasian immigrants have included about 30,000 French refugees from the slave uprising in Haiti at the end of the 18th century, and numbers of European and American immigrants between 1900 and 1950.

Although in the early days of the Spanish occupation there were a few small farmers who worked their own farms, slaves were the basis of the agricultural labor force from the beginning. The native Indians were used first, but as the Indians began to die off, the Spaniards imported African slaves, especially after 1790 when the United States market for Cuban sugar expanded and plantation labor was in great demand. Only about 60,000 slaves were imported before 1762, but by 1817 Africans outnumbered Spaniards on the island. Pre-independence civil uprisings and epidemics of infectious diseases took the lives of many blacks in the mid-19th century, and after independence in 1898 the incidence of intermarriage rose, further decreasing the size of the unmixed African population. A second influx of Negroes occurred from about 1900 to 1932 when about 190,000 Haitians and 121,000 Jamaicans came to work on the sugar plantations as paid laborers.

With the abolition of slavery in 1845, the Spaniards turned to the use of indentured Chinese coolies. A coolie's contract generally ran for 8 years. Upon contract termination, some Chinese returned home while others remained in Cuba, many intermarrying with local women since the ranks of indentured coolies included few females. Those who stayed started small business enterprises, such as restaurants and laundries, or took up truck gardening on the peripheries of the large urban centers. The number of unmixed Chinese Cuban citizens today is only about 20,000.*

Emigration from the island since the installation of the Castro regime in 1959 has been on the order of 400,000-500,000 people. In recent years these emigrés have tended increasingly to be middle class and have included more and more technical and professional people, representing a serious manpower loss to the island. In 1971 Castro put an embargo on the "freedom flights" which were bringing Cubans to Miami, Florida, each week.

Spanish is the official language of Cuba. English is the only foreign language taught in Cuban high schools and is practically a second language. A 1958 census indicated that 23 percent of the population was illiterate and that only 50 percent of the school-age children attended school. In 1970 the Government claimed that the school attendance rate had risen to 96 percent. Since 1969 the Government has placed heavy emphasis on expanding and improving rural schools, partially in an attempt to avert migration of young people to the cities in search of educational opportunities. Rural high school students spend half the day in classes and half the day farming land for which the school is responsible. The food crops grown, e.g., citrus fruit, avocados, beans and coffee, are not consumed by the students but are shipped to provincial warehouses for redistribution. The objectives of this work/study program, according to the director of one school, are to teach the young people "that work is part of education" and to enable the students to make a direct contribution to the economy. In December 1971 there were seven such "schools of the countryside." The students are highly disciplined and have no choice in curriculum. Dissent is not allowed and community spirit rather than individuality is stressed. The same attitude prevails at urban secondary schools.

At the university level, technical education is being emphasized as opposed to the traditionally popular fields of the arts and law. The capacity of institutions of higher learning is said to have doubled between 1961 and 1971. As at the secondary level, discipline at the universities is rigid and there is no room for dissent. One Habana University professor has been quoted as saying, "For the time being, progress and great intellectual freedom are not compatible in Cuba."

D. HISTORY AND GOVERNMENT [38] [24] [67] [22]

The island of Cuba was discovered by Columbus in October 1492. Spanish colonization of the island began in 1511 and the capital city of Habana was established in 1515. Due to Cuba's strategic location at the mouth of the Gulf of

---

*In addition, there are many visiting diplomats, technicians and other personnel from mainland China. Cuba has had trade and diplomatic relations with Communist China since 1959.

Mexico, Habana soon became an important commercial port for Spanish ships on their way to or from other Spanish colonies in the New World. Agriculture began to be developed both in order to feed the resident population and to provide food supplies for the Spanish ships. Manioc, sweet potatoes and plantains were the main crops and livestock-raising was initiated. Gradually, Spanish settlers began moving inland to establish sugarcane and tobacco plantations, using Indian and then African slaves, as discussed on page 00.

Because of the island's strategic position and importance to Spain as a naval base, Cuba became the object of attacks by other European powers during the 17th century, with adverse effects on the economy. Moreover, under the prevailing mercantilist policy, the island was forbidden to trade with any country except Spain and was restricted by the mother country in what it could produce. It was not until the late 18th century that economic prosperity, based on sugarcane, reached Cuba. The island benefited from the American War for Independence and became the primary supplier of sugar for the United States.

Mounting Cuban dissatisfaction with Spanish rule led to a long civil war and eventually to a war for independence which began in 1895 and ended when the United States intervened in 1898 (Spanish-American War). The island was ceded in trust to the United States by the Treaty of Paris. Cuba was under temporary U.S. military rule from January 1899 to May 1902, when a civilian government took power under the constitution of June 1901.

Economically, independent Cuba prospered, thanks to a favorable U.S. sugar market; but politically the country went through a period of insecurity, with threats of further U.S. intervention until 1925 when General Gerardo Machado brought stability through the imposition of Cuba's first dictatorship. Upon Machado's downfall in 1933, Fulgencio Batista gained control of the army and became the power behind the President's chair, making and unmaking the many heads of state who followed and finally attaining the presidency himself between 1940 and 1944. When his candidate lost the 1944 election, Batista left Cuba, but returned to power in 1952 in a bloodless coup. Opposition to his rule increased steadily, and from 1957 to 1959 the country was in a state of virtual civil war, with government forces fighting against guerrillas under the leadership of Fidel Castro.

In 1959, Batista fled Cuba and a new government was set up with Castro as premier. U.S.-Cuban relations began to deteriorate and in July 1960 the United States Congress voted to cut the 1960 quota for Cuban sugar drastically and to reallocate the entire Cuban quota to other countries as of 1961. Castro retaliated by nationalizing U.S. enterprises in Cuba valued at $1 billion. Diplomatic relations were broken in January 1961 and in February the Cuban Government was reorganized along the Soviet pattern. In April 1961, a U.S.-supported invasion force of Cuban exiles attempted to liberate the island but was defeated at the Bay of Pigs. Anti-Americanism was intensified and in December 1961 Castro openly declared himself and his government to be Marxist-Leninist.

In January 1962 the Organization of American States (OAS) excluded Cuba from OAS activities and instituted an arms embargo. In 1964 Venezuela discovered that Cuba had been supplying arms to Venezuelan revolutionaries, and at the request of the Venezuelan Government the OAS foreign ministers agreed to sever diplomatic relations with Cuba, discontinue trade except for foodstuffs and medical supplies, and to cut off all sea transportation to and from the island. This "blockade" is still in effect (see *Foreign Trade*).

The Cuban constitution of 1940 was suspended in 1959 and the country has been ruled by decree since that time. Nominally, executive and legislative powers are vested in a 23-man Council of Ministers, but in fact, the Prime Minister (Fidel Castro, who is also First Secretary of the Cuban Communist Party) wields absolute authority. The country is divided into six provinces (Pinar del Río, La Habana, Matanzas, Las Villas, Camagüey and Oriente), 43 regions and 321 municipalities.

E. AGRICULTURAL POLICIES

Cuban agricultural policies have three main objectives: to consolidate the Government's land reform program; to expand sugar output so as to increase export earnings; and to augment food production.

1. Land Reform [34] [22] [55] [26]

One of the revolutionaries' first manifestos, issued in October 1958 even before the revolution had succeeded, was concerned with land reform and stated the principle of ownership of the land by the tiller. The promulgation of this principle helped the revolutionaries rally the support of the *campesinos*—the rural peasants who were tenant farmers, squatters, hired hands or perhaps owners of fragmented plots. The first Agrarian Reform Law, passed by the new Government in May 1959, tried to steer a medium course between latifundia and minifundia and declared that no person or entity could own more than 402.6 hectares and that no property should be parceled below a minimum of 27 hectares. All land in excess of the maximum was to be expropriated and distributed to the landless or to those owning less than 27 hectares. No holding under 27 hectares could be expropriated. Certain exceptions were made for "model" farms, that is, enterprises producing 50 percent more than the national average in crops or supporting more cattle per hectare of pastures than the national average. A supreme limit, however, was set at 1,342 hectares, beyond which no single owner or corporation could go. The law further stated that only Cuban citizens could own land on the island. A National Agrarian Reform Institute *(Instituto Nacional de Reforma Agraria—INRA)* was established to implement the land reform law and to handle all agricultural production, credit and trade matters.

Although INRA did distribute some of the land confiscated under the first land reform law to over 100,000 former landless farmers, most of the large estates which were expropriated were kept intact. They were first transformed into cooperatives and eventually into state farms. According to Gutelman, the Government does not seem to have intended originally that these cooperatives become state farms, but all too soon the elected cooperative coordinators were overshadowed by INRA-appointed administrators and by 1963 the system of state land ownership and control was stabilized (see *Farms*).

Gutelman (quoting INRA statistics) reports that the total amount of land brought under state control by the first Agrarian Reform Law amounted to 1,199,184 hectares in 1961. Two laws aimed at nationalizing all foreign-owned enterprises, especially American-owned properties, were passed in July and October 1960, adding another 2,172,134 hectares to the holdings of the state. Eventually more individually-owned property was expropriated or confiscated for a variety of reasons, and some was transferred to the state as "donations." By March 1961 state land amounted to 4,438,879 hectares.* By the end of 1962 the state held 44 percent of the national land while 56 percent belonged to private individuals, mostly smallholders owning less than 27 hectares.

In 1961 smallholders were organized into an agricultural syndicate called the National Association of Small Agriculturalists *(Asociación Nacional de Pequeños Agricultores—ANAP)* whose primary role was to counter the counter-revolutionary activities of the large landowners. ANAP quickly began to play an economic role as well as a political one, facilitating the orientation of private agricultural production according to the national plans. Eventually it broadened its functions and became the distribution channel for credit, materials, etc. About 90 percent of the small private farmers now belong to ANAP, which has to a large extent become an agency of the Government to control the private sector.

In October 1963 a second reform law was passed, authorizing expropriation of holdings in excess of 67.5 hectares, thus eliminating medium-sized private agricultural enterprises. These confiscated lands were immediately organized into state farms and added 1.8 million hectares to the state sector, bringing the total to over 6 million hectares, while private holdings dropped to an estimated 2.0-2.5 million hectares. This brought over 60 percent of the nation's sugar fields and 60 percent of the country's cattle into the hands of the state. In 1967 a third major land reform was enacted when a pilot collective farming project was established at San Andreas, but so far, this type of reform has been carried out on a very limited basis, involving only 900 farm families.

According to Dumont, the French socialist agricultural economist, the early

---

*Gutelman's figure. According to other sources, the amount was 4,445,600 hectares (see page 39).

agrarian reforms received a certain amount of support from the population, but enthusiasm soon faded when enforcement of the policies of the INRA was entrusted to the army and when it became clear that the promised compensation* would be paid irregularly. Since the October 1963 reform, the trend has been toward greater and greater centralization and more and more dependence on the rigid structure of the army, with less and less participation in decision-making by the grass roots worker. Policy decisions are embodied in "special plans" concerning both crops and cattle. Such plans command the highest priorities in money, resources and manpower and many times conflict with the efficiency of the daily routine, especially when manpower is removed from one project to be assigned to another of higher priority. Some of these projects are integrated along a "vertical line" from harvest to marketing; others are integrated regionally.

2. Increased Sugar Output [22] [34]

Cuba has been the world's leading producer of cane sugar since 1914 and provides over one-fourth of world sugar exports. One of the early objectives of the Castro Government was to pull Cuba out of the monoculture syndrome by diversifying agriculture and attempting industrialization. However, the industrialization effort failed and in 1965 the policy was reversed; once again sugar was promoted as a means of obtaining foreign goods and currencies. A 1970 harvest goal of 10 million tons was announced and land was diverted from food crops to cane cultivation, but the target was missed by 2 million tons.

3. Augmented Food Production [22] [10]

Food production in Cuba has suffered since the revolution due to many factors, including the dislocation caused by land reforms, mismanagement of land and labor resources, changing priorities, shortages of the means of production, lack of incentives, scarcity of credit, and marketing problems. As a result, there have been serious food shortages on the island since 1962, necessitating the introduction of a rationing system and an increasing reliance on food imports, primarily from the Soviet Union. Since 1965, the Government has been in the self-contradictory position of seeking on the one hand to increase sugar output (and hence acreage) for export, and on the other hand to reach a greater level of

---

*This compensation was based on the estimated value of the holding made by the owner for property tax purposes. It was to be paid in the form of 4½ percent interest-bearing bonds redeemable in 20 years. No compensation was paid to foreign nationals whose property was confiscated or to Cubans who emigrated. It is uncertain just how much compensation has actually been paid to Cuban citizens who remained in the country.

self-sufficiency in food crops. First priority (after sugar) is given to production of milk and dairy products for domestic consumption, with a goal of increasing the output of milk by 400 percent by 1970. Second priority is given to citrus fruit, coffee, tobacco and pineapples, for export, not for consumption. Last priority is given to staple food crops and meat for the local market. At this rate, the goal of self-sufficiency in food will be neither quickly nor easily reached.

According to Dumont, the most recent agricultural map assigns 230,000 hectares of lowlands along the southern coastline, especially the lower valley of the Río Cauto in Oriente Province, to rice cultivation. The clay soils of Matanzas and La Habana are to produce more sugarcane, citrus fruit, coffee and bananas, while other lands in the same area will concentrate on fruits, such as mangoes, and on tubers like manioc.

The power of the central Planning Board *(Junta de Planificación)* has been boosted to the extreme and the Board is confronted with the difficult task of reconciling national priorities with regional potentials and idiosyncrasies. The inevitable result is that decisions are more political than technical and a large amount of efficiency is lost in the process. Confronted by so many problems and disappointments, the growing tendency has been to use the army for various activities alien to its traditional role. This unorthodox utilization of the armed forces was welcome to the ranking military leaders who saw in it an educational as well as a prestige value. As a result, the urban population is now increasingly submitted to the overlordship of the Communist Party and the army.

F. FOREIGN AID

1. Bilateral Aid [33] [66] [42]

The country giving most aid to Cuba is the Soviet Union, whose assistance is mainly in the form of trade. While trade is not normally considered foreign aid, in this instance a large part of the trade *is* aid. The Soviet Union is the world's largest producer of centrifugal sugar, and is herself a sugar exporter, yet she sells Cuba commodities needed in the island in exchange for unwanted sugar, most of which is probably re-exported.

The Soviet Union's aid to Cuba dates to the break between Cuba and the United States in 1960, but according to Gouré and Weinkle, assistance was granted with great caution and even reluctance, even after Castro declared himself to be a Marxist-Leninist (in December 1961). Eventually sugar purchases and shipments of food, agricultural machinery, oil, military equipment and technical advisors were intensified, with the U.S.S.R. never missing an opportunity to emphasize Cuba's dependence upon such assistance. While the balance of trade was favorable to Cuba in 1960 and 1961, in 1962 it became negative and it has remained so ever since. In 1970 the Cuban debt to the U.S.S.R. reached over

$1.7 billion. Russian aid to Cuba went beyond bartering goods for sugar and giving technical assistance. The Soviet Union also opened a $100 million line of credit for Cuba at low interest for the purchase of industrial equipment.

As the mutual cooperation program increased, Moscow promised to purchase more and more sugar, paid for 80 percent in kind and 20 percent in currency. As the United States increased its pressure on Cuba, the Soviet Union increased its assistance, buying more sugar than promised and increasing deliveries of food, oil and machinery. After the ill-fated attempt at industrialization in 1962-63, Cuba found itself with less land for sugar and no other resource with which to pay for goods received from the Soviet Union. An indebtedness had been created which increased while the means for erasing it had decreased; hence, the refocus on sugar production. A long-lasting tie was thus created between the two countries, similar to the relationship between a moneylender and a derelict debtor. Soon Cuba's sugar "sales" to the Soviet Union were balanced by the goods imported from the U.S.S.R. so that Cuba lacked cash with which to purchase commodities from other sources.

Soviet aid to Cuba proved to include machines that did not suit Cuban operating conditions. These were not unlike the stuffed crocodiles that money-lenders of old forced their clients to buy from them in order to increase the value of the IOU's. The Soviet Union is now said to be charging interest against its defaulting customer.

For a while, Communist China also purchased Cuban sugar, and in 1961 opened a $60 million line of credit to Cuba for the purchase of rice.

2. Multilateral Aid [63] [62]

Cuba receives technical assistance from a number of United Nations agencies. The United Nations Development Program has provided $8,791,600 in support of a variety of projects through its Special Fund component. Such projects have included assistance to the Central Agricultural Experimental Station at Santiago de las Vegas (with technical assistance provided by the Food and Agriculture Organization of the United Nations), assistance to the Faculties of Science and Technology, University of Habana (through UNESCO), fishery development (with FAO cooperation) and strengthening of the national Institute of Hygiene, Epidemiology and Microbiology (through the World Health Organization). The United Nations Children's Fund has supported a rural health services demonstration project and an applied nutrition program.

II. FOOD RESOURCES

A. GENERAL [34] [55] [64] [59] [66]

The food resources of Cuba can only be approximated. Estimates of the land devoted to food and cash crops are very uncertain, as are evaluations of the fish landings. Only the quantity of food imports can be discussed with any amount of certainty. Foreign visitors to the island vary in their interpretations of the scarce figures released by the Government or gleaned from a perusal of Cuban journals and reviews. Official statistics given by Cuban delegates to the Food and Agriculture Organization of the United Nations (FAO) are at variance with the estimates of foreign experts, which often seem to be more realistic. Hence, the figures given in this section are tentative and reflect an order of magnitude rather than actual fact. They are indicative enough for the purpose of this study, but no mathematical consistency can be expected.

As has been described, the land in Cuba is shared by the state and the private sector but the private sector is itself controlled by the state to a considerable extent (see *Agricultural Policies*). The state sector combines People's Farms *(Granjas del Pueblo)*, Sugar Farms *(Granjas Cañeras)* and State Farms *(Fincas Estatales)*. In 1961 the probable total land area covered by state-controlled farms was 4,445,600 hectares, distributed as shown in the table below. The private sector was estimated by the most optimistic reviewers to occupy 3.5 million hectares prior to the second reform law in 1963. However, considering the successive changes in the law since that time, the size of the private sector cannot now be estimated at more than 2 million hectares, the balance having been absorbed by state organizations.

Land Use in State-Controlled Agricultural Sector − Cuba, 1961*
(in 1,000 hectares)

Province	Cultivated	Pasture	Fallow	Total
Pinar del Rio	193.7	98.7	31.0	· 323.4
La Habana	139.5	32.2	19.6	191.3
Matanzas	258.9	103.5	38.8	410.2
Las Villas	410.8	153.3	141.7	705.8
Camagüey	729.8	425.4	184.1	1,339.3
Oriente	989.6	399.7	95.7	1,484.6
	2,722.3	1,212.8	510.9	4,454.6

*Although Roberts and Hamour cite these figures for 1968, they are compatible only with
  1961 data given by other sources.

Source: C.P. Roberts and M. Hamour, Eds., *Cuba 1968.*

Similar data on the provincial distribution of privately-owned land by use is not available. The Government has always reserved the right to buy from these owners any land that would facilitate its special projects or land needed to start a new form of agricultural development. The amount of acreage that has thus passed under state control since 1963 is not known, but a 1969 estimate gives the land under private ownership as 20-27 percent of the total farmland available, or probably 2 million hectares. Guardedly accepting the figure of 2 million hectares as representing 20-27 percent of the overall farmland, the total can in turn be roughly evaluated at 7 or 8 million hectares, which is consistent with pre-revolution estimates and not too different from that of 7.4 million hectares reported to FAO in January 1966. However, the private sector must include some nonusable land (in particular some of the scrub forest called *marabu*). The three eastern provinces are the most productive.

Other sources of food include the sea. Cuban fishermen may have landed a catch of about 62,000 tons of fish in 1968 and 15,769 tons of shellfish in 1968.

It has been evaluated that the change in monthly per capita food resources, both domestic and foreign, were as follows between 1958 and 1962:

Monthly Per Capita Food Resources — Cuba, 1958-1962
(in kilograms)

Item	1958	1962	Reduction (in percent)
Rice	6.22	3.00	51.89
Other grains	1.20	.75	37.50
Fats	1.45	1.00	31.04
Meats	6.30	2.51[a]	60.02
[a]Reduced to 1.5 kilos in 1971.			

Sources: University of Miami (Cuban Economic Research Project), *Labor Conditions in Communist Cuba.*

F. Soler, "Cuban Economy's in Dire Trouble, Experts Say."

Fifty percent of the calories needed for survival are imported, mostly from Russia, including 90 percent of all cereals consumed and 85 percent of all fats and oils. Until 1967, rice was supplied by mainland China, but after that year efforts were made to increase domestic production of this essential cereal. Corn is important and second only to rice in the diet, but its production has dropped considerably since 1960, necessitating the importation of 150,000 tons from Russia in 1969. Other food resources, such as dry legumes, roots and tubers (sweet potatoes, yams, malanga, taro and manioc) are grown locally but European potatoes are mostly imported. Whatever their origin, however, these food resources are not always available, and when they are, it is only in small quantities (see *Diets*). Witness the fact that in 1962, for the first time in their history, the Cuban population was subjected to rationing which is still in effect.

B. MEANS OF PRODUCTION

1. Agricultural Labor Force [64] [69] [55] [22] [40] [37a] [59] [43]

The current number of Cubans working in agriculture is difficult to evaluate for several reasons, the main one being the lack of definition of an agricultural laborer. The revolution has replaced individual land ownership with the concept of the worker-owner who exercises his ownership collectively through the bureaucracy of the state. Students at various levels of education, starting with schoolchildren and going up to university students, are commandeered to work in the cane fields at certain times of the year, regardless of their studies. The army has mobilized farmhands, only to assign some to cane cutting duty at harvesttime (at a very different wage from the one they received for the same work as civilians*). According to Fenton Wheeler, in the spring of 1968 more than 1 million urbanites from all walks of life were drafted to help with the cane harvest and thousands were asked to help in agriculture during the weekends. Habana residents are frequently mobilized when needed to keep the fields around the capital in full production. In 1953 the number of agricultural workers was estimated at 818,700 and in 1957 at 855,000. According to figures quoted by Roberts and Hamour (see Table No. 2), the agricultural labor force fell to 297,000 in 1962 and rose to 449,900 in 1968.

The condition of the Cuban worker is no different from that of the Soviet citizen. As many have begun to realize, the situation of the canecutter has not changed much since the revolution and the worker is still the servant of an extraneous authority. Since the state is the sole employer, the laborer cannot choose the nature and location of his work; he can receive promotion only if the state decides he deserves it; he cannot transfer to any other work except by decision of the state. Moreover, the state can force any worker to do any task deemed necessary at any time and has set up forced labor camps at 10 different locations throughout the island.

Unemployment and underemployment existed in Cuba before the revolution, especially during the "dead season" following the sugar harvest. According to a census made by the National Economic Council of Cuba in 1956-57, about 16.4 percent of the labor force was unemployed. No figures for unemployment have been available since, but the acute food shortages which began in 1962 and have compelled the promulgation of a rationing law suggest that there must be an enormous number of unemployed people in agriculture, which may have been a partial reason for the drop in crop returns.

General working conditions do not seem to have improved. Before the revolution, the workweek was limited by law to 44 hours but the worker was paid on the basis of 48 hours. Since 1961 the reverse has been the case: the workweek is 48 hours, paid on the basis of 44. Leisure hours have been restricted or used for "recommended" attendance at political meetings. The Party pressures the workers to deny themselves overtime pay and to work 12 hours for the wages of 8 and even to donate their weekends to the job. There are no sick leave rights. Holidays are celebrated by participating in "special work drives" and it is reported that even North Vietnamese holidays are observed in

---

*The army wage is $7 a month while the civilian canecutter is paid $2.66 a day.

this fashion. Six hundred thousand members (50 percent) of the Central Labor Union are said to have responded favorably to such pressures.

Thanks to these changes, the annual worktime for the average Cuban has increased from 1,854 hours to 2,554 hours, while the contents of his wage packet have diminished. While prior to the revolution Cuba ranked second among Latin American countries in terms of percentage of national income devoted to salaries, after 1962 the island dropped to the level of the seven lowest countries.

Rationing has resulted in a black market, which further diminishes the purchasing power of the already reduced wages. It is estimated that the salary of a canecutter dropped from $3.14 per day in 1958 to $2.66 in 1962. According to Lawson, the overall minimum wage in 1969 was $85 per month. This is more generous than appears at first because many families include two employed workers, although the male population strongly resists seeing their wives work at anything but menial jobs. (Mothers who work leave their children in a state creche.) At the other end of the scale, a maximum wage of $900 per month is also imposed. Incapacitated workers get $60.00 a month plus assistance in the form of free medical care, food and lodging.

That these low salaries are one of the causes of low productivity is possible, but not likely, as the pressure of need would probably overcome at least in part the lack of ambition. In a speech at Habana University on the occasion of the commemoration of the 12th anniversary of the revolution, Castro blamed low productivity on the "bourgeois prejudices of the labor force which showed individualism, self-centeredness, complexes of superiority and vanity." Whatever its cause, this lack of enthusiasm has resulted in considerable absenteeism from the field and factories, to the point where the Government has had to promulgate a "vagrancy law" providing penalties, including prison terms, for insubordinate workers.

The low wages are not entirely offset by the cheap prices of food and other necessities. The INRA cooperative sells food to agricultural workers, marking up the prices 50 or 60 percent. It is reported that while the agency pays 4¢ a pound for white fishmeal, it sells it to the laborers for 10¢ a pound. Moreover, social security, maternity benefits, union fees, income tax and "voluntary" deductions further reduce the worker's purchasing power.

In short, the labor contract is no longer the result of a mutual covenant, but has become a unilateral compulsion. Because work is compulsory, because the state determines what the work should be and because no argument about working conditions is tolerated, it is probable that the conditions of the workingman in Cuba have become far worse than they were before the revolution. The consequences of this change, in terms of status of the agricultural labor force and the nutrition of the population, will be apparent in the following sections.

2. Farms [34] [22] [55] [5] [3] [9]

The revolution brought about considerable changes in the land tenure pattern and the organization of agriculture. According to the preamble of the first land reform law in 1959, the land had previously been distributed (as in most Latin American countries) in a way that placed the smallholder at a disadvantage: 2,236 landowners (1.5 percent of the total) controlled 3.6 million hectares or 46 percent of the national farmland, while another 111,000 farmers (74 percent) occupied 2.3 million hectares, or less than 27 hectares each. Under the first phase of land reform (1959-1961), confiscated land was organized into three types of state enterprises. The first type were called "Cooperatives," but this was a misnomer because the INRA representative (generally a member of the military) practically superseded the elected administrator of the enterprise. The second type were known as "Farm Units Under Direct Administration," and a third type, concerned mainly with the production of sugarcane, were called "Cane Cooperatives." The first type were usually former latifundia that had specialized in some agricultural activity which was incorporated in its post-revolutionary name ("Tomato Cooperative," "Cattle-raising Cooperative," etc.). The "Farms Under Direct Administration" were state-run cattle ranches which came into being when the state bought out small cattle breeders to save them from economic strangulation by the large ranchers. As implied in the descriptive title of these farms, they were administered directly by INRA-appointed administrators. The workers were salaried laborers. The "Cane Cooperatives" operated under a specific statute and were in principle run by a board of directors elected from among the workers who had been employed on the estate from which the cooperative was formed. (These workers were paid on a wage plus profit-sharing basis.) In fact, the coordinator who headed the board of directors shared his decision-making power with an INRA-appointed administrator. The system proved unworkable and eventually power was transferred to the INRA administrator.

After June 1961 the first two types of enterprises, "Cooperatives" and "Farms Under Direct Administration," were merged wherever possible and labeled "People's Farms" *(Granjas del Pueblo)* in which the land was owned by the state and the workers were paid wages but did not share in profits. In other words, they became true state farms. The labor force, previously employed by a landowner, now served a bureaucracy. A year later, in August 1962, the "Cane Cooperatives" became "Sugar Farms" *(Granjas Cañeras),* thus losing their cooperative status and like the others becoming nothing more than state farms. Finally, in 1963, the "People's Farms" and "Sugar Farms" were merged administratively and called simply "State Farms" *(Fincas Estatales).* To simplify the bureaucracy and to take into account the regional potential, these units were grouped by geographical as well as vocational nature under the name "Groupings" *(Agrupaciones)*. In 1966, there were 58 "Groupings" which included 575 "State Farms." The size of the "Groupings" varied from a coverage of 13,000 to 100,000 hectares.

Private farms still exist in Cuba but the authorized acreage has diminished with each agrarian reform. Following the first law of 1959, private farms could encompass up to 402 hectares. After the second law (October 1963) the maximum dropped to 67 hectares. At the same time, some of the land confiscated under the two agrarian reforms was distributed among landless farmers in lots not exceeding 67 hectares each. Thus, after 1963 smallholders were of two categories: old ones and new ones. Some could even be both, if they had owned less than 67 hectares prior to the revolution and had received land to bring the total up to 67 hectares after the reform. Gutelman states that since the revolution, these poor peasants have come to represent 94 percent of the private farm sector. In 1961, smallholders numbered 150,120 and held 3,531,403 hectares or somewhat more than 23 hectares each. Hence, these people were the only landowners who really profited from the revolution since their holdings increased to 67 hectares each.

A few true production cooperatives have survived the tendency toward increasing state control and these operate without direct state intervention in their administration. According to Gutelman, in 1966 there were only 270 such cooperatives, all very small, covering about 20,000 hectares.

In 1967, a third land reform, of smaller scope than the first two, however, came into effect, creating a new type of collective farm in the province of Pinar del Río at San Andreas. There, 900 families have pooled their farms and run them under governmental direction in exchange for promises of new homes, hospitals, recreation areas, etc.

3. Fertilizers [72] [33] [55] [50] [27] [6] [4] [3]

There is agreement among experts that the amount of fertilizers applied per hectare of land in Cuba has increased substantially since 1958. At that time, 220,000 tons were used during the year, 80 percent of which had to be imported. About half of the total amount available was spread on canefields but this was well below the need. According to Wylie, in 1967 imported fertilizers totaled 270,000 tons, including 105,000 tons of nitrogen, 90,000 tons of phosphates and 75,000 tons of potash. Gouré and Weinkle report that in 1968 Cuba imported 287,500 tons of fertilizers from the Soviet Union alone. Local fertilizer production amounts to about 20,000 tons of ground rock phosphate and 30,000 tons of nitrogenous fertilizer. A serious effort is being made to increase domestic fertilizer output. A large plant is being completed in Cienfuegos at an alleged cost of $45 million, financed with British credit and built with the assistance of British engineers. This factory is expected to more than double the domestic output of nitrogenous fertilizer. The Soviet Union is also aiding in the construction of fertilizer plants. Overall fertilizer consumption (both domestic and imported) in 1970 was reported by FAO to total 477,900 tons (178,900 nitrogenous, 115,000 phosphatic and 184,000 potassic).

According to Roberts and Hamour, more than 500,000 tons of fertilizer were distributed on sugarcane fields in 1968 while 300,000 tons went to nonsugar fields. It is not clear what proportion of these inputs came from local production and what from imports. It is highly probable that great attention is given to the state farms but no breakdown is available, except that ANAP members who receive fertilizers from the state are instructed to use them on canefields. According to the *Miami Herald* of August 25, 1970, the fertilizer production plan is in arrears by 32 percent, equivalent to a shortage of 132,000 tons. Transportation difficulties are given as the cause of this delay. On the other hand, Castro complains that the students' lack of enthusiasm for acquiring the technical agronomic skills needed to do a good job results in fertilizers being wasted because the real needs of the soils are not considered.

Worthy of note is the incipient interest shown in using chemicals to get rid of the *marabú* shrub which covers 300,000 hectares of potentially fertile land.

4. Mechanical Equipment [72] [27]

The terrain of Cuba's farmland is favorable for mechanical cultivation. After the end of World War II, farm mechanization in Cuba was intensified, but the increased imports of machines from the United States (tractors, plows and harrows) and the establishment of an assembly plant for imported parts benefited the sugarcane fields and rice farms almost exclusively. Half of the latter were fully mechanized while the other half made use of at least some equipment. After the revolution, all the equipment entering Cuba came from East European countries, mainly the U.S.S.R. and Czechoslovakia. Some domestic production of tractors also began. A combine to harvest sugarcane was introduced recently but is not yet popular, as shown by the tremendous propaganda efforts made to get students and other nonfarm personnel to work in the fields at harvesttime. It also appears that considerable maintenance problems exist, both because skilled Cuban mechanics are few and because replacement parts are in short supply.

Wylie reports that 18,000 tractors were in use in 1963 and indicates that over 5,000 were imported in 1967 alone. By 1971, therefore, there must have been well over 20,000 tractors of all kinds in Cuba. The imported machines are now purchased in Western as well as Eastern Europe. The real questions, however, are: how many of these machines are in working order; how many are actually used for what crops; and what is the efficiency of maintenance services throughout the island?

C. PRODUCTION [27] [51] [22] [59]

There is no doubt that agricultural production in Cuba has dropped drastically during the last 12 years, and that the economic debacle produced by the switch to socialized methods of production has not yet been overcome. FAO's indices show that the per capita agricultural output of Cuba has dropped from an index of 126 in 1952 to an index of 79 in 1968 (1952-1956 average=100). Other Latin American countries also experienced a decline in per capita output during the same period: Argentina, 102 to 92; Chile, 97 to 94; Colombia, 105 to 97; Dominican Republic, 104 to 75; Paraguay, 105 to 95; Peru, 97 to 95; and Uruguay, 100 to 85. However, except for Uruguay, each of these countries saw its gross national product increase during the same period, indicating that the reduction in agricultural production was deliberate and compensated by some developmental effort in the industrial sector. There is no evidence that such a compensatory increase has occurred in Cuba. Moreover, the FAO index of per capita food production for Cuba is still more discouraging: it dropped from 128 in 1952 to 80 in 1968. Only Argentina, Colombia, Paraguay and Uruguay lost ground during the same period, but none as much as Cuba.

Among the many reasons for this decline, the French socialist writer René Dumont gives one in an amusing anecdote. Productivity, he reports, is stimulated by prizes, medals, rewards and election to the elite workers' group. Attracted by the First of May Prize, promised to the cane mill which could crush the highest tonnage, a certain factory organized its supply in such a way that on the assigned day it had on hand several more tons of cane than it receives through its regular delivery system. As a result, the mill won the prize, but it took a week for the factory's wagons, ox carts and other conveyances to be redistributed in such a way as to allow activities to be resumed on the regular basis. The mill won the prize, all right, but when taking the whole picture into consideration, between the day the disruption of schedule began and the day it returned to normal, a substantial production loss was found to have occurred. This kind of disruption, of course, does not suffice to explain the general drop in output that has resulted in the scarcity now prevailing in Cuba. But it is related to a series of adverse measures based on ideological rather than practical factors which handicap productivity in Cuba as well as in most other communist countries. Dumont provides us with another example, based on the operation of a state farm where the permanent staff includes 550 workers (95 percent of them mobilized soldiers), and ad hoc platoons of military personnel numbering 545. Dumont reports that these men show about as much enthusiasm for cutting cane as can be expected of soldiers on "KP" duty.

Prominent among other adverse measures is the inefficiency and scarcity of farm labor which has to be supplemented by incompetent and reluctant "volunteers" from the cities to reinforce the military. All observers agree that too much planning of the smallest operational details by uncoordinated and incompetent bureaucrats is a big factor in causing delays and confusion. The deterioration of such allied functions as transportation, trade patterns and ownership has also contributed greatly to the disruption of the production system. This is more profoundly felt in the agricultural sector because it is the most important of all aspects of Cuban life. While it is true that less than half of the people live in rural areas, more than half depend on agriculture for their livelihood. The extensive rather than intensive character of Cuban agriculture results in multiplying the negative effects of all the changes brought about by the revolution and maximizes rather than minimizes their impact on production.

An estimate of the situation by Soler, published in 1971 and recently confirmed in a private interview, is very pessimistic. Only a few sectors have progressed, notably fishing and rice farming. Rice suddenly surged to a record crop in 1970 after slumping for 12 years, thanks to the sowing of the IR-5* line of seed. But the production and hence availability of meat, bread, milk and corn has lessened to the point where acute shortages are frequent. Even water is in short supply. Countless consumer products, such as clothing, shoes, soap, toothbrushes and tobacco, are scarce. As for sugar, the main crop, in spite of considerable efforts in which "the honor of the revolution" was involved, the record 1970 output did not exceed 8.5 million tons.

1. Food Crops [27] [22] [66] [45] [3] [2] [1] [8] [10] [35]

It is probably true that if food crops are still harvested, it is because between 55 and 60 percent of them come from the private sector, or rather from what is left of the private sector. Table No. 3 gives an idea of what the production figures probably are. In compiling the table, statistics from FAO have been preferred to other data compiled by researchers working outside the island. From our comparison of these various data, the FAO figures appear to be more consistent.

a. Cereals

Only two cereals of importance are cultivated in Cuba: corn and rice. Some sorghum is also grown in small quantities for animal feed. The amount of corn harvested has steadily declined in the last 20 years but more drastically since the revolution. The drop is the more surprising, given the interest of the Government in encouraging livestock production. The area sown was reduced by more than one-half between 1948 and 1970 and so was the harvest, which is now estimated at 115,000 tons per year (see Table No. 3). More than half of the crop is eaten by the populace; the rest is used for animal feed, especially for pigs and chickens. Most of the corn comes from Oriente Province, which produced over 60,000 tons in 1962, but only 16,000 tons in 1966.

Rice is one of the few crops that has increased since the revolution. The area sown has expanded from an average of 63,000 hectares in 1948-52 to 150,000 in

---

*IR-5: "miracle" seed developed at the Rice Institute at Los Baños, Philippines.

1970 and production has risen from 164,000 to 326,000 tons. A goal of 200,000 hectares had been set for 1971. The crop is increasingly grown on state farms which enjoy full mechanization, irrigation, fertilization, pesticides and herbicides. The Honduras short grain variety (Zayas Bazan) was the dominant kind until it was gradually replaced by European seeds and more recently by the Philippine "miracle" IR-5. Since it has been decided to forgo buying rice from China, a special effort is being made to develop the lower Río Cauto into a 67,000-hectare rice field, sown almost exclusively with Philippine seeds. By 1969 about 10,000 hectares were ready but a number of difficulties arose, caused by poor management, defective technology and lack of organization. On the other hand, in some places modern methods are combined with defective ones. Pesticides are sprayed with the help of Russian Antonov planes designed for that purpose, whose efficiency seems to counterbalance the failures of other sectors of technology. The work is done with the help of cowboys taken away from their cattle and army officers taken away from their camps to drive tractors. Yet, substantial progress has been made against heavy odds, as proved by the result of the good crop harvested in 1970.

b. Roots and Tubers

Roots include sweet potatoes and yams, manioc, malanga (*Xanthosoma* spp.), taro and European potatoes. Sweet potatoes and yams have always been popular with the local peasantry and even with the lower income groups in the urban areas, but production seems to be on the decline. Taros are found everywhere, but more so in Oriente where production was said to have tripled in the last 8 years, and in Camagüey where it has increased six times. Manioc production has also risen, according to FAO, while the area sown has decreased compared to 1948-56. It is quite believable that this root, which is easily grown in a wide variety of soils and keeps in the ground for over 18 months, is increasingly popular in a country where, except for rice, better food resources are dwindling. European potatoes are greatly appreciated, especially in the cities, and harvests have increased (see Table No. 3). The foci of production are in La Habana and Matanzas provinces, although some fields can be found almost everywhere. Domestic output has risen slowly, reaching 120,000 tons in 1970. An additional 30,000 tons are imported from the Soviet Union each year.

c. Legumes

Legumes are part of the basic Caribbean diet. Black beans, red beans, peas and lentils are either grown locally (22,000 tons a year) or imported from Russia (55,800 tons a year) to meet the demand. The black bean, the most popular of all these pulses, is still grown in Cuba, but in lesser and lesser amounts. This good source of protein is gradually being replaced by manioc in the daily fare, and it is disturbing that the area sown in beans should have been reduced by almost half and the crop by one-third since the revolution. Beans are grown in Camagüey, Oriente and Las Villas provinces.

d. Fresh Vegetables

Fresh vegetables, especially tomatoes, onions, cucumbers, cabbages, eggplant, carrots, peppers and garlic, are grown in Cuba, mainly by a labor force of 10,000 women. Asparagus and onion cultivation was started in a large scale project in 1967 in the Escambray Mountains, together with grape and strawberry production. The focus of these crops is the Bañao area in Las Villas Province and the objective is massive production for export. The area is well-watered and has easy access to the sea. The surface sown in asparagus was said to cover 535 hectares in 1967 and was scheduled to increase. Cultivation is mechanized. Tomato and cucumber production falls short of local demand, necessitating imports to supplement domestic output—a change from pre-revolution days when there was a surplus of these vegetables for export. It is believed that domestic production of garlic and onions covers about 50 percent of the domestic demand, and that some of the imports come from Spain.

The Government is encouraging the private sector to concentrate on fresh vegetables. All provinces grow some, but as could be expected, La Habana Province is at the top of the list, especially in tomato production. In 1969, the gardens around Habana produced about 70,000 tons instead of the 90,000 tons harvested in 1967. This resulted in an acute shortage of fruit and vegetables, except for priority ration card holders. Dumont tells the story of a contract sought by a French importer of fresh vegetables who needed 5,000 tons of tomatoes to meet part of the French demand between December and April. He found that in order to export one box of fresh vegetables, the coordination of over 13 different offices had to be secured and that this could not be done in less than 6 months. Needless to say, he gave up the project.

e. Fruit

Cuba grows a wide spectrum of tropical fruits, which at one time found a market in the United States. No doubt if and when the agricultural house of the island is restored to order, a similar market could be found in Eastern Europe. For the time being, production of these fruits is decreasing for some (bananas and pineapples) and increasing for others (citrus). Oranges and grapefruit are among the favorite special projects of Dr. Castro. In 1969 the plan originally provided for planting 270,000 hectares of citrus fruit with an ultimate target of 5 million tons of fruit in 1985. In 1969, after overcoming serious shortages of water supply, inadequacy of the soil and careless plantings, 140,000 tons of oranges and tangerines and 15,000 tons of grapefruit were harvested (see Table No. 3). Most citrus fruit is grown in Camagüey Province or on the Isle of Pines.

Other fruits include mangoes (which amounted to an unusually large crop in

1965, some of which had to be fed to pigs for lack of machinery to deal with the surpluses), guavas and melons (both of which could be exported in the future). Strawberries and grapes are grown in the Bañao area as part of the earlier mentioned project of intensive cultivation for export. It is said that this is the first time that strawberries have been grown successfully in Cuba. They are used for making jelly and flavoring ice cream. Five harvests are expected every year on 668 hectares, making the area sown therefore equivalent to 3,000 hectares. Grapes have also been experimented with since 1960.

2. Cash Crops [22] [7] [72] [33] [9] [30] [39]

As long as fruits and vegetables have not regained a significant foreign market, sugarcane remains the most important cash crop and much as been sacrificed in its favor. Tobacco and coffee are listed second and third in importance.

Sugarcane is, of course, a dominant resource. It is the key to the success of the revolution and to future development. Since 1965, the production of sugar has been in the hands of a special department, the Ministry of the Sugar Industry *(Ministerio de la Industria Azucarero—MINAZ)*. This agency cooperates with INRA to establish production goals and standards of quality from the cane to the finished product which is then exported through the Cuban Export Company for Sugar and Its Derivatives *(Empresa Cubana Exportadora de Azúcar y sus Derivados)*. With the exception of the record year of 1952, during which the crop yielded 7.2 million tons of sugar, the annual output has averaged between 5 and 6 million tons of sugar extracted from about 50 million tons of cane. In 1970, however, a new record of 8.5 million tons was set. The 1971 output was estimated to be 5.7 million tons of centrifugal sugar. To be certain of meeting export commitments, sugar had to be rationed within the island, albeit at the high level of 6 pounds per person per month.

Cane grows in all provinces, but the three easternmost, led by Oriente, are the most productive. The plantations in the three eastern provinces are reported to be of unequal value: some are quite creditable, but many are ill-kept and located on unsuitable soil. Two crops are harvested every year: one in the spring and another in the winter. The latter is planted on about 40 percent of the total acreage. A sizable amount of the sugarcane crop comes from the private sector: 33 percent in 1964, 31 percent in 1965 and 27.7 percent in 1966. Moreover, the reassignment of sugarcane lands to industrial development between 1960 and 1968 gradually limited the acreage in sugarcane until 1970 when its precedence was reestablished.

Given the background, it was certainly overambitious to have predicted 10 million tons of sugar in 1970. Such a total had never been reached and there was no reason why it could have been reached at that time. Oriente Province was to carry the major part of the burden, supplying 30 percent of the total expected. The top production for Oriente in the past decade had been 15 million tons of cane in 1965, yielding around 1.8 million tons of sugar. Moreover, it is reported that to reach the desired 1970 total, part of the 1969 crop, which did not exceed 54 million tons of cane and 4.3 million tons of sugar, had been set aside to bolster the 1970 output. This maneuver resulted in a glut of canes in sugar mills, which in turn caused delays in crushing and loss of sugar content. By combining the two crops, the total output did not exceed 8.5 million tons. In 1971 production returned to the average level of about 6 million tons a year.

Sugarcane is still planted mostly by hand. Diminished productivity of the labor force and shortages of canecutters and other workers have resulted in the creation of volunteer brigades whose efficiency is still lower than that of the regular field hands. They are blamed for wastage and losses in the output of sugar. In 1965 only an estimated 2 percent of the crop was harvested by machine and the situation has remained the same ever since. In the three following years, in spite of increasing applications of fertilizers, which have multiplied 5 times since 1958, the yield seems to have diminished and some researchers believe that the fertilizers have been applied at the wrong time. Be that as it may, the trend up to 1968 seemed to be toward less yield per hectare than in 1958.

The major significance of sugar is that it is still the only agricultural product that can buy the developmental equipment so badly needed. The lack of consumer goods, the food shortages, the many hardships imposed on the citizenry, make it imperative to develop economically as fast as possible. The proportion of sugar consumed domestically does not exceed 5 percent of the total crop. Until 1961, exports to the United States brought privileged prices. By 1961 Cuba had committed itself to providing 2.2 million tons to Eastern European countries and 4 million tons in 1962. After January 1964, the communist countries agreed to take 4.9 million tons of sugar annually, 3 million of which were to go to the U.S.S.R. On several occasions the deliveries did not reach the target and new contracts had to be written. After 1968, a new international agreement was established which allowed Cuba to sell 2.1 tons of sugar on the free market. This was intended to allow Cuba to earn some hard currencies to pay for its industrialization. According to Gouré and Weinkle, this was made necessary by the fact that Russian payments were made in goods rather than in cash. It became obvious that between the U.S.S.R. and other communist countries, Cuba was more and more committed to produce only sugar, sinking deeper and deeper into the monoculture type of economy which the revolution had opposed.

Cuba has not yet solved the problem that handicaps its sugar harvests. Bernstein lists them as follows: breakdowns at the mills, absenteeism, low productivity, delays in transporting the canes from field to mills, and the fact that it has not yet been possible to mechanize the industry.

Tobacco has been a traditional Cuban cash crop and Habana is the home of the most famous cigars in the world. Tobacco is still the country's second most valuable export, and production seems to be increasing on a fairly constant amount of land (see Table No. 3). Tobacco is grown mostly in Pinar del Río. Ninety-six percent of the crop is cultivated by about 40,000 private farmers under government supervision. However, the traditional methods of production and marketing have been changed, with a consequent drop in quality. After 1965, the Cuban Tobacco Enterprise *(Empresa Cubana del Tabaco—CUBA-TABACO)* was reorganized and made responsible for all phases of tobacco growing and marketing. Cigarettes and tobacco are now rationed at 2 packages of the former and 2 cigars daily. What may be an economic constraint, however, fails to be a health benefit because it is too liberal.

Cuba could probably regain a 12,000-ton annual coffee quota which it lost in 1968 when it withdrew from the International Coffee Agreement. At present, the crop is reported to be around 30,000 tons, part of which is consumed at home under ration cards and part of which is exported to nonquota countries. Coffee has been produced in southern and eastern Oriente, in small areas between Cienfuegos and Trinidad, and also in Pinar del Río. New plantings around Habana have met with little success.

3. Animal Husbandry [72] [22] [27] [55] [57]

a. Livestock and Poultry

Livestock could probably become the second major resource of Cuban agriculture—after sugarcane and before tobacco. Yet, the industry has known many vicissitudes during the first years of the revolution. In the early 1960's indiscriminate slaughterings occurred, resulting in a loss of animals. In 1962 a law was passed requiring permits to slaughter cattle for sale or for home consumption. In 1964, a special registry for livestock operations was established to carry out the regulations formulated for the protection and expansion of the herds.

Hogs and sheep are of mediocre quality, as the climate does not favor their development. The pigs fend for themselves and get little corn. Sheep, which graze on what is left after the cattle have been fed, are used for meat rather than wool. Goats are traditionally kept for milk and meat by the poorest families. Mules and donkeys are still in widespread use as pack animals and for individual transportation. Table No. 4 gives the approximate numbers of livestock existing between 1948 and 1970. It is well known that animals surviving in the remaining private sector have not been accurately assessed.

Cattle are for the most part located in Oriente, Camagüey, and Las Villas provinces. The majority of the animals were originally Zebu strains *(criollos)*, well-adjusted to the local climate, providing reasonably good meat but poor supplies of milk. Since the revolution, Cuba has encountered problems in feeding its animals because the supply of concentrated feeds from the United States has disappeared. After the revolution an attempt was made to grow the grain needed for feed but it was soon abandoned as impracticable. Procuring grain from

THE REPUBLIC OF CUBA

Canada was possible but very costly, so it was finally decided to expand the pastures and to introduce a system of rotating grazing for 7 million cattle in the country. This implied fencing which, according to Dumont, was to extend over 500,000 kilometers and was formidably expensive as well as unnecessary in many places. The amount that was actually installed is not stated, but is considered to be far too much for the goal to be achieved. Moreover, the scarcity of competent managers has caused the grass to be misused and wasted.

Eventually, a program to provide molasses feed was adopted. To a certain extent, this supplied the energy normally expected from grain, but posed problems in terms of mineral and vitamin nutrition, as well as increased water consumption. The latter was especially serious since there was not a constant and sufficient supply. Eventually, the diet settled on was a combination of good quality grass and molasses, but it is agreed that this is an ill-balanced fare which gives the animals too much grass in the rainy season and too little during the dry months. The cattle are therefore much less productive than they could be. Since the possibility of feeding them grain is precluded, the present diet is likely to remain the same with the hope that the amount of sugar involved will help fatten the beef lines for the export market.

Castro has given much attention to the improvement of the quality of the herds. While Santa Gertrudis and Brown Swiss animals were imported before the revolution, Short Horn, Holstein, Charolais and Hereford cattle have been brought to the island since. In 1967, an artificial insemination program was started with the establishment of 11 insemination stations. The pastures began to improve and to expand at a rate of 270,000 hectares a year. The best animals are sent to feed lots in Camagüey which cover 175,000 hectares planted with pangola grasses. These are divided into smaller lots of 27 hectares each, shaped in a quadrangle. Four lots usually surround a shelter, a water tank and a molasses tank. Young bulls arrive there at the age of 8 months weighing 180 kilos and are sold back to the Government at age 24 months weighing 425 kilos. Unfortunately, brucellosis, tuberculosis and cysticercoses are widespread, and foot-and-mouth disease is still prevalent.

According to Dumont, the plan for improving Cuban cattle is assigned to a number of army officers whose responsibility is to supervise the feedlots. Each of these functionaries is in charge of a number of ranching families, say 10,000, each owning 7-8 animals. These people have three choices: 1) they can remain as they are, operating their farms on their own (Dumont reports that no one has chosen to do this); 2) they can pledge themselves to follow the directives of the Plan (then they become eligible to be entrusted with a few young bulls for fattening); or 3) they can accept the solution recommended by the army man in charge, which is for the rancher to sell to the Plan all of his holdings except for 2-3 hectares which he may keep for his own use, and work as a cowboy on his former ranch. The overwhelming majority of these families, of course, knowing what was good for them, have followed the recommendation of the Government's representative. Dumont remarks that through this system, the Party's ideas are effectively conveyed to the masses.

Chickens also seem to have suffered from excessive slaughtering following the revolution, but the Government has introduced a chicken and egg policy which may begin to show results after 1970. Between 1965 and 1970 poultry production averaged about 7.5 million birds annually. For the present, both chickens and eggs are on the ration list and are frequently unavailable.

b. Meat, Milk and Eggs

According to Dumont, the highest priorities after sugar are milk and egg production, followed by export crop production, meat output, and finally food crop production. The amount of meat available in Cuba is known only approximately. Based on the ration of 330 grams per week allotted to each citizen in Habana, and 220 grams per week outside Habana, the following amounts would have to be available in order to meet the ration requirements:

Habana	330 grams × 2 million people × 52 weeks =	34,200 tons
The rest of the country	220 grams × 6 million people × 52 weeks =	68,640 tons
Total:		102,960 tons

Dumont gives the following figures:

            1963 = 72,800 tons
            1965 = 97,700 tons
            1967 = 99,700 tons
            1968 =110,800 tons

However, reports from visitors to the island indicate that the ration allotment is seldom met.

FAO gives a very optimistic picture which, if it were accurate, would certainly permit the fulfillment of the ration card's promises. According to this source, which reflects official Cuban information, the following amounts of meat are available annually:

Beef and veal	195,000 tons
Pork	50,000 tons
Total	245,000 tons

Wiley reports that a heavy slaughter in 1959, which brought 200,000 tons, was followed by a decline in consecutive years and a new increase from 1964 to 1967.

While the amount of poultry meat produced is not known, it has certainly increased in recent years, especially in the countryside where the number of chicken farms is growing in implementation of Castro's policy to increase egg consumption.

Milk is the object of one of the grandiose projects which, according to experts, have foundered on the hard rocks of reality. The Consolidated Enterprise of Milk Industries *(Empresa Consolidata de Indústrias Lactéas)* has released the following figures which are difficult to reconcile with Castro's expectations.

Gross Production of Cows' Milk — Cuba, 1962-1968
(in 1,000 liters)

Year	State Sector	Private Sector[a]	Total
1962	–	–	219,414.3
1963	60,323.8	157,113.7	217,437.5
1964	134,554.4	91,423.5	225,977.9
1965	148,850.2	85,348.0	234,198.2
1966	235,874.7	93,629.8	329,507.5
1967	–	–	324,119.8
1968	–	–	302,102.2

[a]It is interesting to note the steady decrease of the private sector's contribution.

Source: C.P. Roberts and M. Hamour, Eds., *Cuba 1968.*

In May 1967 Castro promised that Oriente Province would produce 1.3 million liters of milk a day, but in 1969 the provincial production was only 310,000 liters. Yet, it was still believed that by 1970 milk production could be multiplied 4 times. The basis for this expectation seems to have been the success of the artificial insemination program, which resulted in a large number of heifers of good stock. Five hundred thousand were expected to lactate for the first time in 1970. With good care, each of these animals could deliver 3,000 liters a year or 1.5 million tons which, added to the 300,000 said to be available in 1969, would amount to a total of 1.8 million tons. Dumont asserts that one could reasonably expect another 525,000 tons from the Camagüey area, bringing the total for the country to about 2.3 million tons a year, if everything goes well. From this total, the preemption of milk for calves and for the food industry to manufacture cheese, butter and evaporated milk, as well as some unavoidable wastage, should be deducted, The milk ration is 1 liter per family per day. On the basis of 1.6 million families of 5 people each, the requirements would be 584,000 tons. The margin seems wide enough to insure satisfaction of the ration card. One wonders why, then, there have been so many reports of shortages. The only explanation is that production has not reached the 2.3 million tons estimated.

According to FAO estimates, the number of eggs produced in 1970 was 1.1 billion, weighing 49,500 tons. The ration is 12 eggs per capita per month in Habana but no rationing is in force in the countryside. If the figures given by FAO are accurate, and if the Government honors the urban ration quota, the inhabitants of the city would feast on about 288 million eggs a year, leaving 762 million to their 6 million rural compatriots, who would then each have about 12 eggs a month.

4. Fisheries [18] [13] [11] [12] [15] [16] [17] [20] [25]

Fishing has long been the livelihood of a small section of the population. However, according to information originating from the State Fishing Authority *(Empresa Estatal de Pesca)* which regulates the fishing industry, pre-revolutionary fishing was carried out by a fleet of 3,000 small boats, each operated by one or two men, fishing the coastal waters. Very few vessels, none more than 80 feet in length, were sailing the high seas and none had modern equipment. In 1970, the total tonnage of the Cuban fishing industry was over 21,000 tons distributed among 300 vessels of different sizes and types, 130 of them manufactured and equipped abroad. Ninety shrimp trawlers have been delivered from Spain as well as three older Spanish factory vessels. Thirty more ships, which are refrigerated and have 50 tons frozen storage capacity, have been ordered from France and are now presumably delivered. Italy has also sold two carrier mother ships built in La Spezia, reputed to be the fastest and best equipped vessels of the Cuban high seas fleet.

The vessels now in operation make up a more than respectable fleet. The Caribbean shrimp fleet was expected to bring 10,000 tons of shrimp in 1970 and 60,000 tons of fish to be processed into fishmeal. This fleet is scheduled to operate out of Cienfuegos Bay where land facilities, including an ice plant, a fishmeal plant and more warehouses, will be built. No evidence has been seen as yet that these plans are on the way to completion. The so-called Gulf fleet plies the waters of the Gulf of Mexico. It is less well-equipped than the shrimp fleet, operating mostly with Cuban-built wooden ships, but it possesses some modern electrical and electronic equipment. Other small boats operate on the continental shelf. A coastal fleet continues to fish the home waters under a special agency responsible to the *Empresa.* Domestic fishing areas are divided into four zones as follows:

From Punta de Maisi (Oriente) to Cienfuegos (Las Villas)

From Cienfuegos to Cabo San Antonio (Pinar del Río)

From Cabo San Antonio to Punta de Guanes (Matanzas)

From Punta de Guanes to Punta de Maisí

The catch of the coastal fleet is distributed within the province where the vessel is based. Habana sends some of the catch landed at its fishing port to the interior consumption centers.

The substantial effort to expand fishing is assisted by a fishery research center in Habana where tuna, lobster, shrimp, oyster and other marine fishery studies are carried out. More important, an educational effort has been made to develop a taste for fish among the population in view of the shortage of meat. Per capita fish consumption is said to have doubled since pre-revolution days. Export markets for Cuban fish exist in Western Europe (France, Italy and Great Britain) and Eastern Europe, making it possible to earn foreign exchange with which to buy hardware and develop industry.

All of the state-controlled landings in 1961 were the result of cooperative activities and amounted to 18,578 tons. By 1968, the total catch (state and private) came to 66,032 tons. The largest catches always come from La Habana, which dominates the other provinces by threefold. According to a statement made in April 1970 on the occasion of a Cuban delegation's visit to the International Fishing Fair in Peru, the total catch landed by Cuban fishermen was expected to reach 175,000 tons in 1970. This prognosis has not yet been confirmed. In 1958, the year before the revolution, a total of 21,900 tons of seafood were recorded. It seems reasonable to estimate a threefold increase during the 1958-1968 decade, and an output of over 80,000 tons of fish and shellfish after 1971.

The *Empresa Estatal de Pesca* was established in 1963 with the assistance of the Soviet Union. It directs the activities of the Cuban fishing fleet and governs the port of Habana, the cooperatives, the warehouses, a ship-building facility, canning plants, the research center at Habana and an export company (see *Food Industries*). In March 1967, a Fish Culture Department was created within the *Empresa* and it has established stations throughout Cuba for the purpose of developing freshwater fish in inland waters. The main species raised are *Ctenopharyn godon idellus* (white amur) and *Hypophtalmichtys molitrix*) (white tenca), plus some species of carp. Freshwater turtles are also raised.

D. FOOD INDUSTRIES [22] [39] [55] [19] [14] [18] [21]

The Cuban Revolution, contrary to a view often expressed, is not based on a gigantic transformation of an agricultural economy into an industrial system. After yielding for a short while to Guevara's insistence that Cuba be industrialized, Castro adopted the policy of concentrating on what Cuba knows best how to do: grow and process sugarcane. The accent is now on the development of agriculture since the major source of income is sugar. It is notable that almost all the promises made by the Prime Minister refer to agricultural products: a fourfold increase in milk production: 15 percent annual increases in other agricultural products, etc. While these promises have not been and could not have been implemented, no similar targets seem to have been considered in the industrial sector.

In 1966, the food processing industry provided the largest share (22.4 percent) of total industrial output. It has held this position since the revolutionary government began publishing statistics in 1963. As expected, the second largest share of industrial output is contributed by the sugar industry, which is shown separately from food processing (see Table No. 5). The sugar mills and refineries are by far the most important single plants in the country. There are, in all, 152 sugar mills, unequally distributed among the six provinces. Las Villas has the most and Pinar del Río the least, according to the following table.

Distribution of Sugar Mills by Province – Cuba, 1968

Province	Mills
Pinar del Río	8
La Habana	12
Matanzas	22
Las Villas	47
Camagüey	24
Oriente	39

Source: C.P. Roberts and M. Hamour, Eds., *Cuba 1968*.

Some of these mills are operational. Many are under par, dating from pre-revolution days, needing repairs and lacking the needed spare parts.

The present tendency is to burn the canes before cutting them. This facilitates harvesting but destroys the valuable foliage which could be used as fodder. Also, if any delay occurs in crushing the cane (which should take place 48 hours or less after harvest), substantial quantities of sugar are lost. Refineries in Cuba yield about 16-17 percent refined sugar from the raw cane.

The fishing industry is next in importance in terms of its extension, although not yet in terms of financial returns. The Government hopes to make Cuba one of Latin America's leading seafood exporters. Some experts, however, wonder if the investments made so far do not exceed the potential returns. The Cuban fishing industry has received considerable aid from the United Nations, the Soviet Union and from a number of European countries. The fishing port of Habana covers 13.7 hectares and cost a theoretical $35 million. It was built with U.S.S.R. technical assistance and has eight storerooms fully refrigerated with a capacity of 11,500 tons of fish, an ice plant that can produce 40 tons of ice per day, and a floating dry dock that can handle ships of 2,500 tons.

A salted cod industry has been established, which should eliminate the need to import this traditional food. In 1969 existing salting facilities had an annual capacity of about 5,000 tons of dried salted cod. A new plant at Antilla was expected to bring total production up to 20,000 tons which was the amount imported in 1969. Fishmeal production is a goal of the Cuban industry, but to date no data have appeared on this undertaking. Tuna, shrimp, lobster tails and canned lobster meat are processed on the island, primarily for export.

The milling and baking industries are not as progressive as the fishing industry. The output of flour in 1968 was reported to be 137,600 tons, the same amount as in 1967. About 163,000 tons of bread were produced in 1966 (or only 2 kilos per capita), and no figures are given for subsequent years. About 54,200 tons of biscuits were manufactured in 1966 and 42,000 tons of pasta in 1968. This would amount to about 17 kilos of cereal flour in various forms a year per inhabitant, a very spartan ration.

Preserved fruits are produced, yielding 5 kilos per capita per year. Canned tomatoes could yield almost 2 kilos per capita per year if not exported.

The milk industry pasteurizes about 10 percent of the milk output, processes around 0.2 percent into condensed and evaporated milk, and manufactures small quantities of yogurt, cheese and butter, the latter amounting to a maximum ratio of 170 grams per capita per year.

There are few figures for Cuban-produced rum and other alcoholic beverages. The 1966 output of rum was probably as much as 119,000 hectoliters. This would mean about 12 liters for every 8 inhabitants per year or about 1 1/2 liters per capita, a very reasonable consumption if the figures are correct.

E. TRADE

1. Domestic Trade [22] [55]

Domestic trade now consists chiefly in the distribution to the population of the goods purchased abroad by the Government or collected from local state farms, cooperatives and small private farms. In addition, there is a small amount of trade taking place among citizens themselves on the black market. According to Dumont, this last is quite developed and there is a schedule of black market prices to which most adhere.

The list and amounts of food distributed by the Government in honoring the ration cards is shown in the table below for the years 1963-1966. Crediting the table with some degree of accuracy, the food products mentioned can be divided into two groups: those which were on the increase in terms of availability and those on the decrease during the 3-year period considered.

Rationed Foods – Cuba, 1963-1966

On the Increase	On the Decrease
Refined vegetable oil	Canned meat
Crude sugar	Smoked meat
Refined sugar	Roasted coffee
Onions	Fruit preserves
Beans	Canned vegetables
Condensed milk	Flour
Pasteurized milk	Shrimp
Lard	Cheese
Pastas	Garlic
Fish	
Plantains	
Table salt	

Source: Compiled from various sources.

At a glance it appears that with the exception of fish, the availability of which is on the increase, the distribution of protein-rich foods, such as meat, and good cereals, such as wheat flour is on the decrease while most empty-calorie foods or starchy foods like sugar and plantains, are on the increase.

All these rationed goods are traded in an estimated 20,805 outlets distributed among six government agencies as follows:

Commercial Outlets for Food Distribution, by Agency – Cuba, 1968

Agency	Number of Outlets
Ministry of Domestic Commerce	4,889
National Tourist Institute	1,649
Ministry of Public Health	1,334
Ministry of Transportation	268
Regional Administration	12,665

Source: C.P. Roberts and M. Hamour, Eds., *Cuba 1968.*

These outlets are themselves supplied by nonretail stores performing the function of wholesale dealers. In 1966 there were 893 of these.

2. Foreign Trade [33] [66] [71] [22] [72] [29]

Prior to the revolution, the United States had been Cuba's traditional primary trading partner. Even in 1959, the year Castro came to power, 68 percent of Cuba's trade was with the United States. The reorientation of Cuba's foreign trade away from the Western Hemisphere and towards the communist bloc began in earnest in February 1960 when Cuba signed its first trade agreement with the Soviet Union. The U.S.S.R. promised to purchase 5 million tons of Cuban sugar during the next 5 years, 20 percent to be paid for in hard currency, 80 percent in goods. The Soviet Union pledged not to resell the Cuban sugar so as to protect its price on the world market. At the same time, a $100 million line of credit was opened for Cuba for the purchase of Russian industrial equipment.

In 1960 the United States still purchased a fairly high proportion of Cuban exports—52.8 percent—and the communist countries purchased 24.2 percent; but in 1961 the U.S. share dropped drastically to 4.8 percent and the communist bloc level rose to 71.6 percent. In 1962 the communist countries (primarily the Soviet Union) purchased 82 percent of all Cuban exports and provided 82.8 percent of the island's imports (up from 18.7 percent in 1960). At present, this trade is unfavorable to both sides. Cuba sells its sugar to Russia but cannot sell enough to meet the cost of what it buys, thus incurring a debt of about $150 million per year. On the other hand, Russia sells more than she buys but pays an exorbitant price for Cuba's sugar and cannot reasonably expect ever to receive repayment for the credit extended. The benefits both sides receive from this operation are obviously political rather than commercial.

The Soviet Union's gradual increase in sales to and purchases from Cuba began as a rescue operation to bail out the Cuban economy, hit first by the U.S. blockade of Cuba and then by the OAS endorsement of this blockade (see page 34). In order to frustrate these practices, the U.S.S.R. found itself engaged in operations of greater and greater magnitude as years went by. Goure and Weinkle believe that at the beginning the Soviet Union did not anticipate the extent its involvement was to reach. As the policy of the U.S. tightened vis-à-vis Cuba, the Soviet attitude softened, its sugar purchasing program was enlarged, and its aid support was expanded to include steel mills, oil refining and mining equipment, and power generators. In 1964, a second trade agreement was signed but this one was based strictly on barter arrangements and excluded the prohibition on Russian resale of the sugar purchased from Cuba. The Soviet Union did agree, however, to barter goods at a rate exceeding the world market price for sugar, thus in effect subsidizing the Cuban sugar crop.

A study of the shipments from the U.S.S.R. to Cuba reveals enormous quantities of food exports. About 500,000 tons of grain are shipped every year to the island to keep the population alive (see Table No. 6). In terms of calories, the U.S.S.R. certainly holds the survival of Cuba in her hands since with her grain alone she supplies almost 450 calories per capita per day to the Cuban population. Moreover, 20,000 tons of fish, millions of boxes of preserved meat, 52,000 tons of potatoes, and almost 300,000 tons of flour explain the extent of the black market that ultimately allows the population of Cuba to survive as it could not do on the scanty rations described under *Diets.*

The Soviet Union is, of course, the most important of all Cuba's present trade partners. In addition to food, in 1969 the U.S.S.R. sold to Cuba virtually all its requirements in fuel oil (5.7 million tons), mineral fertilizers, trucks, tractors (4,619 in 1968), agricultural machines (9,741 units in 1968), etc.* Suchlicki** thinks that in 1970 Cuba occupied sixth place (just ahead of Rumania) among the U.S.S.R.'s major trading partners. The total cost of machinery sold to the island in 1969 rose to about $235 million. All this, naturally, is exchanged for sugar*** at the equivalent of 6¢ a pound, which is well above the world market

---

*Many of the Russian goods exchanged for sugar are reported to be unsatisfactory. Agricultural machines, for instance, must be adjusted to the length and width of Cuban planting rows before they can be used. Moreover, the steel components rust quickly in the island's subtropical climate and spare parts are difficult to obtain. Breakdowns are frequent, representing a 60-80 percent loss of operating time.

**Private communication.

***In January 1964 the Soviet Union signed an agreement with Cuba which provided for the following shipments of sugar to Russia, acting for COMECON countries as well.

Year	Million tons
1965	2.1
1966	3.0
1967	4.0
1968	5.0
1969	5.0
1970	5.0
	24.1

price. In 1965, for instance, the Soviet Union paid Cuba 5 times the world market price of 1.32¢ per pound for sugar. In 1968 the world market price was 3.38¢ per pound. The cost is apparently worth the leverage it gives the Soviet Union over Cuban foreign policy. Other communist countries—Czechoslovakia, East Germany, Rumania, Hungary, Bulgaria and Poland—have opened trade credits for Cuba, all offset to some extent by sugar imports which amounted to 796,000 tons in 1969 but left Cuba with an unfavorable trade balance.

Cuba assumes that the Soviet Union will continue to buy at the equivalent of 6.1¢ a pound large amounts of sugar which it could easily produce itself or could purchase elsewhere cheaper at 3¢ a pound. Moreover, if the "honor of the revolution" had materialized in 1970, which it did not, this would have meant selling 4-5 million tons of sugar outside the saturated Russian market, a questionable possibility at best. It is reported that all trade with COMECON * countries goes through the U.S.S.R. as general contractor, thus adding to Russia's total control of the Cuban economy. Trade with COMECON countries is oriented towards procuring the wherewithal needed to reconstruct the Cuban sugar industry along modern lines.

Understandably, Cuba is trying to expand its trade outside the communist world, especially since most of the commerce with the Soviet Union is in the form of barter, thus failing to produce the hard currencies needed to pay for a flexible list of purchases. On the noncommunist side of the world, Cuba trades with France, Spain, Canada, Japan, Italy, Holland, West Germany, Mexico and the United Kingdom.

After sugar, tobacco is Cuba's most important export. Before the revolution, the United States purchased 65-70 percent, by value, of the yearly crop. Now, Eastern and Western European countries are the primary customers. However, exports of unmanufactured tobacco are reported to have declined from 26,000 tons in 1960 to a present annual average of about 14,000 tons, although it has been difficult to make precise estimates since 1960 due to the unreliability of statistics.

The fall in sugar production in certain years has to be offset by the export of other products so as to recoup the loss in foreign exchange earnings. In 1968 Cuba exported 540 tons of spiny lobster to France worth $1.45 million. In the same year meat valued at $2.25 million was shipped to England, and Spain promised to buy $1 million worth of beef. Large amounts of citrus fruit and coffee are traded to Western Europe in order to buy industrial and military items.

If one looks at data on Cuban food imports, perhaps the most startling fact which emerges is the continuous need for basic cereals and flour. Wiley reports

---

*Council for Mutual Economic Assistance (sometimes referred to as CEMA): the communist bloc trading organization.

that 55,000 tons of rough rice were imported in 1965 from Communist China and 96,000 tons in 1967 paid for with 556,000 tons of sugar. After 1968, an increase in homegrown rice replaced imports of the Chinese grain.

F. FOOD SUPPLY [22]

That the Cuban food supply is inadequate is made obvious by the fact that it is rationed. The reasons for this inadequacy are multiple. The most important is certainly the complete dependence upon the sale of sugar to purchase the food needed every day by the population. At the same time, the amount of land available for food crops has decreased during the last 5 years, partly because of the return to expanded sugar production. A second reason for scarcity lies in the agrarian reforms which have drastically limited the number of privately-owned farms in favor of state farms or cooperatives. These types of farms have proved disappointing, both because of the incompetence of the administrators placed at the head of the enterprises and because of the lack of enthusiasm of the workers, who are more anxious to do justice to their small personal plots than to the common crop in which they will never share. A third cause for scarcity is lack of interest in work due to the unavailability of consumer goods and private property on which to spend earned income. The result is a high rate of absenteeism. A fourth reason for scarcity is that most of the production plans to increase the output of food are poorly prepared. Dumont lists a number of such errors in planning: vegetable gardens are sown on iron-rich lands which are too porous and too eroded to serve the purpose for which they were chosen; coffee is planted on lands receiving less than 1,000 millimeters of rain a year; costly experiments are made with vegetables sown to float on fertilizing solutions; vineyards are burned by too much fertilizer while other fields go begging for more; citrus, pineapple and banana plantations are sown on inadequate ground and are poorly maintained by incompetent workers led by unskilled army officers. Finally, the universal scarcity prevailing in all aspects of the economy— the extensive rationing of practically everything, and the frequent absence of goods promised by the ration cards—has resulted in a general discouragement, lack of interest and lack of incentive to improve. The situation is best exemplified by the crowds lining up until midnight for a mediocre supper at a restaurant, or queuing up for 3 hours in the hot sun to buy ice cream cones (many to be disappointed at the time they finally step into the store), or lining up for hours just for the privilege of sitting at an outdoor café, where no coffee or beer is available but where one can sit sipping a sugary fruit juice while others move slowly down the line. There seems to be no doubt that the excessive strain of everyday life, this constant major effort to achieve nothing, decreases stamina and productivity.

A serious and valuable effort has been made to create regional food supplies.

Given the length of the island and the losses incurred when bananas, for example, have to be hauled from Oriente Province to Habana, it seemed logical to create a vertical organization for the commercialization of foods from producer to consumer within each province rather than a horizontal organization (e.g., growing the bananas in Oriente, and processing them in Habana).

1. Storage

With the exception of the information given in the section on fisheries, no up-to-date information is available on storage facilities in each region, and there is all possible evidence that foods do not spend any length of time in government storage; but warehouses are said to exist in all provinces, both for the collection of food and for their distribution. Agents of the Government collect the produce from state farms, cooperatives and private farmers and store it before it can be distributed again to retail outlets. In all of the six provinces, however, finding food is a major preoccupation.

2. Transportation [24] [22]

Transportation in Cuba is not a problem. A railroad line joins the southeast-ernmost point of Guantánamo to La Fé, the most extreme western point. Santa Clara, about midway, is a junction station where a line to Mientras on the north coast branches off and another links Habana to Cienfuegos. There is a central trunk road following almost the same design as the railroad, and branches of this main highway link the primary inland urban centers to the sea.

III. DIETS

A. GENERAL [22] [69]

So long as Russia provides Cuba with food, no one will really starve, but the diets are mediocre, both in quantity and quality. The fact that the foods are rationed and that many rationed goods are not available does not brighten the picture. Normally, the Cuban conforms to general Caribbean food tastes and customs. Rice and beans, salted cod, plantains and *viandas* were the basis of the pre-revolution diet. This diet was remarkable only because it was more abundant in meat and milk than is usually the case in the Caribbean. Now the Cuban eats what he can get. Thirteen years after the revolution, food shortages remain a chronic problem. Most Cubans try to supplement their rations if and when possible at restaurants, although long lines are formed to gain entry. The cost of these meals adds an additional 30-35 percent to the family food budget, but there is no point in saving since practically nothing else can be purchased. The cost of food on the black market is also an important aspect of the expenditure, and can bring the family food bill up to 60-70 percent of the salary. According to Wheeler, reporting in October 1968, the average family budget allocates 17 percent for restaurant meals, pastries and pizzas, 43 percent for rationed goods, and 4 percent for black market coffee.

B. RATIONS [22] [52] [73] [53] [23] [59] [36]

The rations allowed by the Government probably provide 1,427 calories per capita per day. Through restaurant and black market purchases it is estimated that the average citizen can raise this total to 1,800 and perhaps to 2,200 if he has enough money. The following table presents a comparison between the availability of certain foods in 1945 and the authorized rations of 1971.

Food Availability – Cuba, 1945 and 1971
(grams per capita per day, unless otherwise stated)

Item	1945 Availability[a]	Estimated 1971 Ration	Sources of Information for Estimated 1971 Ration
Milk	200	200	Dumont
Eggs	1/2 egg	1/3 egg	Porterfield
Meat	150	40	Edmonstone, Dumont
Fats	60	15	Winfrey
Green & yellow vegs.	120	–	–
Citrus fruits	120	–	–
Other fruits	82	–	–
Sugar	75	88	Dumont
Tubers	300	–	–
Cereals	200	50 (rice)	Soler
Bread	130	72	Edmonstone
Beans	–	23	Dumont
Butter	–	2	Winfrey
Coffee	–	6	Winfrey
Fish	–	31	Dumont

[a]Source: O. Pereira Calzadilla, " Que Ocurre con el Gandul en Cuba?"

The supply of milk is reserved primarily for children and adds up to 1 liter per day for infants up to 2 years of age and 1/2 liter per day for children between 2 and 7 years of age. None is allowed for those over 7. Old people and pregnant women have a special ration card allowing them some milk. Vegetables are very scarce, occasionally available in November and December (lettuce, cauliflower and cabbages). None are found the rest of the year. Fruits, such as citrus, suddenly appear and cause crowds to assemble. Oranges are scarce but occasionally are distributed to children: the equivalent of one small orange per child or half a big one. Tomatoes also occasionally appear in shops. City hotels offer a lunch consisting of fish soup, a meat croquette, a plate of rice, salad and beer. The cost of such a meal in 1971 was the equivalent of $7.00 to $8.00.* On the black market, coffee sells for $40 per 460 grams, black beans for $12 per 460 grams, chickens for $25 each, pork for $9 per 140 grams and beer for $7 per small bottle. Running water is rationed at 2 hours per day and the problem of providing enough drinking water is serious.

On the basis of the figures given by the ration cards, the following daily calorie and nutrient ration can be computed.

Estimated Calories and Nutrients in the Daily Ration – Cuba, 1971

Item	Quantity per day (g)	Calories	Pro-teins (g)	Fats (g)	Calcium (mg)	Iron (mg)	Vitamin A (mcg)	Thia-mine (mg)	Niacin (mg)	Ribo-flavin (mg)
Meat	43	40	7	2	4	15	44	.5	1.0	.05
Fish[a]	31	100	27	1	15	1.2	–	.03	3.3	.15
Eggs	20	15	2	2	10	.5	25	–	.07	.07
Beans	23	80	8	–	16	–	–	–	–	.24
Butter	1.5	8	.2	.5	–	–	9	.07	.1	–
Oil or lard	14	112	–	14	–	–	–	–	–	–
Bread	220	675	20	1.6	70	3.7	–	.20	.12	.03
Rice	41	149	3	.3	4	–	–	.04	.6	.02
Sugar	80	248	–	–	–	–	–	–	–	–
Milk										
Total		1,427	67.2	21.4	119	20.4	78	.84	4.65	.56

[a] Assumed to be dried fish.

Sources: Computed on the basis of information provided by various sources.

In addition to the official per capita ration, Dumont reports that each family may get the following supplements every month.

Supplements to Per Capita Ration – Cuba, 1970

Item	Amount
Pasta	1 package
Tomato paste	1 can
Detergent	1 box
Toothpaste	1 small tube
Cigarettes, or	1 pack
Cigars	1
Toilet paper	1 roll
Soap	2½ cakes

Source: R. Dumont, *Cuba: Est-Il Socialiste?*

---

*A simpler meal of soup, spaghetti, ice cream, coffee and beer costs $4.50.

Still in addition, small amounts of flour may come one's way when the shipment from Russia arrives and 1 cup of yogurt may be distributed every month. Roots and tubers may occasionally show up for a few hours in certain shops. Other items that can make an occasional temporary appearance are bananas (never more than one at a time per person), ears of corn (never more than two apiece), avocados (two at a time), and a few small lemons.

Speaking of prices makes no sense. The peso is officially considered to be equivalent to 1 U.S. dollar but cannot be bought or sold outside Cuba while a dollar cannot be legally introduced into the country. The price fetched by $1 on the Cuban black market amounts to 5 or 6 pesos, but this has little significance, either. What might give an idea of the income situation is a comparison between the minimum wage paid in Cuba and the cost of a satisfactory ration, if such were available. Given a family of 5 and a basic monthly wage of 85 pesos for the head of the family and perhaps 50 pesos for the wife (not all wives work full-time and many do not work at all), a budget of 135 pesos per month would be available. The cost of the ration diet mentioned above is, according to Dumont, 1/4 peso per day or 1.25 pesos per day for the entire family, or 37.5 pesos per month, to which the monthly supplements listed above should be added. Quite clearly, the margin is sufficient to cover the cost of rationed goods and a substantial surplus is available for the restaurant, the pastry and the pizza. At the other end of the salary scale, a maximum is set at $900 per month for skilled engineers, or highly paid government officials.

C. SPECIAL DIETS [22]

In addition to preschool children, pregnant women and old people may also get certain privileges. Expectant mothers are entitled to milk, which they may or may not get, and to one chicken a month but the joke is common that a pregnant woman will have to wait until the fetus goes to school to receive her "pregnancy chicken." Old men also have minor privileges and canecutters may receive additional rations. (It was noticed that their work was slow and inefficient because of undernutrition.) There is a group of privileged few (probably Party members, etc.) for whom certain well-supplied restaurants function but where admission requires a card delivered by the Government which bears an identification number.

IV. ADEQUACY OF FOOD RESOURCES

Obviously, Cuban food resources are inadequate since they have to be supplemented by considerable imports. Importing expensive food from half a globe away is no economic crime per se if the income of the country can bear it. One may wonder about the wisdom of a policy which results in the living conditions described not only by Cuban refugees but also by residents interviewed by visitors, and which may be regarded as subjecting daily rations to the goodwill of a foreign country. Given the most favorable rice crop, estimated at 326,000 tons in 1970, supplemented with a 90,000-ton import, the total would yield a daily ration of 142 grams per capita if nothing were wasted or used for seed. Dry beans, the next food staple on the list, have been in constant decrease because of efforts at industrialization and the increasing demand for land for cash crops. The daily per capita availability could not exceed 7 grams a day and the ration is 23 grams. Corn has also lost ground in drastic proportions and according to 1970 figures provides a daily per capita availability of 40-45 grams. No wonder the people eat manioc, yams and malanga for the filling effect.

The picture is worse when it comes to good proteins, which are more severely rationed than other foods and are often not available at all, even with a ration card. Meat, official meat, that is, was available at the rate of 7 grams per capita per day in 1969, fish at the level of 27 grams and eggs at the rate of 2 grams, making a total of 36 grams of animal protein and 67.2 grams of total protein.* This is short of the minimum daily requirement (1 gram per kilo of body weight) which is probably not met, regardless of the little additions alert people can find for themselves or their families. The increasing availability of fish already makes a welcome difference. Fish is not rationed but it is hard to come by in the interior. Given a catch of 60,000 tons a year, which does not include shrimp and lobster tails reserved for export, it is conceivable that about 7.5 kilos of fresh fish are, or will soon be, available per capita per year, delivering probably 5 kilos of edible meat. This could cast a new light on the level of nutrition of the population.

The vitamin intake is certainly inadequate, or at best very irregular and unevenly distributed. Obviously, those who have a couple of citrus trees or a mango tree on their plot are better off than the rest. Vitamin pills are occasionally distributed to pregnant women and to children.

V. NUTRITIONAL DISEASE PATTERNS

No nutritional surveys have been made in Cuba since the revolution. The last ones, dating back to 1958 and 1953, are obsolete, given the changes that have occurred. All the information available comes from individual reports made by emigrant physicians who have left Cuba in large numbers and are now established in Florida. According to several interviewed in 1971, signs of hypoprotinemia are common, but none mentioned the word "kwashiorkor" or even protein-calorie malnutrition. This may mean that these practitioners have not observed

---

*We have assumed that the fish is dried salted cod which provides more protein and calories per 100 grams than fresh fish.

the disease or that the deficiency is not sufficiently acute to create a visible problem. Anemia is reportedly very common, but no one can say whether its cause is nutritional or due to blood or intestinal parasites, or a combination of all. Average findings of hemoglobin levels per 100 ml of blood appears to stand at 10-12 grams, obviously low but not deficient. Signs of vitamin A deficiency were reported by at least one physician interviewed. All agree that riboflavin deficiency is prevalent, as evidenced by angular cheilosis. Pellagra was not mentioned. The weight of newborn babies continues to be between 6 and 7 pounds. This is not unusual under such conditions, since the mother bears the brunt of the impact of malnutrition or undernutrition.

VI. CONCLUSIONS

There seems to be no doubt that the ability to provide indigenous food for the people has substantially deteriorated in Cuba since the revolution. This is due to physical, psychological and political causes. The most important physical reason for the present situation is the intensification of the policy of concentrating the agricultural effort on sugar production. It is true that a significant promotion of the livestock industry and of rice cultivation has also taken place, but there is little evidence that the returns from these investments are as yet of sufficient magnitude to restore the country to the minimum of independence that usually goes with freedom from want. To implement this "sugar first" policy, much land that could have been used for food crops has been preempted for cane.

The lack of skilled technicians in all fields of production affects the availability and the distribution of foods. While it is true that, frightened by the revolution, many educated people and technicians have left the island, it is also true that a great educational effort seems to have been undertaken by the new regime. Why is it, then, that in almost 13 years it has not been possible to create a new squadron of the most essential skilled laborers to assure at least the production of acceptable diets and their distribution?

The psychological reasons for the present scarcity can be found mostly in the lack of interest of the people in improving their lot. This negative frame of mind is born from the certainty that the task is impossible and that nothing can really be done. At a time when initiative is considered with suspicion because it implies a lack of agreement with official policies, when expressing an opinion that is slightly different from the party line may result in classifying one among the enemies of the state, and when additional exertions in toeing the official line may bring one a medal but not an ounce more of rice, a certain "take it easy" attitude becomes understandable.

The question of "material stimulus" is frequently discussed by communist theoreticians. It is usually shyly and covertly given some consideration. Not so in

Cuba where the idealism of Guevara, who thought the revolution could create an ideal man free of the bourgeois appetite for earthly comforts, has not been overtly repudiated. The futility of money, with which only a little more food can be bought on the black market at a certain risk, destroys any interest in work. Moreover, the availability of a minimal although inadequate diet at a price all can afford further muffles energy and results in a high level of absenteeism, while the low caloric intake also contributes to weak productivity. So far, no physical coercion seems to have been used to bring the workers back to the fields or to the lathe, but it is hard to see how it could not be forthcoming. If and when it comes, it might increase "presence" but hardly productivity.

The political causes for scarcity are just as obvious. The dominant impression received from a study of Cuban nutrition is the realization of the quasi-total hold the Soviet Union has over the economy of the country and over the vital minimum of food needed for the population to survive. There seems to be no way open at present for this economic bondage to be shaken off. While it is conceivable that Cuba might wish to return to a subsistence economy owing nothing to anyone, it is inconceivable that such a change could be made in the face of the formidable repression that would naturally ensue.

The sugar monoculture which existed before the revolution did not carry the potential of enslavement to a foreign power that the present condition entails, regardless of anti-American propaganda claims. The main difference is that in earlier days the major part of the sugar industry belonged to United States enterprises which returned a portion of the earnings to the island in the form of salaries, taxes, road building, health and community services, education, etc. At present, although the Soviet Union does not own the industry, it does own practically all of its output, which is equivalent to owning all of its purchasing power. If the crop failed in pre-revolutionary days, the U.S. lost, but Cuba suffered only insofar as it received fewer benefits. Domestic food production could supply most of the local needs and money from previous years' harvests could be used to purchase additional necessities abroad. If the crop were to fail now, the country's entire economy would be in jeopardy and the Government might not be able to buy food anywhere, having no means of payment. The quasi-monopoly on the island's production held by the communist bloc makes it impossible for Cuba to find other trading partners on short notice. It is difficult to see how under the present setup Cubans can be fed adequately except at the sufferance of the Soviet Union.

For all these reasons, the conclusion that the ability of Cuba to feed itself has considerably diminished since the revolution, cannot be avoided. The long range picture is hard to perceive. Most of the factors involved in food production are favorable; left to itself in a free economy there are no reasons why the island could not enjoy a safe and plentiful diet. The land and climate are good and the capital needed to restore agricultural production to a well-balanced structure could conceivably again be made available again. One is hard put to understand the rationale of the present policies on a scientific and economic basis.

BIBLIOGRAPHY

1. *ANAP* (Habana), January 1970, 20-22.
2. _____, February 1970, 22-27.
3. _____, May 1970, 20-22.
4. _____, July 1970, 18-22.
5. _____, August 1970, 18-20.
6. _____ , September 1970, 21.
7. Bernstein, L.A. "Cuba's Record Sugar Output." *Foreign Agriculture,* 1970, VIII (46), 6-8.
8. Bohning, D. "Cuba's Mango Supply Provides a Unique Dilemma—a Surplus." *The Miami Herald,* July 8, 1965.
9. Buck, W.F. "Cuban Agriculture Ten Years Under Castro." *Foreign Agriculture,* 1969, VII (1), 2-4.
10. _____ . "Cuba's Agricultural Output is Lagging Despite Shifts in Farm Policy." *Foreign Agriculture,* 1968, VI (5), 2-4.
11. *Commercial Fisheries Review,* 1968, 30 (10), 67.
12. _____ , 1969, 31 (3), 40.
13. _____ , 1969, 31 (5), 50.
14. _____ , 1969, 31 (6), 62.
15. _____ , 1969, 31 (8-9), 66.
16. _____ , 1969, 31 (10), 63, 66.
17. _____ , 1969, 31 (12), 56.
18. _____ , 1970, 32 (2), 49-50.
19. _____ , 1970, 32 (5), 54.
20. _____ , 1970, 32 (7), 50, 63.
21. Cuba, Government of (Ministerio de la Industria Alimenticia). *Industria Alimenticia.*
22. Dumont, R. *Cuba Est-Il Socialiste?* Paris, Edition du Seuil, 1970.
23. Edmonstone, W. " 'Things Are Very Disorganized Here.' " *The Miami Herald,* January 12, 1971.
24. *Encyclopedia Britannica.* Chicago, William Benton Publisher, 1970.
24a. Espinosa Figueroa, M. *Informe al Gobierno de Cuba Sobre un Programa de Nutrición Aplicada de la FAO.* CEP Informe No. 54. NU:TA/68/19. Rome, FAO, 1968.

25. Fagen, R.R. and Fagen, P.W. "Revolution for Cuba's Lobster Industry." *The Geographical Magazine*, 1970, 42, 867-875.

26. Food and Agriculture Organization of the United Nations. *Country Report of the Cuban Delegation to the Food and Agriculture Organization on Land Reform.* RU:WLR/C. Rome, FAO, 1966.

27. _____. *Production Yearbook 1969.* Volume 23. Rome, FAO, 1970.

28. _____. *Production Yearbook 1970.* Volume 24. Rome, FAO, 1971.

29. _____. *Trade Yearbook 1969.* Volume 23. Rome, FAO, 1970.

30. *Foreign Agriculture*, 1971, IX (42), 12.

31. Gendler, E. "Holy Days in Habana." *Conservative Judaism*, 1969, 23 (2), 15-24.

32. González, A. "The Population of Cuba." *Caribbean Studies*, 1971, 2.

33. Gouré, L. and Weinkle, J. "Soviet-Cuban Relations—The Growing Integration." *Cuba, Castro and Revolution*, J. Suchlicki, Ed., Coral Gables, University of Miami Press, 1972.

34. Gutelman, M. "The Socialization of the Means of Production in Cuba." *Agrarian Problems and Peasant Movements in Latin America.* R. Stavenhagan, ed. Garden City, Doubleday Anchor, 1970.

35. Harding, T. and Bray, D. "Urban Farmers: The Green Belts of Cuba." *The Nation*, 1968, 207, 107-109.

36. Harker, D. "Food Outlook Brightening for Average Cuba Housewife." *The Miami Herald*, May 24, 1965.

37. *Industria Alimenticia* (Habana).

37a. Iñigo, R. "Un Fracaso." Munich, Centro de Informaciones Periodisticas, October 15, 1969.

38. James, P.E. *Latin America.* Fourth Edition. New York, The Odyssey Press, 1969.

39. Lawson, H.G. "Castro May Produce A Record Sugar Crop, But Problems Remain." *The Wall Street Journal*, March 7, 1969.

40. _____. "Fidel's Experiment—Most Cubans Appear Content With Castro's 10-Year-Old Regime." *The Wall Street Journal*, February 5, 1969.

41. Leontief, W. "Notes on a Visit to Cuba." *New York Review of Books*, 1969, 13, 15-20.

42. Losman, D.L. "The Economics of Bloc Aid and Trade with Cuba." *Marquette Business Review*, 1970 (Summer), 68-77.

43. Mesa-Lago, C. *The Labor Sector and Socialist Distribution in Cuba.* New York, Praeger, 1968.

44. _____. *Revolutionary Change in Cuba.* Pittsburgh, University of Pittsburgh Press, 1971.

45. *The Miami Herald*, July 20, 1967.

46. _____ , October 24, 1968.

47. _____ , August 24, 1969.

48. _____ , February 6, 1970.

49. _____, February 14, 1971.

50. _____, August 25, 1970.

51. *Monthly Bulletin of Agricultural Economics and Statistics* (FAO), 1971, 20 (7/8).

52. Pereira Calzadilla, O. " Que Ocurre con el Gandul en Cuba?" *Agrotecnica de Cuba,* 1966, 4 (4), 16-25.

53. Porterfield, W.R. "Barren Havana Rations Even Toilet Tissue." *The Miami Herald,* September 18, 1969.

54. _____ . "Returning Visitor Discovers 'Drab Anthill' Under Castro." *The Miami Herald,* September 14, 1969.

55. Roberts, C.P. and Hamour, M., Eds. *Cuba 1968—Supplement to the Statistical Abstract of Latin America.* Los Angeles, University of California at Los Angeles, 1970.

56. Roche, M. "Notes on Science in Cuba." *Science,* 1970, 169, 344-349.

57. Ryder, W.D. "Feeding Cuba's Livestock." *New Scientist,* September 18, 1969.

58. Simons, M. "Cuba Forming 'Socialist Man' in New Countryside Schools." *The Washington Post,* December 12, 1971.

59. Soler, F. "Cuban Economy's in Dire Trouble, Experts Say." *The Miami Herald,* February 14, 1971.

60. _____ . "Havana: 'The Saddest Sight . . . A Flicker of Candles.' " *The Miami Herald,* December 2, 1968.

61. United Nations (Department of Economic and Social Affairs). *Demographic Yearbook 1969.* New York, UN, 1970.

62. United Nations Children's Fund. *Digest of Projects Aided by UNICEF in the Americas.* New York, UNICEF, 1969.

63. United Nations Development Program. *Projects in the Special Fund Component as of 30 June 1971.* DP/SF/Reports Series B, No. 12. New York, UNDP, 1971.

64. University of Miami (Cuban Economic Research Project). *Labor Conditions in Communist Cuba.* Coral Gables, University of Miami, 1963.

65. Valkov, E.V. "Fertilidad Sabanas del Oeste de Cuba." *Agrotécnica de Cuba,* 1967, 5 (2), 22-27.

66. *Vneshnaia Torgovla SSR za 1968 i 1969 g.,* p. 287.

66a. Waltenberg, K. *Informe al Gobierno de Cuba sobre Alimentación de Colectividades.* Serie de Informes de Consultores sobre Nutrición No. 17. Rome, FAO, 1970.

67. West, R.C. and Augelli, J.P. *Middle America: Its Lands and Peoples.* Englewood Cliffs, Prentice Hall, 1966.

68. Wheeler, A. "Housekeeping Headaches Plague American Wife in Havana." *The Miami Herald,* November 3, 1968.

69. Wheeler, F. "Food Remains Chronic Problem in Cuba Economy." *The Miami Herald,* October 18, 1968.

70. _____ . "Hunger Increased in Cuba." *The Miami Herald,* June 18, 1967.

71. _____ . "U.S. Cuban Blockade Costly to Castro but Ineffective." *The Miami Herald,* August 23, 1968.

72. Wiley, K.H. *A Survey of Agriculture in Cuba.* ERS-Foreign 268. Washington, D.C., U.S. Government Printing Office, 1969.

73. Winfrey, L. "What Cuba Doesn't Ration Isn't There." *The Miami Herald,* April 28, 1966.

LIST OF TABLES

LIST OF MAPS

TABLE NO. 1

Population Distribution by Province – Cuba, 1967
(estimate)

Province	Population
Pinar del Rio	603,500
La Habana	2,102,600
Matanzas	467,900
Las Villas	1,257,600
Camagüey	842,000
Oriente	2,663,600
TOTAL	7,937,200

Source: C.P. Roberts and M. Hamour, Eds., *Cuba 1968 – Supplement to the Statistical Abstract of Latin America.*

TABLE NO. 2

Distribution of State Sector Employment and Average
Annual Wage, by Activity — Cuba, 1962 and 1968

| | 1962 | | 1968 | |
Activity	Employees (1,000's)	Wage (dollars)	Employees (1,000's)	Wage (dollars)
Agriculture				
Sugarcane	123.5	950	222.0	1,020
Nonsugarcane	117.6	830	130.0	904
Livestock	47.6	1,200	82.3	1,289
Forestry	2.9	1,103	5.3	1,132
Fishing	0.6	1,400	2.5	2,280
Agricultural services	4.8	1,500	7.8	1,872
Industry	267.0	1,941	323.4	2,063
Construction	104.0	1,700	118.0	1,803
Transportation	62.0	2,227	71.5	2,336
Communication	11.9	1,983	11.1	1,937
Commerce	132.4	1,360	235.0	1,502
Other productive sector	0.0	1,110	6.7	1,884
Housing & community services	14.3	1,413	28.5	940
Education	74.0	1,672	109.4	1,711
Culture	15.4	1,844	12.9	1,899
Public health & social assistance	41.4	1,635	62.0	1,715
Sports & recreation	3.4	1,676	4.8	1,708
Research and development	—	—	10.0	2,400
Administration & finance	60.4	1,825	53.0	1,928
Other nonproductive	—	—	21.1	1,891
Total	1,083.2	1,593	1,517.3	1,601

Source: C.P. Roberts and M. Hamour, Eds., *Cuba 1968 — Supplement to the Statistical Abstract of Latin America.*

TABLE NO. 3

Area and Production of Crops – Cuba, 1948-1970
(in 1,000 hectares and 1,000 tons, unless otherwise stated)

Crop		Annual Average 1948-52	Annual Average 1952-56	1964	1965	1966	1967	1968	1970
Corn	A	275	175	132	120	127	121	130	120
	P	243	174	129	117	127	120	127	115
Rice	A	63	107	71	38	45	57	93	150
	P	164	206	123	55	68	94	182	326
Sugarcane	A	1,204	1,010	1,055	979	1,039	1,000	1,000	1,745
	P	50,466	58,765	50,695	36,846	50,882	44,000	39,000	64,000
Potatoes	A	10	9	8	8	9	9	8	9
	P	84	107	75	83	104	105	101	120
Sweet potatoes and yams	A	99	92	65	60	60	60	62	62*
	P	290	278	300	250	240	230	240	240*
Manioc	A	55	60	30	30	30	30	30	33*
	P	179	180	200	200	200	200	200	220*
Onions	A	1	1	2	2	2	3	3	3*
	P	2	5	8	6	11	15	16	22*
Tomatoes	A	6	3	9	9	10	13	13	8*
	P	40	44	112	120	133	164	132	90*
Cucumbers and gherkins	A	–	–	1	1	1	1	1	1*
	P	–	–	10	15	12	13	13	12*
Melons	A	–	–	2	3	1	2	2	2*
	P	–	–	15	32	13	26	26	22*
Dry beans	A	60	46	40	35	35	35	35	35
	P	32	26	27	25	23	22	22	22
Grapefruit	P	7	7	12	11	13	14	15	15
Oranges & tangerines	P	46	64	94	91	127	123	130	140
Other citrus	P	2	4	6	9	7	9	9	10

TABLE NO. 3 (continued)

Area and Production of Crops – Cuba, 1948-1970
(in 1,000 hectares and 1,000 tons, unless otherwise stated)

Crop		Annual Average 1948-52	Annual Average 1952-56	1964	1965	1966	1967	1968	1970
Bananas	A	4	4	4	4	3	3	3	3*
	P	39	42	33	36	29	27	30	30*
Pineapples	P	120	90	42	26	20	17	20	20*
Groundnuts	A	16	13	20	20	19	15	15	15
	P	14	8	18	18	17	18	15	15
Cottonseed	A	–	–	3	4	3	4	4	4
	P	–	–	2	2	1	2	2	2
Coconuts	P	10	10	12	13	12	11	10	23*
(in million nuts)									(1969)
Coffee	A	89	–	–	–	–	–	–	–
	P	31	38	32	23	33	34	30	33
Cocoa beans	A	6	8	–	–	–	–	–	–
	P	3	2.6	2.6	2	1.5	1.5	1.5	1.2
Tobacco	A	52	59	55	57	60	54	54	54
	P	32	36	43	43	51	45	45	45

A=area
P=production
*1969 figures.

Source: Food and Agriculture Organization of the United Nations, *Production Yearbook 1969* and *Production Yearbook 1970.*

TABLE NO. 4

Livestock and Poultry – Cuba, 1948-1970
(in thousands)

Animal	Annual Average 1948-52	Annual Average 1952-56	1964	1965	1966	1967	1968	1969	1970
Cattle	4,333	4,103	6,378	6,611	6,700	6,774	7,172	7,250	7,100
Pigs	1,315	1,330	1,540	1,747	1,810	1,670	1,531	1,500	1,490
Sheep	177	194	148	170	240	245	260	270	280
Goats	147	162	65	71	80	81	82	82	84
Poultry	7,190	7,146	7,450	7,500	7,500	7,600	7,700	7,500	7,600

Source: Food and Agriculture Organization of the United Nations, *Production Yearbook 1970.*

TABLE NO. 5

State Industrial Production by Sector and
Percentage Share – Cuba, 1963-1966

Sector	Percentage Share			
	1963	1964	1965	1966
Minerals	2.0	2.5	2.4	2.1
Metallurgy & mechanical	5.7	4.5	3.5	4.1
Construction material	5.0	3.9	5.3	5.8
Petroleum & derivatives	7.8	9.4	9.8	10.3
Chemicals	9.2	9.6	8.3	8.8
Textiles & leather	11.4	11.4	9.7	9.6
Sugar	15.3	15.8	20.1	15.6
Food products	21.1	20.5	20.2	22.4
Drinks & tobacco	10.3	11.2	10.4	10.9
Electric energy	3.7	3.5	3.4	3.7
Other	8.5	7.7	6.9	6.7

Source: C.P. Roberts and M. Hamour, Eds., Cuba 1968 – *Supplement to the Statistical Abstract of Latin America.*

TABLE NO. 6

Soviet Food Exports to Cuba, 1968-1969

		Quantity	
Kind of Food	Unit	1968	1969
Fish flour	1,000 tons	9.0	10.0
Grains, total	1,000 tons	480.9	525.9
Wheat	1,000 tons	279.0	375.0
Barley	1,000 tons	42.0	28.7
Oats	1,000 tons	6.1	8.2
Corn	1,000 tons	153.8	114.0
Starches	1,000 tons	3.6	3.6
Meat	Million boxes*	51.7	45.1
Dry milk	Million boxes*	43.8	43.5
Cheeses	1,000 tons	2.0	2.0
Fish (fresh and frozen)	1,000 tons	19.9	22.1
Fish (salted)	1,000 tons	10.1	10.1
Fish (preserved)	Thousand boxes*	936	566
Flour	1,000 tons	294.9	297.5
Peas and beans	1,000 tons	24.4	55.8
Vegetables	1,000 tons	39.0	38.6
Fresh potatoes	1,000 tons	31.5	32.1
Vegetable fats	1,000 tons	52.6	53.5
Wine	100 hectoliters	167.3	151.1

*Capacity not indicated.

Source: *Vneshnaia Torgovla SSR za 1968 i 1969 g.*

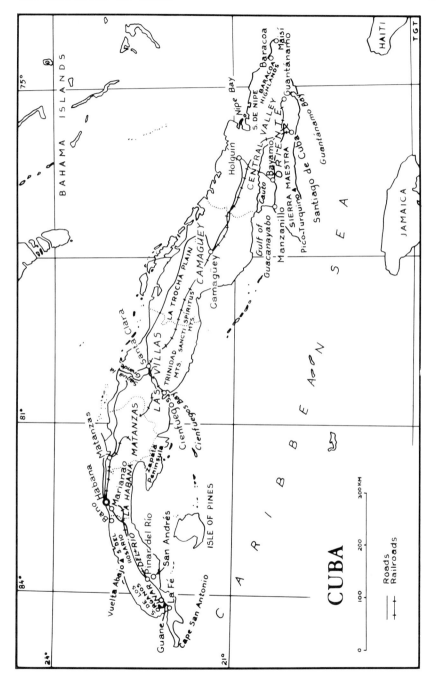

MAP NO. I.

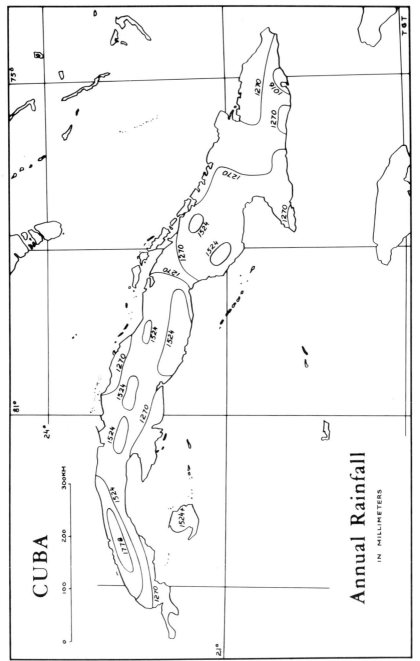

CUBA

Annual Rainfall

IN MILLIMETERS

MAP NO. 2.

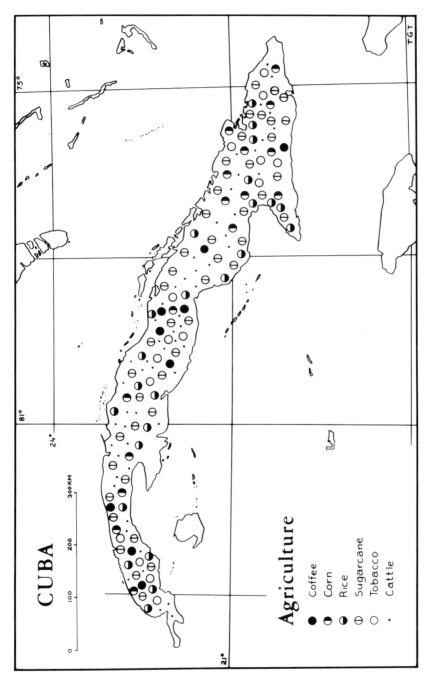

MAP NO. 3.

CUBA

Agriculture

Coffee ●
Corn ◖
Rice ◑
Sugarcane ⊖
Tobacco ○
Cattle ·

JAMAICA

TABLE OF CONTENTS

JAMAICA

I. BACKGROUND INFORMATION

A. PHYSICAL SETTING [11] [31] [13] [55]

The island of Jamaica lies in the Caribbean Sea 150 kilometers south of Cuba and encompasses 10,960 square kilometers, making it about the size of the state of Connecticut. It is the third largest island of the Greater Antilles, following Cuba and Hispaniola. Jamaica is 240 kilometers long on its east-west axis and 80 kilometers wide from north to south. The smaller islands of Morant and Pedro Cays which lie to the south belong to Jamaica but they are uninhabited and serve mainly as sources of guano and sea birds' eggs. Jamaica is a link in the relief system extending from the Yucatán Peninsula through the Antilles to South America. It is part of a succession of islands forming the northern limit of the Caribbean Sea.

An east-west interior chain of jagged mountains forms the backbone of the island from which valleys emanate, creating a ring of plains at sea level. The highest elevation is found at Blue Mountain Peak (2,450 meters) in the eastern Blue Mountains. The contiguous John Crow Mountains, still farther east, rise to 1,250 meters and form a rugged limestone plateau. The eastern mountains are cut by deep valleys and narrow ravines. The central and western areas comprise a heavily dissected plateau of deep-sea white limestone which Preston James describes as "honeycombed with caverns and pitted with sinks." In the northwestern Cockpit Country (see Map No. 1) these sinks are innumerable, steep-sided (some as deep as 180 meters) circular hollows which make the intervening land take the form of conical-shaped hillocks. This area is extremely hard to traverse and hence is practically uninhabited.

There are several large solution basins in the plateau, filled with fertile red soils which make up some of the island's most productive agricultural land. These basins, such as the Rio Minho Valley, Lluidas Vale and St. Thomas in the Vale (near Linstead), are densely settled. A layering of bauxite, which occurs over most of the western two-thirds of the island, is one of Jamaica's important natural resources, earning a good foreign exchange income.

In the north, in many places the plateaus or uplands extend right to the sea, ending abruptly in high cliffs, while in other places the land slopes steeply to a coastal plain up to 8 kilometers wide. The Queen of Spain Valley near Montego Bay is one of the island's productive agricultural zones. In the south, the lowlands extend farther inland. The Liguanea Plain around Kingston covers an area of about 340 square kilometers and initiates a lowland which extends to the District of Vere in southern Clarendon Parish. The Black River Valley and the Parish of Westmoreland are other major lowland regions. The soils of the southern coastal plains are composed of alluvial sands, gravels and loams, making these areas well-suited to large-scale commercial agriculture and hence foci of concentrated settlement.

The island's vegetation is mostly tropical, with mangroves lining the sheltered coasts and herbaceous swamp and marsh forest covering some of the low-lying land. The humid northeastern section was originally covered by a luxuriant rain forest but little of it remains except on the higher mountain slopes. A reforestation program has been started in some areas in an attempt to control erosion and leaching of the soil. Evergreen and deciduous limestone forests characterize the central and western highlands.

More than 100 rivers and streams, most of them unnavigable, traverse the island of Jamaica. The principal ones are shown on Map No. 2. Most of the watercourses originate in the mountain spine, and run north or south to the sea. During the rainy season many of the rivers, especially in the hilly eastern region, become torrents and some, like the Yallahs, the Rio Grande, the Rio Cobre and the Wag Watter, can cause serious flood damage. Rivers in the southern and western parts of the country dry up between rainy seasons, causing a serious water supply problem for both urban and rural inhabitants.

Jamaica enjoys 16 harbors, the most important of which are Port Morant, Kingston, Old Harbor, Lucea, Montego Bay, Falmouth, St. Ann's Bay, Port Maria and Port Antonio.

B. CLIMATE [11] [31] [13]

The island has a tropical maritime climate characterized by consistently high temperatures. Variations in both temperature and rainfall are governed by altitude. At Kingston (near sea level), the temperature in January ranges from a mean minimum of 20.2°C to a mean maximum of 31°C and in July from 23°C to 33°C, while at Cinchona in the Blue Mountains (at an elevation of 1,632 meters) the January range is from 12°C to 20°C and the July variation from 16°C to 23.9°C.

Rainfall is irregular in both amount and frequency. Precipitation is more pronounced on the northeast (windward) side of the island, where over 2,500 millimeters of rain are received annually (see Map No. 3). Total precipitation on the more exposed slopes of the Blue Mountains exceeds 5,000 millimeters a year, causing considerable erosion. The southern coastal lowlands, which lie in the rain shadow of the interior mountains, receive less than 1,250 millimeters annually. At Kingston the yearly average is 750-875 millimeters. In these areas, widespread irrigation is necessary for survival of both crops and livestock.

Jamaica experiences two periods of heavy rainfall: the main rains occur from September to November and the lesser rains fall in May and June. Hurricanes are a constant threat between June and November and can do considerable damage to crops.

C. POPULATION (13) (45) (36) (28) (42) (29) (46) (26) (15)

The 1970 population of Jamaica was estimated at 1.9 million (see Table No. 1) with an annual growth rate of about 1.5 percent. Overall density is about 178 persons per square kilometer, with considerable variation from parish to parish. The Kingston-St. Andrew urban and suburban areas comprise the most densely populated zone of the country, accounting for almost 30 percent of the total population. The heavy density and rapid population increase present major problems for the country since jobs, housing, educational facilities, health and social services cannot keep pace with population pressure. Some relief is provided through the outlet of emigration; about 20,000 Jamaicans (or 1 percent of the population) emigrate each year, mainly to the United States (about 17,000 in 1969) and the United Kingdom. It is, of course, the educated and skilled workers who find it easiest to obtain work abroad (as shown in the following table), exacerbating the island's shortage of skilled manpower.

Migration of Jamaican Workers to the United States and Canada, by Occupation – 1968

Occupation	Number	Percent of Total
Professional and technical	2,068	13.5
Administrative, executive, managerial	165	1.1
Clerical	1,754	11.5
Sales	185	1.2
Craftsmen, production process	1,616	10.6
Laborers	137	0.9
Service, sports, recreation	8,251	53.9
Other	1,132	7.4

Source: Government of Jamaica (Central Planning Unit), *Economic Survey of Jamaica 1968.*

The present birth rate is around 3.4 percent and the 1968 infant mortality rate was 35 per 1,000 live births (compared to 22 in the United States). The relatively high infant death rate is due to poor nutrition in some areas and to lack of knowledge about proper child care practices. About 45.9 percent of the population is under 14 years of age, making one-half of the inhabitants more or less dependent upon their families for subsistence. Life expectancy at birth is said to be 62 years for males and 66 years for females. Since 1966 the Government has supported a family planning program in an effort to curb population growth. The program, which is coordinated by the National Family Planning Board, is aimed at reducing the Jamaican birth rate from 38.8 live births per 1,000 population in 1966 to 25 per 1,000 by 1976. By 1968 the rate was estimated to have dropped to 34.3 per 1,000. Between 1968 and 1971 the Board undertook to establish 160 centers throughout the island capable of providing family planning education for 75,000 persons. The Government allocates about $500,000 per year to the program.

Most of the population is still rural. At the time of the 1960 census, it was estimated that only 23 percent of the inhabitants lived in urban areas; however, in recent years there has been an ever-increasing drift of population from rural areas to the cities and it is likely that by 1970 this figure had risen to 30 percent. The majority of the city inhabitants live in urban St. Andrew or in the Parish of Kingston. As in most developing countries, the influx of people to the cities has not been matched by a parallel expansion of the urban job market, housing, education and social services. As a consequence, urban slums, typified by illegal squatters, have mushroomed and social unrest has increased. The Government is attempting to halt the population flow to the cities by trying to improve the economic situation in the rural areas (see *Agricultural Policies*).

English is the official language of the island. More than 85 percent of the population over age 10 is literate. About 86 percent of the children in the 6-11 age group attend primary school (grades 1-6). Secondary education consists of two cycles: grades 7-9 and grades 10-13. Enrollment in the second cycle, which is primarily academic and scientific in orientation, includes only about 9.3 percent of the 15-18 year-old population. With the help of the World Bank and the United States, the Jamaican Government is attempting to reform the secondary system to accommodate more students and to give greater emphasis to vocational and technical training.

Most of the people are Christian, belonging to one of the Protestant sects or to the Roman Catholic church. There are also small numbers of Hindus and Moslems.

About 77 percent of the Jamaican people are of unmixed African descent, 17 percent are mulattoes, 2 percent are of East Indian extraction, 1 percent are of European ancestry and the remaining 3 percent include miscellaneous ethnic groups such as Chinese and Lebanese. The people of African or mixed heritage are descendants of slaves brought to the island over a 300-year period—first by the Spaniards, later by the British—to work the large plantations. They now form the backbone of the Jamaican rural peasantry. East Indian indentured laborers came to Jamaica toward the middle of the 19th century following the emancipation of the African slaves, and it is from these forebears that most of the present East Indian population is descended. The Chinese and Lebanese are also descended from immigrants who appeared on the scene in the 19th century, mainly to enter the commercial sector as merchants.

The social pattern of the rural peasantry has a profound influence on the nutrition of the preschool child and is hence worth describing here. According to L.S. Fonaroff, it is characterized by fragmented matriarchal families, widespread illegitimacy and marital instability. The lack of stable marital relationships undoubtedly has its roots in the slavery period when African family life was disrupted. In present day Jamaica, the accepted sexual pattern of behavior for rural women permits successive relationships in adolescence, then progresses to concubinage, and only culminates in legal marriage at 30-40 years of age, usually after several illegitimate children have been born (71.6 percent of all births were illegitimate in 1962). During the adolescent period of successive mating, the young woman—together with any offspring she may have—continues to live with her mother. After having several children, she usually goes to live with her current mate but legal marriage does not take place until a man is able to guarantee economic security. Should a concubinage relationship end, the woman either returns to her mother's home or remains by herself until another liaison is established.

This pattern has an adverse effect on the status of infant nutrition, for even when a man is present, the woman is expected to work when needed to help support the household and she may have to work when one union dissolves and before another is established. When the mother works, her infants are left with an older child, a neighbor or a relative who often knows little about infant care and feeding. Even the young mothers themselves tend to be undereducated concerning proper child care and nutrition. This situation contributes to a high rate of protein-calorie malnutrition (see *Nutritional Disease Patterns*). Moreover, the number of offspring desired and produced (the average woman desires four) is not at all related to ability to provide adequately for them.

The instability of family life is further exacerbated by the uneconomic size of the holdings on which most rural families live, which requires the men to seek supplementary wage work, often as migrant laborers. Thus, near the large plantations which attract the migrant workers on a seasonal basis, relationships are likely to be short-lived, terminating with the work.

D. HISTORY AND GOVERNMENT [11] [8]

The island of Jamaica was discovered by Columbus in 1494 and was christened Sant' Jago. The Spanish established their first settlement at Seville on the north coast in 1509. The original Arawak Indian inhabitants (who called the island *Xaymaca,* meaning "isle of springs"), were soon annihilated by the effects of disease and forced labor. The Spaniards began importing Negro slaves from West Africa in 1517 to work the haciendas where vegetables, sugar and beef were produced for shipment to the colonies in Central and South America.

Following decades of raids on the island, the British captured Jamaica in 1655 and by 1660 they had completely expelled the Spaniards. The Spaniards' African slaves, later known as Maroons, fled into the mountains, especially the Cockpit Country, and from there resisted British domination until the end of the 18th century. For 10 years following the expulsion of the Spanish, the island served as a haven for buccaneers operating in the Caribbean. Finally, in 1670, the Treaty of Madrid recognized British sovereignty over the island and the Government launched a successful campaign to suppress the pirates. Immigration of European planters was encouraged and with the growing importance of sugar and coffee as cash crops, more and more slaves were introduced. The African slave population rose from 3,000 in 1655 to 300,000 in 1800. Slavery was finally abolished in the West Indies in 1838 and with emancipation, most slaves left the large estates and established their own small farms. This massive exodus from the plantations led to a decline in sugar production and necessitated the importation of indentured East Indian laborers to work the lowland estates. It also led to the development of the present day peasant society living on dispersed and fragmented small holdings.

Bananas were introduced to Jamaica in the late 19th century and, cultivated by small growers as well as on large estates, soon replaced sugar as the island's most important export crop. Farmers also began turning to coconuts, coffee, cacao, pimento, ginger, tobacco and cotton as cash crops.

Jamaica became a British Crown Colony in 1866. In 1944 a new constitution was approved which gave a substantial measure of self-government and in 1957 the island achieved virtual independence in internal affairs. In 1962 Jamaica attained full independence as a member of the British Commonwealth of Nations. The British sovereign is the nominal head of the Jamaican Government but, as in Great Britain, the real head of government is the Prime Minister, who is the leader of the majority party in Parliament. The Queen appoints a Governor General on the advice of the Jamaican Prime Minister, and a Privy Council of six members is appointed by the Governor General after consultation with the Premier. The Prime Minister governs with a Cabinet of not less than 11 other ministers appointed by the Governor General on the recommendation of the Premier.

The Jamaican Parliament is bicameral, consisting of a House of Representatives whose 53 members are elected by universal suffrage and a 21-member Senate appointed by the Governor General, 13 members on the advice of the Prime Minister and eight members on the advice of the Leader of the Opposition. The normal life of Parliament is 5 years. An independent judiciary serves the juridical needs of the country.

Jamaica is divided into three counties and 13 parishes: St. Andrew, St. Thomas, Portland, St. Mary, St. Ann, Trelawny, Westmoreland, St. James, Hanover, St. Elizabeth, Manchester, Clarendon, St. Catherine. The capital city is Kingston.

E. AGRICULTURAL POLICIES [46] [29] [26] [20] [17] [39]

Soon after independence, Jamaica adopted The Five Year Independence Plan (1963-1968), to stimulate industrial and agricultural development. In April 1968, at the end of the Plan period, a Second Five Year Plan (1968-1973) was drawn up but never formally approved. The aims of the first plan were extended into the second. A new plan covering 1970-1975 is being reformulated.

In 1969 two new ministries were created to replace the former Ministry of Agriculture and Lands: 1) the Ministry of Agriculture and Fisheries, which is now responsible for the administration of rural cooperatives, the Agricultural Marketing Corporation and the Agricultural Credit Board; and 2) the Ministry of Rural Land Development which administers the Agricultural Small Holdings Law, manages the Farmers Development Programs, Rural Youth Clubs and Farmers Training Programs, controls the 13 Regional Land Authorities and the Land Development and Utilization Commission and manages the Water-Shed Protection Commission. The 13 Land Authorities are the principal decentralized agencies for implementing the development programs of the new Ministry of Rural Land Development. It is intended that each Land Authority should develop a character of its own, adapted to the resources and needs of the region which it serves (see Map No. 2).

The major objectives of the Government of Jamaica in the agricultural sector are:

1. To increase agricultural production in order to meet domestic food needs so as to reduce dependence on imported food while maintaining the level of foreign exchange earnings from export crops.
2. To achieve full and efficient use of all agricultural land.
3. To improve the rural economy and raise the standard of living in the countryside.

In order to implement these goals, the Government has undertaken a number of activities which can be categorized under five main headings: farm and livestock development, agricultural education, land reform, irrigation and nutrition.

1. Farm and Livestock Development

Under this program the Government is providing loans and grants (through the Agricultural Credit Board) and technical assistance (through the Extension

Services) to farmers in order to help them develop their holdings, with emphasis on expanding the number of medium-sized farms at the expense of small uneconomical units. Assistance is available for the improvement of farm water supplies and minor irrigation works, farm buildings, fish farming facilities and pasture improvement. "Enabling schemes" are aimed at rehabilitating several of the poorer areas in St. Thomas, upper Manchester and Clarendon parishes. Agricultural research efforts are being redirected away from export crops to food crops for local consumption, a very unusual but extremely commendable step.

Dairying is being encouraged with the aim of doubling milk production in 10 years. Through loans from the Agricultural Credit Board, farmers are able to purchase in-calf heifers from the Government's two demonstration dairy farms at Rhymesbury and Goshen. A corps of new dairymen is being trained at the demonstration farms at the rate of 40 per year. Cooperatives are being encouraged as a means of establishing the basic facilities for bulk buying and storage of farm supplies as well as group collection, packing and storage of produce. Farmers who organize themselves into cooperatives are assisted with a subsidy of 50 percent of the cost of establishment.

An Agricultural Marketing Corporation has been created to stimulate production of specific crops (primarily root crops, vegetables and fruits), offering an assured market and guaranteed prices at rural buying stations. The Corporation also provides grading services and market information.

An Agricultural Development Corporation (ADC) has been in existence since 1952. On previously undeveloped land purchased by the Corporation, the ADC has initiated rice production, sugarcane and banana cultivation and beef cattle husbandry. Since its genesis, the Corporation has brought over 2,000 hectares of land into production, 800 hectares of which were originally swampland. Other activities of the ADC include: creation of farm machinery pools where needed; propagation and distribution of plant material for farmers; establishment of pilot food preservation projects (canning, processing, etc.) in conjunction with the Industrial Development Corporation; purchase and milling of locally produced paddy; demonstration of fish farming on a commercial scale; experimental production of selected crops; establishment of 160 medium-sized dairy farms.

2. Agricultural Education

Agricultural education is being promoted and/or intensified at all levels. The Ministry of Education and the Ministry of Agriculture and Fisheries are working together to redesign the country's educational system, which previously emphasized a classical British education, in order to relate it to the needs of the island's rural economy. Several training centers are being established at strategic points where production potential is high so that farmers can attend intensive short courses in crop production methods and animal husbandry practices. Emphasis is on crops suited to the areas served by the centers and for which there is a good foreseeable demand. There is a Jamaican School of Agriculture (founded in 1910) whose activities are being expanded.

3. Land Reform

In 1965 the Government estimated that 60,000-80,000 hectares of cultivable land (out of a total of 650,000 hectares) were idle or grossly underutilized, mostly on farms of over 40 hectares in size. A Land Development and Utilization Act was passed in 1966 which authorized a special commission to require owners of underutilized properties of more than 40 hectares either to prepare plans for bringing the land into production or to sell the land to the Government for redistribution to small farmers. By the middle of 1968, over 1,600 such underutilized agricultural holdings had been identified.

As part of the land reform program, the Agricultural Development Corporation is establishing the 160 dairy farms previously mentioned (involving about 1,600 hectares) on suitable lands owned by the Corporation. The land will be made available to the corps of dairymen being trained at the demonstration farms mentioned previously, on a 25-year installment purchase plan.

4. Irrigation

Lack of year-round water supply is a major inhibitor to agricultural and livestock development in Jamaica, hence the Government's concern with irrigation projects. The island's first irrigation scheme was initiated in 1950 in the mid-Clarendon region north of the Vere Plains where approximately 5,200 hectares now support sugarcane, rice and dairy farming. The St. Dorothy Plains Irrigation Scheme services 1,300 hectares where sugarcane and vegetables are being cultivated and pastures have been improved. New schemes under way include the Harker's Hall Multipurpose Reservoir Project, the Black River Irrigation and Drainage Project, the Rio Minho Multi-Purpose Reservoir Project, the Negril Agriculture Development Project and the Queen of Spain Valley Irrigation Project.

5. Nutrition

The Government is concerned with ways to improve the nutritional status of the population through better utilization of local resources. In 1962 a Nutrition Consultant from the Food and Agriculture Organization of the United Nations (FAO) advised the Jamaican Government that cultural and economic causes of malnutrition on the island were exacerbated by inadequate local production of protein foods and lack of knowledge on the part of the populace as to their importance to good health. Following the consultant's report, the Nutrition

Committee of the Scientific Research Council established a Human Nutritive Research Unit. The Unit has sponsored work on the development of a vegetable protein supplementary weaning food, has undertaken an assessment of the effects of local processing methods on the nutritive value of the foods concerned, and has begun an investigation of the dietary pattern and nutritive value of the diets of preschool children. Other projects under way or planned for the future include: collection of data on heights and weights of the Jamaican population by age groups; an evaluation of supplementary child feeding programs, such as the Milk Distribution Scheme and the school feeding program; a study of the possiblity of increasing production of pulses and oilseeds (sesame, groundnuts and coconuts) and incorporating them into the population's dietary pattern; and an investigation to determine the advantages to be derived in terms of working efficiency from instituting well-balanced canteen lunches in local industries.

The 1963-1968 Development Plan proposed to establish a national Nutrition Center where research could be carried out on the island's main nutritional problems, and where plans could be developed for coping with them. The Center was to be given the role of coordinating the training in nutrition for all community development officers, teachers, public health personnel and agricultural extension officers and the nutrition education programs of all agencies concerned with nutrition.

F. FOREIGN AID

1. Bilateral Aid [45]

Jamaica has two major sources of bilateral foreign aid: the United Kingdom and the United States. British aid has totaled more then $38 million since 1960. As of 1968, the United States had provided economic assistance in the amount of $55.9 million, including $22.3 million under Title II of the Food For Freedom (Public Law 480) program, $11.6 million in loans, $7.8 million in grants, and $3.2 million to support a Peace Corps contingent. Canada provided $2.7 million between 1960 and 1967.

2. Multilateral Aid [25] [26] [27] [43] [45] [44]

Multilateral aid has come from the World Bank, the Inter-American Development Bank (IDB), the United Nations Development Program (UNDP) and the United Nations Children's Fund (UNICEF). Loans from the World Bank have included $5.5 million for road construction, $23.0 million for education, $2.0 million for family planning activities and $3.7 million for an agricultural credit program. The IDB has provided loans in the amount of $6.2 million for farm improvements through the Farmers Development Program and $4.7 million for a student loan fund to finance graduate study in key fields such as agriculture. UNDP assistance has included $810,100 for a groundwater survey, $945,200 for forestry development and watershed management, $110,400 for food crop development and a marketing feasibility survey, and $1,162,800 for development and management of water resources, all carried out with the technical assistance of FAO. UNICEF has supported a $370,000 project aimed at intensifying health education activities, increasing the supply of pure water in rural communities and establishing a dental auxiliary service for children. Many of these organizations, but especially UNICEF, provide infant foods, such as nonfat dry milk, through government channels.

II. FOOD RESOURCES

A. GENERAL (16) (50) (56) (39)

The land surface of Jamaica totals 1,000,096 hectares, of which 241,000 hectares were planted in crops and 247,000 hectares were used for pasturage in 1965. The Five Year Independence Plan (1963-1968) estimated the total cultivable area at 688,000 hectares or less than 1 hectare per rural inhabitant. The balance is usable only as woodland and pastures.

For centuries agriculture has been the most important pillar of the Jamaican economy. In recent years (1963-1968) Jamaica's agricultural output has risen by 9 percent but the relative importance of this activity, compared to all other economic sectors, has dropped from 12.3 percent of gross domestic product to 9.2 percent, slowly conceding to bauxite processing and other industries. During the same period, food production remained below the level of increasing demand. Jamaica has a long history of dependence upon food imports for its survival. When the island became a major sugar producer, its export crops received priority over its food cultures and the laborers who produced the cane were fed cod imported mostly from North America. During the American Revolution, this trade was interrupted long enough to cause 15,000 Jamaican slaves to die of famine between 1780 and 1787.

The usual picture of conflict between food and cash crops is in evidence in Jamaica today. The largest farms producing for export enjoy the best land and the best equipment while the smallest, usually producing for domestic consumption, have little or no equipment and are located on the periphery of estates, on hillsides, or in remote valleys away from the urban markets. However, the Government's present policy is to promote the domestic market and minimize dependence on foreign purchases of food. To this end, the Government of Jamaica has initiated an interesting program of assistance to small farmers (see *Agricultural Policies*).

Surveys of expenditures for food revealed that it cost $1.02 per capita per week in the rural areas to keep a person alive and $2.69 in Kingston and St. Andrew Parish. This must be seen in conjunction with the fact that food commodities sometimes do not sell for as much as they cost to produce, a situation which is not found in the cash crop sector. This contempt for locally produced food is surprising, given the fact that output is inadequate to meet the demand for foodstuffs, which would normally lead to a rise in prices. Yet, according to McKigney, one-half of the calories and two-thirds of the protein consumed in Jamaica are imported at prices that have quintupled during the last three decades. Thus, there are a number of paradoxical circumstances: food production is inadequate in spite of the existence of demand; prices for most locally-produced foodstuffs are low and non-remunerative to the producer in spite of overall food shortages; on the other hand, the price of some local products (broilers, for example) is higher than equivalent imports due to the fact that foreign producers enjoy economies of scale; food necessities (such as cereals, flour, meat and fish) are imported at prices which, while regulated by a Control Board, are still high enough to compel the population, whose incomes are inadequate, to spend 60-90 percent of their budgets on these imported foods.

The reasons for this situation are multiple. The local prices of the food produced in the subsistence sector are not remunerative because the holdings are too small to be economically exploited and the outlets are too few to stimulate greater production. Because the returns are poor, the farmers have to devote much time to earning cash wages and cannot do justice to the land they own. The agricultural areas where this type of miniproduction takes place are difficult to reach, hence these farmers find themselves outside the city commerical circuits; on the other hand, because the cities and towns cannot count on the small farmers to supply them, their stores are stocked with relatively high-priced imports. The output of the local industry is high-priced, partly because it is confronted with a small market while imports originate in highly sophisticated enterprises whose market is the world. On both counts the local customer is faced with prices he cannot afford. Thus there seem to exist side by side two food circuits which overlap only marginally, leaving many people underfed and a few overspent.

B. MEANS OF PRODUCTION

1. Agricultural Labor Force [54] [24] [36] [15] [33] [53]

In 1960 the potential Jamaican labor force, that is, all those between 14 and 65 years of age, comprised 606,823 persons. Salary and wage earners numbered 357,407 and represented almost 59 percent of the total. It is estimated that 84 percent of the men in Jamaica and 43 percent of the women are part of the labor force at any one time. Agriculture occupied 43.8 percent of the force in 1943 and 37.9 percent in 1960. Mining and quarrying had jobs for 0.1 percent in 1943 and for 0.7 percent in 1960, a slow increase because of the use of automatic devices and machines. Manufacturing employment rose from 11.7 percent of the work force to 14.8 percent over the same period while domestic employment dropped from 16.5 percent to 14.5 percent. Figures for the decade ending 1970 are not yet available. While the percentage of people employed in agriculture dropped in relation to the total labor force, it remained at about 229,700 individuals, the most numerous body of workers in all sectors.

Except in agriculture, mining, fishing and forestry, most of the labor force is employed in Kingston and St. Andrew. To a large extent, this labor force is unskilled or semiskilled. Another interesting trend is that the female contribution to the agricultural labor force is decreasing. Only 17.3 percent of the female labor force was working in agriculture in 1960 against 24 percent in 1943. The same decline in female employment was observable in the domestic servant category: 38.6 percent of the females were employed in this activity in 1943 against 32.9 percent in 1961. It is the manufacturing sector which, according to 1960 figures, has benefited most from the trend. Figures for 1970 were not available at the time of this writing but there are indications that the trend away from agriculture and domestic work toward factory employment is increasing among women, especially in the parishes of Kingston and St. Andrew. Thirty-four percent of all male wage earners and 43 percent of all female workers are residents of these two parishes; over 20 percent of the male wage earners are in Kingston and 24 percent in St. Andrew. Fifty-nine percent of the males employed in rural parishes earn less than $280 annually and female workers probably fare worse. Another interesting trend is the excess of males (51 percent) over females (49 percent) in the self-employed category of farm workers.

There is a Minimum Wage Law which provides for advisory boards of the Ministry of Labor to recommend pay rates. In 1964 wages in agriculture ranged from $22.40 weekly for supervisors and technicians down to $7.00 for unskilled workers. On the sugar estates the pay is sometimes higher, ranging from $37.52 weekly for supervisors to $11.20 for unskilled hands. Some factories subsidize canteens or cafeterias but they are not compelled to do so. There are no sickness, unemployment or maternity benefits.

The state of nutrition is not good among agricultural workers. It is reported by FAO that (in spite of the fact that male members of the family are privileged to help themselves first at the dinner table) the average percentage of satisfaction of nutritional requirements among the workers is low.

One of the major problems confronting Jamaica is the choice between unemployment and efficiency. The latter cannot be achieved without the aid of machines, but machine-intensive enterprises generate unemployment. A surplus of unskilled workers alongside a serious shortage of skilled ones characterizes the labor situation in Jamaica, as it does in most developing countries. With a population which must by now exceed 2 million (it was estimated at over 1.9 million on January 1, 1970–see Table No. 1), and with a continuous increase in the younger age groups, each year the labor force grows faster than the number of jobs. Neither the bauxite works nor the large plantations can absorb the inexorably rising manpower pool which seems to prefer half-starvation in the cities to subsistence agriculture and boredom in the rural parishes. In 1960, 18-25 percent of the labor force was unemployed and the rate is estimated to have reached as high as 30 percent in recent years. The problem is most acute among the younger element of the force. The solution would seem to be an emphasis on labor-intensive enterprises, including manufacturing activites.

The rate of growth of the work force is slower than that of the overall population due to changes in the age structure of the population and emigration of workers. According to the 1960 census, many workers labor only a few days a week. In 1970 it was reported that only 70.8 percent of the labor force had 5 to 7 days' weekly employment, 20.3 percent worked 3 or 4 days a week, 5.4 percent worked 1 or 2 days, and 3.5 percent were on leave, on strike or prevented from working by bad weather. These conditions have led to both permanent and seasonal emigration. Until recently, permanent emigration was United Kingdom-oriented with smaller groups trying to go to the United States or Canada or to other Caribbean islands. At its peak, the United Kingdom was receiving 20,000-40,000 immigrants a year, including the most skilled ones. However, in 1962 the British Parliament tightened its immigration regulations while the United States eased its own limitations. Now the U.S. is the recipient of most Jamaican immigrants. Internal seasonal manpower migrations are directed wherever a demand for labor seems to exist.

It is against this background that the "sugar crisis" presents itself with its ominous consequences. The cane industry has become unpopular for ideological and sociological reasons against which hard economic facts cannot prevail. The industry is viewed as a remnant of the plantation way of life and a leftover of the days of slavery. The wages paid do not compare with the wages even unskilled workers receive in the bauxite sector, and the plantations offer an antiquated way of life in primitive huts of corrugated iron, wood and banana leaves. Some cane cutters, especially the younger ones, leave the fields and go to the cities to wait for jobs rather than apply for work on the sugar estates. While outlets for Jamaican sugar seem reasonably secure for the time being at the prevailing price, the industry cannot survive if it has to offer bauxite or oil pay scales to its labor force. On the other hand, if it modernizes and automates, a large number of unskilled workers will join the ranks of the unemployed, creating an incendiary social problem.

2. Farms [29] [16] [50] [28] [10]

As indicated in the section of *Agricultural Policies*, it was the purpose of the Five Year Independence Plan to try to eliminate holdings smaller than 2 hectares and to concentrate on developing farms of 2-6 hectares, depending upon location, type, and quality of land. The Government hopes that such farms will offer job opportunities and a chance to use mechanical equipment.* These enterprises should be able to yield an income of about $25.00 per week from a selected range of export crops and foodstuffs (roots and vegetables) for local consumption. A few livestock and minor crops would be needed to supply subsistence for the family, and about one-half hectare could be devoted to tree crops. Some of these resettlements have already taken place, but with what success was not known at the time of this writing.

The total number of farms and farmers certainly is on the decline as the attraction of the cities deprives the rural areas of youthful manpower. This fosters a number of changes, the most important of which is the expansion of large estates producing exports for cash at the expense of small holdings devoted to subsistence crops. A small number of large estates (over 200 hectares each) produce sugar, bananas and coconuts on 40 percent of all the farmland (see table page 102) while 70 percent of all farms work less than 2 hectares of poor land each. The small farms which shelter about one-third of the population are either tightly agglomerated in villages or scattered over wide areas. These farms grow pineapples, plantains, manioc, yams, green and red kidney beans, cowpeas, pigeon peas, tomatoes, turnips and a variety of other vegetables. Since 1964, the output of these crops has considerably increased while that of sweet potatoes, rice and corn has decreased.

The system of land tenure does not encourage improvements. Most small farms are occupied by tenants holding one-year leases with no renewal guarantees. Others are held jointly under the freehold principle by the entire family, with the result that individuals are reluctant to cultivate or improve the land since all members of the family, whether they contribute to output or not, are entitled to share in the produce. Such conditions give impulse to the persistent drift from the land to the cities which in turn results in swelling the crowds of petty entrepreneurs who lead a substandard life in the money economy, awaiting the day when luck will place temporary jobs in their paths.

The distribution of farms by size in 1954 and 1961 was as follows:

---

*This seems to some extent contradictory. Mechanization of agriculture in a country where there is an excess of unskilled labor and a high rate of unemployment should be approached with a great deal of caution and gradualism.

Number and Area of Farms by Size Groups – Jamaica, 1954 and 1961

		Under 2 Ha	2-9 Ha	10-39 Ha	40-200 Ha	200+ Ha	Total of All Farms
Number of farms per	1954	139,043	45,024	4,650	881	332	189,93
size group	1961	113,239	40,769	3,803	779	351	158,941
Number of hectares per	1954	100,835	172,864	77,898	82,644	289,906	724,147
size group	1961	81,404	158,078	64,635	73,416	313,249	690,782
Average number of hectares per	1954	0.7	3.8	16	94	892	3.6
farm per size group	1961	0.7	3.8	18	96	864	4.3

Source: Government of Jamaica, *Five Year Independence Plan (1963-1968)*.

The table shows the trend toward larger farms and fewer small ones, yet the large amount of land still in the hands of very small holders as well as the reduction of amount of land used for agriculture since 1940 is evident. Edwards finds that the total cash income derived from farming these undersized holdings, as well as that coming from other activities, is usually small, hence canceling any possibility of capital formation. The high cost of food absorbs the major part of the household's resources while the concentration of population on small acreages throws the carrying capacity of the land into a spin, with dangerous social consequences.

In 1956 Edwards found that the average number of people living on these small farms was 4.45 per household, of whom less than half were under 15 years of age and that the yearly income of the group was less than $288 a year in both cash and kind. Moreover, the instability of marriage in Jamaica threatens the economic efficiency as well as the security of the families. As a result of the conflict between new and old values a very somber picture emerges of incipient economic distress which cannot but lead to violent upheavals.

The modernization of this sector of the economy is a tremendous task. The policies of the Government are oriented to accomplish this transformation but the pace is by necessity slow. To accelerate the rhythm of improvement, in 1969 the Government established a Ministry of Rural Land Development and 13 land authorities (see *Agricultural Policies*). The activities of the newly-created Ministry include raising the farmer's technical competence, improving rural infrastructure and giving farmers certain development incentives, such as low-cost, long-term credit. In connection with this last item, the Ministry is instituting the self-supporting Farmers' Development Project which will provide low-interest, long-term capital as well as technical assistance to the recipients of loans.

3. Fertilizers and Irrigation [16] [29]

The consumption of fertilizers in Jamaica is small and practically limited to the large estates. A total of 13,000 tons of nitrogenous, 5,000 tons of phosphatic and 10,000 tons of potassic fertilizers was used for the 1969 crop, an increase from a yearly average of 3,100 tons, 300 tons and 1,300 tons, respectively, during the period 1948-1952.

Together with encouraging fertilization through a demonstration program, the Government facilitates the distribution of farm water supplies. Subsidies up to $700 a year are available to farmers who wish to build tanks, spring catchments or facilities for storing piped water. In 1961 the pattern of water and fertilizer usage was as shown in the following table.

Number of Farms Using Irrigation and/or Fertilizers – Jamaica, 1961

	Under 2 Ha		2-9 Ha		10-29 Ha		40-200 Ha		200+ Ha	
	Number of Farms	%	Number of Farms	%	Number of Farms	%	Number of Farms	%	Number of Farms	%
No irrigation	110,629	97.6	39,344	96.5	3,500	92	688	88.3	279	79.5
Hand watering	2,490		1,108		84		22		6	
Irrigation	120		317		219		69		66	
No fertilizer	89,265	78.8	29,527	72.4	2,284	66.9	354	45.4	106	30.2
Farmyard manure	12,477		5,992		538		126		56	
Inorganic fertilizers	13,933		9,405		1,305		368		229	

Note: Discrepancies in the total number of farms between this table and the table on page 102 are due to the fact that some farms are included in both irrigation statistics and fertilizer statistics.

Source: Government of Jamaica, *Five Year Independence Plan 1963-1968.*

The table shows that not even among those farms with over 200 hectares is there 100 percent use of fertilizers, and that 78.8 percent of farms with less than 2 hectares, 72.4 percent of those with 2-9 hectares, 66.9 percent of those with 10-39 hectares, 45.4 percent of those with 40-200 hectares and 30.2 percent of those with more than 200 hectares use no fertilizer at all. The moisturization of crops is left mostly to rainfall since 79.5 percent of even the largest estates have no irrigation systems while 97.6 percent of the farms with less than 2 hectares depend upon the weather to stimulate the growth of their food crops.

The Government is establishing a number of demonstration plots on farmers' holdings to prove the advantages of scientific fertilizing, concentrating efforts on food crops (see *Agricultural Policies*). Together with the demonstration, the

Government is making available free plant materials, with the exception of citrus seedlings, to farmers competent to cultivate their crops in accordance with accepted practices, provided the fields are suitable for the seeds handed out.

4. Mechanical Equipment [16]

The Agricultural Development Corporation (see *Agricultural Policies*) has undertaken to create implement pools in areas where few or no services of this kind are available. In some cases, private contractors rent or lease simple tools as well as more complicated ones to farmers who can pay. The farm machinery pools will be set up first in three or four parishes where the nature and morphology of the soil lends itself to motorized practices. The number of tractors grew from a known 1,030, both wheel and crawler type, in 1948 to 4,900 in 1966. No reliable figures are available for more recent years. Understandably, about 66 percent of these are on farms of more than 200 hectares, but the machine stations provided for in the Plan may bring the use of mechanical equipment within the orbit of the small farmer.

C. PRODUCTION [16] [28] [50] [20] [26]

In 1964, agricultural output accounted for 13 percent of Jamaica's gross domestic product, but by 1969 agriculture's share of GDP had declined to 9 percent. As already stated, the production of food crops is still inadequate to feed the population in spite of the Government's efforts to encourage small farmers and to limit food imports as much as possible. The conflict between the need to support local production on the one hand and the demands of the large tourist trade on the other has already been stressed.

In its *Economic Survey* of 1969, published in 1970, the Central Planning Unit of the Government of Jamaica reported indications that the output of root crops, pulses and vegetables for the domestic market had declined in 1968 due to repeated droughts since 1966 which affected the smallholders who produce the country's food crops. Further declines were reported in 1969. The output of cash crops such as citrus fruit and that of expensive quality proteins like meat, milk and eggs increased in 1969, indicating recovery from the effects of drought and reflecting the adoption of improved techniques and practices.

1. Food Crops [51] [16] [35]

The preferred food crops of Jamaica are rice, yams, taro, plantains and beans. Meat, expecially goat's meat, fish and chicken, and dairy products are also available for domestic consumption but in smaller quantities and at higher prices than the field-grown food stuffs.

a. Cereals

Rice and corn are the only cereals produced in Jamaica, although not in sufficient quantities to meet the demand. Thirty thousand metric tons of rice were consumed in Jamaica in 1958 but only 9,800 tons of rough rice were harvested. In the following years, the area sown, which had reached 6,000 hectares per year in 1952-1956, shrank to 2,000 hectares in 1964 and to 1,000 hectares in 1966 where it has remained (see Table No. 2). Production is now around 2,000 tons (see Table No. 3), leaving a considerable amount to be imported. The demand is estimated to have reached 42,000 tons per year in the 1968-1970 period and is expected to reach 48,000 tons in 1975. The reasons for the steady decline in production are not clear except that Guyana, another member of the Caribbean Free Trade Association (CARIFTA—see page 116) is in the process of expanding its own rice production to meet the demands of other member states.

The area sown in corn also fell from an average of 17,000 hectares per year between 1948 and 1952 to 4,000 hectares in 1968, but production, assisted by better seeds and techniques, did not decrease as rapidly. Until very recently, corn was the subsistence crop of small farmers operating hillside farms. Yields per hectare, which were given at 0.75 tons in 1948, are now about 1 ton per hectare. In recent years modern techniques and hybrids have been introduced which may result in drastic changes in the future of corn in the island. The demand is expected to increase to about 35,000 tons in 1975, up from 23,000 tons in 1958. This increase is in answer to the greater needs of the livestock and poultry industries which have experienced some growth in recent years.

Wheat, oats and barley are not produced in Jamaica and the demand for these commodities must be met through increasing imports. The total demand for wheat and wheat flour, computed in terms of wheat equivalents based on an extraction rate of 0.73, amounted to 108,858 tons in 1958 and is expected to rise to 178,488 tons in 1975.

b. Roots and Tubers

Jamaica has a small potato acreage which remained stable at 1,000 hectares until 1969 when the area sown was doubled. Production now amounts to about 13,000 tons of potatoes annually. Sweet potatoes and yams have been on the increase since 1948 when 16,000 hectares were planted. The area planted in these roots rose to 45,000 hectares in 1969. Production has increased considerably from 64,000 tons per year during the 1948-1952 period to 210,000 tons in 1969. Manioc is less popular than the previously mentioned tubers. The crop covers 4,000 hectares but the yield is low at 10,000-11,000 tons a year. Manioc production is not expected to increase in the future because the population is increasingly favoring an American or European type of diet. The demand for

European potatoes is expected to rise more rapidly than that for tropical roots and tubers and to reach 230,000 tons in 1975.

c. Vegetables and Pulses

Vegetables form the staple of the Jamaican diet, yet production suffers from competition with bananas and lack of fertilizers on small farms. No attempt is made to produce improved varieties. The combined production of all fresh vegetables was estimated at 54,000 tons in 1970 and should rise to 59,000 tons in 1975. Demand is expected to reach 72,700 tons by 1975, necessitating the importation of 13,700 tons.

The most important pulses grown in the West Indies and especially in Jamaica are: the cowpea *(Vigna sinensis)*, also known as the black-eyed pea; the pigeon pea *(Cajanus cajan)*, also called gungo pea or Congo pea; and the lima bean *(Phaseolus lunatus)*. The pigeon pea is probably the most commonly grown and eaten pulse in Jamaica as well as in the rest of the Caribbean islands. It is used in many forms—fresh, dried and canned. Dry beans are quite popular in Jamaica and are called "red peas". Other pulses, such as garden peas *(Pisum sativum)* and soybeans *(Glycine max.)*, are imported in canned, frozen or meal form, or as ingredients in special preparations. It is hoped that a soybean industry may be developed in the West Indies, especially in view of the damage caused to the coconut crop by yellowing disease, but so far it has not been attempted.

The amount of pulses produced in Jamaica in 1964 was given as 2,000 tons, mostly pigeon peas and dry beans. Domestic production did not meet demand and over 4,000 tons had to be imported. In recent years production has risen slightly to 3,000 tons, grown on 7,000 hectares (see Tables 2 and 3). The demand is much higher than the output and is expected to increase even more in the 1970 decade when it is estimated that daily consumption could rise to about 15,000 tons. These projections are well-recognized by the Government and research is being carried out at the University of the West Indies on ways to increase the production of beans, pigeon peas and soybeans.

2. Cash Crops [16] [35] [5a] [51]

Cash crops consist essentially of bananas, sugar, citrus fruit, pepper and pimentos.* There has always been some fluctuation among these crops, governed by world prices and the availability of labor. The competition between banana and sugar for first place has also been conditioned by disease. Sugarcane averaged 46,000 hectares between 1948 and 1952, rose to 60,000 hectares between 1964 and 1968 and fell back to 55,000 hectares in 1969 and 1970 (see Table No. 2), covering about 23 percent of all permanent cropland. Production

---

*Acreages and production figures are not available for pimentos.

followed the same trend and dropped from almost 4.8 million tons of cane (yielding 497,000 tons of raw sugar) in 1964 to about 4 million tons (377,000 tons of raw sugar) in 1969 (see Table No. 3). The drop in production of this important cash crop in recent years is ascribed to the late maturation of cane, a shortage of field workers at the time they are needed (see *Agricultural Labor Force*) and a scarcity of transportation to take the cane to factories. Production is divided between individual farmers growing small quantities of cane and large sugar estates. The output from the two types of holdings is about the same: in 1969 the small farmers produced 2,012,000 tons and the sugar estates produced 1,988,000 tons. In that year, however, the sugar content of the cane was far below the previous crops, resulting in less sugar from more canes. The slow harvesting of cane in the early stage of maturation resulted in a great volume being reaped during the rainy period when the sugar content is reduced.

Bananas have known a succession of good years and bad. When world sugar prices were high and Panama disease was rampant on the banana plantations, this fruit's role in the economy dwindled. Later, a glut of sugar on the world market, together with the introduction of the Lacatan disease-resistant variety of banana, restored it to predominance. The present trend again seems to be unfavorable because of the long-term effects of the 1966-1968 drought. The drought was largely responsible for the drastic fall in banana production from 330,000 tons in 1966 to 210,000 tons in 1968 and a reduction even further to an estimated 145,000 tons in 1970. From an average 29,000 hectares cultivated between 1948 and 1952, the area rose to 38,000 hectares in 1968 but fell back to 30,000 hectares in 1969 and 1970. At the same time, the industry is meeting increasing local demand for green bananas or plantains.

The price of export bananas is controlled by the Banana Board and the Government subsidizes growers when needed. During 1969 the Government initiated an advance guaranteed price to growers. The formation of a Commonwealth Banana Association is being considered by Jamaica and a group of the Windward Islands. The specific objective of this association would be to control the banana market in the United Kingdom.

Sweet oranges, grapefruit, tangerines and bitter oranges are all produced in Jamaica. One plantation grows citrus on a large scale; sugar estates produce the rest of the crop. Production fluctuates widely from year to year, probably because citrus competes with sugar for land and attention. Between 1948 and 1952 the yearly average production of oranges and tangerines was 54,0000 tons. Output rose to 87,000 tons in 1966 but dropped to 62,000 tons in 1968. In 1970, production was estimated to have recovered to 75,000 tons. Other citrus fruits, such as grapefruit and lemons, have shown a sustained increase. However, an interesting fact is revealed by looking at Table No. 5. It can be seen that only a small fraction of the citrus crop is being exported and that these exports have declined considerably since the peak year of 1963. The explanation offered is that domestic demand for these fresh fruits has been increasing rapidly at prices which are on the average 90 percent above export prices. In 1969, the Citrus Growers Association set up a commission to the study problems of citrus farmers and to work out an expansion program which would take advantage of the market opportunities.

The coconut industry continues to suffer from the ravages of the 1966-1968 drought and from yellowing disease and is now going out of favor. Copra production fell from 17,500 tons in 1968 to 16,800 tons in 1968 and 11,800 tons in 1970. All the copra produced goes into the local manufacturing industry which is supported by the Government, as are the growers. Annual production of processed copra has remained at more or less the same level since 1964. The production and export of frozen coconut meat continues to increase, although the harvest of nuts declined from 125 million in 1966 to 115 million in 1969 (see Table No. 3).

The Government encourages farmers to replace diseased trees with the Malayan dwarf variety, which is disease-resistant. The Malayan variety also begins to bear earlier and produces a higher yield per hectare than the Jamaican type. In 1967 the Board distributed 157,000 seedlings of Malayan dwarf trees where the yellowing disease had appeared. This was increased to 245,000 in 1968 and in 1969 a total distribution of 345,000 seedlings was reported. In addition to the effects of disease, drought and labor problems are cited as factors which have held back the growth of this industry recently. Coconut trees tend to produce fewer and smaller nuts after a period of drought. The labor supply is one of the industry's problems since there is a seasonal diversion of labor away from estate work into more lucrative employment.

As for the other export crops, cocoa suffered in 1969 and production was down 36.4 percent over the 1966-1968 period. The heavy rains which followed the drought brought an extra amount of damage to the young fruit of the trees. Cocoa products increased in value between 1963 and 1966; thus, there is a potential for revenue from this crop if it can be revitalized. The Board guarantees a minimum price to growers. A Cocoa Rehabilitation Program is intended to improve cultivation practices and to increase yields per hectare, with a target of raising production from the present level of approximately 2,000 tons per year to 3,500 tons over a 5-year period at a cost of $365,000.

The coffee crop is small at 1,000-1,400 tons a year. A growing local demand for instant coffee as well as an opportunity to sell to CARIFTA countries (see page 116) has already resulted in an expansion of Jamaica's coffee-processing industry. In 1969 the Coffee Industry Board had to import 500 tons of unroasted coffee for local processors as compared to only 6 tons in 1968. At present, the instant coffee processed in Jamaica is sold almost exclusively on the local market. In 1969 the Coffee Industry Board launched an intensive expan-

sion and resuscitation program to revitalize coffee production. Increased acreages, control of pests and disease, training for participating farmers and fertilizer
subsidies of 33 percent over and above the Government's fertilizer subsidy
scheme are part of the program.

The harvests of pepper and pimento have remained steady over the past few
years. The amount exported in 1969 was 43.6 percent above the 1968 figure of
2,200 tons. Demand on the world market has increased and growers enjoy a
minimum price support.

3. Animal Husbandry [35] [16] [50] [28]

a. Livestock and Poultry

Cattle-raising has been a feature of Jamaican plantation enterprises since the
beginning of colonization when there was a need for animal transportation and
traction. This in turn created the need for pastures which took up a large
amount of land. Recently, better management and the use of better grasses have
resulted in improved herds. Feed lots which have been introduced are also
contributing to the development of a modern cattle industry. This is just a
beginning but it may eventually result in lessening dependence on imports of
quality beef for the tourist patron. The cattle herds have increased from 240,000
head in 1966 to 250,000 in 1970. The number slaughtered every year is about
61,000. The herd included 32,000 cows in 1969, a drop from 45,000 in 1948,
but these are now mostly younger cows, kept primarily for their milk.

The number of pigs has increased from 145,000 in the 1948-1952 period to
180,000 in 1970 and the number of sheep has fluctuated from 17,000 during
the 1948-1952 period to 10,000 between 1961 and 1967, to 13,000 in 1970.
Goats are the most numerous of all livestock in Jamaica. There were about
360,000 in 1970, representing an increase from 312,000 in 1966. Chickens on
the island have increased from 1,867,000 in the 1948-1952 period to 2,170,000
in 1970, due mainly to an expansion of the broiler industry. There are also
17,000 ducks, 4,000 geese and 10,000 turkeys.

b. Meat, Milk and Eggs

In 1969 total meat production was estimated to reach 32,000 tons compared
to the 1948-1952 average of 15,000 tons per year. Larger poultry production
has accounted for most of the rise. The output of broilers increased from
approximately 4,800 tons (eviscerated weight) in 1964 to about 12,000 tons in
1969. On the basis of a population of 2 million, the overall availability of meat
provided about 44 grams per person per day in 1969. Of course, there are
considerable imports in meat but most of this is consumed by the tourists.

The following short table indicates the number of cattle and other livestock
slaughtered between 1965 and 1969.

Slaughter of Indigenous Livestock – Jamaica, 1965-1969

Item	1965	1966	1967	1968	1969
Cattle	61,200	61,600	61,100	61,251	61,481
Hogs	79,113	71,983	85,524	105,855	128,994
Goats	164,900	164,565	210,000	202,984	134,911
Sheep	1,908	2,067	2,122	2,221	1,853

Source: Government of Jamaica (Central Planning Unit), *Economic Survey – Jamaica 1969.*

While the number of cattle slaughtered between 1965 and 1969 has remained static, meat statistics indicate that the amount of beef available from local production has increased by 5.9 percent from 1968 to 1969 due mainly to an increase in the weight of the cattle slaughtered. At the same time the number of animals slaughtered in the rural areas dropped from 46,000 head in 1968 to 45,000 head in 1969. This is consistent with the trek of rural people to the cities.

The production of pork and its processing for local consumption has also increased. In 1969, it was reported that 128,994 pigs were slaughtered and this increase, contrary to the situation with cattle, occurred mostly in the rural areas, reflecting a trend which could be interpreted by saying that as people drift to the cities they eat more beef, while the people in the rural areas eat more pork in compensation.

In 1968, less reliance was placed on local supplies of goat's meat and more on the importation of mutton and the increased slaughtering of local sheep. In 1969 the number of goats slaughtered continued to decline, but it also became apparent that the supply of sheep was not sufficiently elastic to meet the increased demand for lamb and mutton. The number of goats slaughtered fell by 33.5 percent while the number of sheep butchered fell by only 16.6 percent.

Production of poultry meat continued to expand, largely in response to technical improvements and increasing consumer demand. From a level of 9,900 tons of such meat in 1968, production rose by 21.1 percent to 12,000 tons in 1969. In April 1969, a government subsidy on poultry and dairy feeds was removed* and the subsidy on hog feed was lowered from 33.1 percent of the cost to 20 percent.

An estimated 98 million eggs were produced in 1970 compared to an average of 20 million per year between 1948 and 1952. Milk production in 1969 was estimated to have expanded to 48,000 tons from a yearly average of 35,000 tons in the 1948-1952 period. This increase is ascribed to the recovery from the 1966-1968 drought and to the adoption of improved methods of husbandry and grass cultivation practices by dairy farmers. Supplies to the Jamaica milk

---

*Probably reflecting progress on the road to self-sufficiency.

products industry increased to 7,000 tons from a previous level of only 6,000 tons.

From this short review of animal resources, it would seem clear that the policies recommended in the Five Year Independence Plan (see *Agricultural Policies*) have brought some results. The expansion of the dairy industry to supply the island's milk needs, the continued research on livestock breeding, pasture management and nutrition, artificial insemination services, – all these and many more factors must have had some effect on the weight and productivity of these animals, if not on their numbers.

4. Fisheries [52] [9] [29]

The search for animal protein.in Jamaica could certainly be rewarded by increasing the amount of fish consumed. Large untapped resources exist in kingfish, snapper, mackerel, whiting, bonito and tuna. Freshwater fish include perch and mullet. Between 1955 and 1965 fish production rose from 6,500 tons to 15,000 tons and could be augmented still more.

In contrast to other Caribbean islands whose coastal waters do not favor large-scale commercial fishing, Jamaica has a number of offshore banks within reasonable distance. The industry is equipped with small craft, some of which have engines but most of which operate under sail or with oars. As a result, their range is limited and so is the catch. Since 1967 and with the assistance of FAO, the Jamaica Fisheries Division has extended its operations to more peripheral banks and islands. Large vessels like the FAO-owned *Alcyon* are showing the way.

In the past, development of marine fisheries has been aimed at mechanizing the traditional small canoes used in order to allow them to move farther offshore. In addition, the fishermen have been provided with duty-free gasoline and have been trained in improved fishing methods and the elements of navigation. However, the fishing industry needs further modernization, such as the introduction of trawlers and equipment which would allow boats to reach more lucrative commercial fishing grounds. More up-to-date fishing techniques are also needed. The Government plans to help fishermen's cooperatives acquire deep-sea vessels and to provide training. The Government is also seeking permission to fish off Honduran and Colombian coasts.

Inland fisheries development has been successful. In 1965 there were nearly 500 fish ponds and tanks, covering approximately 305 hectares. They were stocked primarily with *Tilapia mossambica* (African perch). In addition, there were at that time more than 600 hectares of natural waters where African perch were produced. The Black River marsh and river system, estimated to cover 3,500 hectares, has been stocked with young African perch on a phased plan.

In 1968 the per capita availability of fish amounted to 14.6 kilograms per annum and it had been estimated earlier that the figure would rise to 23.7 kilograms in 1970. However, this does not imply an actual per capita increase in consumption since much of the increment will undoubtedly be consumed by visiting tourists or exported in response to foreign demand for Jamaican fish. It is rather interesting to see that the reliance on fish among insular populations is inversely proportionate to the size of the island. In the Caribbean area the highest consumption of fish occurs in the Leeward and Windward islands but is much smaller in Jamaica, Trinidad and Puerto Rico. It is also interesting to note that fresh fish represents only a fraction of the fish consumed. The most popular form of fish in Jamaica is canned.

D. FOOD INDUSTRIES [50] [28] [21] [12] [17]

Through the Ministry of Trade and the Jamaican Industrial Development Corporation, the Government encourages private enterprise and stimulates the growth of industry in general, although food industries have a lower priority than others. By the end of 1968, there was a total of 181 industries covering a broad range of activities. Those devoted to processing locally-grown or imported agricultural products numbered approximately 30, but represented a limited spectrum. Jamaican food manufacturing industries include: dairies, sugar refineries, coffee and cocoa plants, breweries, vegetable and fruit canneries, bakeries, and firms processing vegetable oils, spices, coconut, beef and pork. In addition, there are three feed mills. United States Department of Agriculture experts remark that American and other foreign interests have significantly penetrated the Jamaican food processing industry. There are over 100 small bakeries of small to medium size but one of the large ones, along with its single flour mill, is a subsidiary of an American company. Two large broiler companies which together produce 90 percent of Jamaica's broiler output are owned in part by American firms. The coconut and vegetable oil processing plants are owned by the Government of Jamaica. Most food importing firms also own control of local food processing plants. As a result, much of the food industry is dependent upon imported goods so that eventually only a small share of the food industry is both completely Jamaican and independent.

Most of the food processing plants are small and yet operate below maximum capacity, as shown in the following table.

Estimated Percent of Operating Capacity Reached
by Jamaican Food Industries in 1969

Industry	Percent of Capacity
Dairy products	33
Confectionery and syrup	39
Food and vegetable canning	48
Coffee	50
Meat processing	63
Vegetable oils	13

Source: U.S. Department of Agriculture (Economic Research Service), *Prospects for U.S. Agricultural Exports to Jamaica.*

Although operating below capacity, the Jamaican food processing industry has been expanding, resulting in the importation of raw materials instead of finished or semifinished commodities. A reclassification of some items which were formerly included in the food group has placed them in the raw material category, e.g., unmilled wheat which was imported at the rate of 34,000 tons in 1968 and 54,000 tons in 1969. As mentioned earlier (see *Trade*), the constant rise of food imports has inspired the Government of Jamaica to create a Food Technology Division to assist the local food processing industry. The policy of this agency is to concentrate on the handling of local food products not yet manufactured in Jamaica, especially tropical products which have export appeal. In addition, a Food Processing Committee has been set up to determine how a regular flow of agricultural raw material to processing plants in Jamaica can be insured. Subcommittees will concentrate on the three main aspects of the problem: marketing, agricultural production, processing and packaging.

The Government has assisted in the establishment of Jamaican Frozen Foods, Ltd., which repackages frozen vegetables and other imported items under its own brand name, "Jamaica Way." This firm also prepares frozen dishes, especially typical local recipes, made with local foods which it tries to export. To offset the shortages which occur between harvests and to prevent waste at the time of harvest, this company also produces banana and breadfruit flour, which it hopes to mix with proteins for good nutrition all year round.

A special conference to study the problem of bringing good but cheap protein mixtures to the Caribbean area met at Georgetown, Guyana, in July 1968. While it is believed that at least 10 mixtures of protein foods grown in Jamaica could serve as the basis for a weaning food industry, the prospects for the establishment of a national or regional infant foods industry are somewhat limited. The reasons given are: the smallness of the market, which is confined to a total of about 300,000 infants of weaning age for the whole Caribbean region; the need for subsidization if the unit price, given the small market, is to be kept low; the limited amount of protein-rich foods left after auto-consumption needs of the population have been satisfied; and the added cost of inter-island freight for distribution of the product. Hence it is unlikely that even with the trade facilities offered by CARIFTA a regional infant food industry will be established in Jamaica or elsewhere in the area.

Salaries in food processing plants do not exceed 45¢ to 50¢ an hour. This is to be viewed in the context of a highly protected market where the lower cost of labor is an indispensable asset. Without this compromise between high cost of imported raw material and low cost of local manpower, there might not be a food industry at all; hence, more unemployment and less processed food.

E. TRADE [29]

The absence of an organized and efficient internal marketing system has been the main hindrance to increased production of local food crops in Jamaica. The

Agricultural Marketing Corporation is a statutory body which was established in 1963 and is responsible for providing and maintaining an efficient marketing organization for agricultural produce. The Corporation's primary activities are:

1. The initiation of stipulated price contracts with farmers, cooperatives and other producer organizations so that the Corporation can, in turn, enter into contracts with hotels, supermarkets and retail institutions for the sale of agricultural products. The Corporation also seeks to make contact with buyers in overseas markets when there is a surplus of any commodity.

2. The provision of a guaranteed outlet for selected crops at stated prices in order to assure producers of a market.

3. Participation in open market trading in order to meet shortfalls in contracts or to supply the demand when it is in excess of contracts.

The Food Technology Division was established in 1965 with the goal of assisting the development of food products not presently manufactured in Jamaica. The Division's interest is in exotic products whose technology has not yet been developed. These locally produced foods could replace imports and because of their originality have a high export value. The Division also processes more commonly known foods like tomatoes and carrots and Jamaican specialities like ackee and codfish, curried goat's meat, rice and peas. The Division utilizes the surplus harvest which otherwise would be wasted due to inadequate storage space and lack of knowledge of preservation techniques at the farm or community level.

1. Domestic Trade [50] [29] [20]

Most of Jamaica's domestic trade consists of the local distribution of foods imported from abroad, which represent two-thirds of the proteins and half of the calories consumed on the island per year.* Eight large firms distribute the foreign foods together with some of the locally produced food and feeds. These firms work through small wholesalers. Most of the imported food is the output of foreign manufacturers and is distributed by local intermediaries under their own trademarks, sometimes after final processing at local plants. The island has many retail food shops but their numbers are diminishing since they cannot compete with the supermarkets which now number more than 50 and differ in size and scope. Some supermarkets in the Kingston area carry as many as 5,000-6,000 items, most of them from the United States.

Small old-fashioned food stores, quite a few operating in floor space of less than 25 square meters, sell canned goods, flour, beans from 50-kilogram bags

---

*By whom—tourists or local people—cannot be determined.

and some household utensils. There were 17,926 such small stores in 1964, all of them supplied by the importer-wholesalers who are better equipped than the retailers to obtain the required import licenses.

At a still lower retailing level, we find the higglers (a distortion of the word "haggler"). These higglers are known for driving a hard bargain when selling small items from their stalls or stands (often reserved or numbered) or from mats on the ground. They fill the marketplaces of Kingston and other towns by the thousands. Most of them are farmers' wives selling the output of their own orchards or small quantities of foods bought from others. Higglers crowd the buses to and from the market centers, where some go to vend their produce at the market itself, while others peddle their goods from house to house. Most important from the point of view of nutrition are the fruits which, thanks to the higglers, are now consumed in greater and greater quantities. As mentioned earlier, the export of oranges has suffered from this growing domestic consump- tion at higher prices. The existence of the higglers is linked to the continuation of the small farms which supply them. When these farms are absorbed into larger estates, the higglers will disappear and the quality of the diets of their clients will probably drop.

By withholding import licenses, the Government brings considerable pressure on the tourist hotels and restaurants to acquire their foodstuffs locally, but the problem is one of reliability and quality. If farm produce could be made safe and could be delivered on time in sufficient quantities, a considerable step would be made towards the development of Jamaica since some of the income from the tourist trade would eventually reach the local food producer.

2. Foreign Trade [50] [18] [28] [40]

On the foreign side of the trade picture, the Agricultural Marketing Corpora- tion is in charge of meeting shortfalls in the food requirements of the local and visiting population by means of imports. It is proposed to establish a marketing intelligence service at the Ministry of Agriculture and Fisheries which would provide information on a regular basis on such matters as current prices, trade practices in neighboring countries, supplies in the principal markets, storage stocks for each major commodity and seasonal or annual changes in such factors as acreages, yields, production and prices. Most of the foreign trade is first United States-oriented, then directed to the United Kingdom and Canada. In 1968 the U.S. supplied 38.6 percent of all Jamaican imports, the U.K. 20.4 percent and Canada 9.6 percent. The U.S. bought 39.2 percent of Jamaica's exports, the U.K. 23.7 percent and Canada 14.4 percent. The main imports consist of machinery and transportation equipment plus a variety of manufac- tured goods and foods.

It is customary to say that the rate of economic growth of Jamaica during the decade following 1950 was phenomenal. This, however, was simply the result of the discovery of bauxite and the exploitation of this resource and does not connote any improvement in nutrition for the majority of the population. The agricultural sector has not followed pace, mostly because the demand for food on the part of the richest part of the population and the 500,000 tourists who visit Jamaica annually, is satisfied only through imported foods. The best hotels and restaurants buy their meat from the United States. The meat wholesalers and retailers get some of their supplies from Australia, New Zealand and even Canada where lower prices prevail due to economies of scale.

Table No. 4 gives a quantitative idea of the nature and quantities of imported food. Cereals, 50 percent of which comes from the United States, represent the major portion of these imports and are virtually the one imported food which could contribute significantly to the daily diet of the population. Table No. 6, which should be compared with Table No. 4, shows the cost of these imports by item and by year. Among cereals, imports of rice increased to 26,000 tons in 1969 compared to 24,000 tons in 1968 but were below the 33,000 tons imported in 1967. The import bill for vegetables in 1969 showed a slight increase over 1968. Larger quantities of seed potatoes, beans and peas, fresh and dry vegetables and preserved vegetables and vegetable preparations of all kinds were imported in 1969 than in the previous year. Agricultural exports are limited to bananas, raw sugar, citrus fruit, pepper and pimentos. Table No. 5 shows the yearly changes. Most items seem to have reached a plateau. Citrus fruit, once a successful export item, appears to have lost vigor in recent years but is said to have shown a modest improvement in 1969. Banana exports have been declining since 1967.

The picture of Jamaican external trade will change considerably in future years as the Caribbean Free Trade Association develops. CARIFTA was created in May 1968 and includes Trinidad and Tobago, Antigua, Guyana, Barbados, Dominica, Grenada, St. Christopher-Nevis-Anguilla, St. Lucia, Montserrat, St. Vincent, Jamaica and British Honduras. The last joined in 1971. Among CARIFTA's main provisions is the stipulation that 22 agricultural commodities may not be imported from outside the area until all internal supplies have been utilized and that 50 percent of a finished product's value must be added locally to qualify for the free trade area benefits. Obviously these arrangements will provide a greater market (totaling 4-5 million customers) for local farm output and will encourage local finishing industries and food processing enterprises. Moreover, it is considered by some as the first step towards a Caribbean economic community which will ensure that the different resources and skills of the members are harmonized efficiently into producing and trading organizations.

F. FOOD SUPPLY

1. Storage [13]

The food supply of Jamaica is for the most part either on ships bringing it to the wholesalers from producers abroad or in the ground of the many small and few large farms, or on the citrus, banana and coconut trees. To be sure, after harvest a very small amount of the locally grown food is stored in boxes and baskets in the family's dwelling place or in the warehouses of the Agricultural Marketing Corporation and its subsidiaries or associated farms. The AMC maintains buying stations in the rural areas. Thus the Government is attempting to build its food supply from local production in an effort to slow down the costly imports of foods. This is in wise contradistinction to the policy frequently adopted in developing countries of basing food supplies upon imports paid for with exports of cash crops. While Jamaica is still heavily dependent upon food imports, the policy of the Government seems to be in the right direction. However, some critics feel that the cost of domestic agricultural development is high and has not brought the expected returns; but it must be remembered that the activities of an Agricultural Marketing Corporation comprise a long-range investment which brings dividends only after considerable social changes have had time to occur.

In addition to the supplies of the AMC, more food is stored in the warehouses of the eight most important wholesalers who release it according to the contracts they have with distributors. No figures on capacity of this storage space are available.

2. Transportation [52]

Transportation is a problem in certain areas of Jamaica. It is still difficult to gain access to the villages of the central mountains because of steep slopes and primitive roads. In 1968 the island had over 4,200 kilometers of government-maintained roads and over 11,000 kilometers of secondary roads kept up by the parishes. There is a continuous ring of major roads circling the island along the coast and linking all major towns and harbors. Some of the main roads also cross the central mountains in a north-south direction. A program of road expansion is being carried out with the financial assistance of the World Bank. Secondary roads are being improved and connected with the main arteries to increase the outlets of agriculture and industry. Much of the food is transported on these roads by bus or truck from the producing areas to the distribution centers and vice versa insofar as imported food is concerned. Imports arrive by sea at one of the six first-class ports, in practice through the main port of Kingston. A few kilometers west of the old Kingston docks a modern complex is being finished which includes substantial cold storage facilities. Outgoing bananas, sugar and molasses are loaded at some of the second-class harbors.

There are two international airports, one at Palisadoes, 18 kilometers from Kingston, and another at Montego Bay. There is no evidence that food supplies are moved by air. Jamaica has 390 kilometers of railroads. One main trunkline links Kingston and Montego Bay. From Spanish Town a line goes to Port Antonio via Linstead and Annotto Bay while another branch links May Pen and Christiana. The railroads are important because they carry the domestic supplies of food from production to consumption centers.

III. DIETS

A. GENERAL [15] [5] [50] [30]

Jamaican diets are understandably low in animal proteins and high in carbohydrates as a consequence of low production of domestic proteins and the high price of imported ones. This is due to a lack of understanding of the importance of proteins, a situation which is common to all of the developing world and to a good section of the developed one. Following the 1962 visit of an FAO consultant, the Nutrition Committee of the Scientific Research Council set up a Human Nutrition Research Unit whose mandate has been described on page 96. It is hoped that the work of the Unit will have a positive influence on the diets of pre-school and school-aged children, especially.

The basic foods eaten by Jamaicans are rice, roots, coconut products, plantains and, in increasing quantities, oranges and other tropical fresh fruits. Meat and fish are eaten when available, but usually not in adequate amounts. When possible, the diet is supplemented by canned foods which have a prestige rather than a nutritive value due to the small quantities people can afford.

L.S. Fonaroff has made a valuable study of the causes of these inadequate diets, with emphasis on malnutrition in infants and on the pattern of rural settlement as a cause for this malnutrition. According to him, the distribution to emancipated slaves of small holdings, often located at the periphery of large estates, created dispersed households with two major consequences: 1) because the holdings were uneconomical, a need to supplement subsistence production with wages was created; and 2) corollary to this, members of the family were reduced to part-time labor on their own land, which resulted in even more inefficient utilization of the limited amount of ground available. The road patterns also influence malnutrition. Fonaroff makes the penetrating remark that the hardships of bad roads are overcome to go to the markets, to church or to social gatherings, but not to go to clinics.

Another important factor contributing to malnutrition is the fragility of the family pattern, which is characterized by high illegitimacy rates, marital instability and households consisting almost solely of unwed mothers who must work, leaving their infants in the care of relatives who have neither the knowledge nor the means to provide the children with balanced diets (see page 91). This pattern may slowly disappear as rural people move to cities where the population gradually adopts the moral values of the middle class; but there they will suffer from the urban type of malnutrition caused by acute lack of money, which can be far worse than the rural type because it occurs on a year-round basis and yields to nothing but increased income.

In 1968 Ashworth confirmed earlier unpublished results obtained by Cruickshank and Fox showing very low caloric intakes in some Jamaican rural communities. Testing these people in a metabolic ward, the investigator found ratios of 41.8 kilo calories* against 59.1 kilo calories for male controls, and 34.4 kilo calories versus 41.2 kilo calories for female controls. The samples used for the study had significantly lower weight/height ratios than controls, implying the existence in Jamaica of pockets of malnutrition due to very low caloric intakes.

The existence of these pockets is in contrast with an estimated overall availability of 2,600 calories per capita per day as shown in Table No. 8. This computation also shows that each Jamaican could consume 66.7 grams of protein and 64.4 grams of fat. Obviously, in the light of the studies just mentioned, this is not the case, pointing to a faulty distribution of food, added to generalized lack of nutrition education. As it is, the table shows that 76.4 percent of the calories come from carbohydrates, 11 percent come from fats and only 12.6 percent from proteins. This was in 1964, and most 1970 production figures have changed for the worse (see Table No. 3). The rice crop has declined and corn has remained static. Corn imports may have filled the production gap in 1966, but comparing production and import figures (Tables 3 and 4), it appears that rice imports diminished substantially after 1965 so that the cereal deficit must have been met partially by costly wheat and wheat flour imports, little of which is likely to have found its way into the pockets of malnutrition discussed above. The increased imports of vegetable oil may also have helped to bridge the calorie gap.

Economists, however, may not agree with this picture. It is stated in economic reports that food consumption in Jamaica has risen and is likely to continue increasing significantly in the years ahead in response to increases in population, income and tourism. While this is probably true, the beneficiaries of these increments are not defined and no indication is given as to which part of the population is likely to eat more. It is currently stated by the U.S. Department of Agriculture that milk, cheese and butter are in greater demand in 1968 than they

---

*The amount of energy needed to raise the temperature of 1 kilogram of water from 15°C to 16°C.

were in 1959 (see table below) but this should be seen against an increase in the tourist trade of 107 percent during the same period. The table below must be read with these factors in mind.

Consumer Food Expenditures by Major Food Groups –
Jamaica, 1959-1968
(in percent)

Food Group	1959	1963	1968
Bread and cereal, including rice	24.2	22.8	22.0
Meat	16.6	18.3	18.2
Fish	8.8	8.4	7.4
Milk, cheese, eggs and butter	12.5	14.1	16.5
Oils and fats	4.1	3.8	3.8
Fruits, vegetables and pulses	16.9	16.7	16.2
Root crops	9.2	6.5	7.1
Sugar, preserves and candies	4.4	6.1	5.1
Coffee, tea, cocoa and herbs	2.2	1.9	1.9
Other foods	1.1	1.4	1.8
Total	100.0	100.0	100.0

Source: U.S. Department of Agriculture, *Prospects for U.S. Agricultural Exports to Jamaica.*

This table shows that, indeed, expenditures for cereals are declining and those for meat, milk, cheese, eggs and butter are rising. What it does not say, however, is that the people who contributed to an increased demand for these rich foods are probably the tourists, and not the people on the mountainsides who continue to live as they have for centuries—except less well because of the crowding in their midst and the rising cost of imported basic foods. Meanwhile, there is no doubt that a small number of enterprising people have moved to higher income and educational levels and imitate the American type of diet to a greater extent than they did before. However, the change from small farmholder status to slumdweller continues and it is only the habitat, not the numbers or the percentage of the malnourished that is significantly changed.

B. CHILDREN'S DIETS [23] [22] [32] [17]

As always in the developing world, the children are those whose diets are most defective. Grantham-McGregor and Back have studied a representative sample of 300 infants of working mothers in the city of Kingston and found that most of these children were breast-fed to age 6 weeks, following which some bottle feeding was added up to 5 months. Then the switch to complete bottle feeding occurred and the child was weaned. Among nonworking mothers, breast feeding was extended for a longer period. Weights were found to be higher during the breast feeding period than during the bottle feeding period, when gastroenteritis was also more frequent and increased as breast feeding diminished.

Fox, Campbell and Morris found that children from 6 months to 3 years of age consume little protein of poor quality. Between 3 and 6 years the protein intake is low but the diet is more diversified. This may fill the need for nutrients. The investigators indicate that a variety of mixtures based on soy, sesame, cowpeas, groundnuts, cashews and red beans, or any combination of them with corn or wheat flour, are available. These mixtures could go a long way toward upgrading the diets of the preschool children, if they were available in sufficient quantities, which is not the case. All of these pulses could be grown and processed in Jamaica, making a substantial contribution to improved nutrition. The same investigators made a survey based on a sample of 665 children and found that most children obtained less than 63 percent of their protein and energy requirements. The older children (3 to 6 years of age) had 80 percent of their protein requirements filled, the 1- to 3-year-olds 68 percent, and the younger group (weaning tots to 1 year of age) received only 55 percent of their protein needs. The diets of these younger children consisted of cornmeal, condensed milk and sugar. Occasionally they were given bread and butter and a sip of orange juice. After 3 years of age, the regimen more and more resembled the adult diet in kind but not in quantity. These diets involved 17 different items of food. Comparing children of the same age groups in urban and rural areas, the same investigators found that the rural children managed a more satisfactory, although less diversified diet than the urbanites. Animal protein represented 61 percent of the total protein intake in urban areas but only 51 percent in rural areas.

W.P.T. James confirms that the length of breast feeding in Jamaica is between 5 and 8 months. One-half of the mothers feed their first child longer than they do successive ones. This may be due to the increased burdens on mothers as the number of their children increases. Both children and a need for cash compete for their time. Daytime feeding is discontinued first, obviously because of the demands of work on the mother. Nighttime feeding is continued, but at greater intervals: the number of feedings drops from three to two, and then to one. As a result, the mother's milk production dries up.

James reports that while urban mothers have a better chance to receive medical advice and education at hospitals where they are delivered or at postnatal clinics than do rural mothers, this advice is often accompanied by free samples of proprietary mixtures given by manufacturers' agents who are known as "milk nurses." The prices of these mixtures are several times higher than the cost of ordinary nonfat dry milk available to the Jamaican children. Once the pattern is established, the mothers feel they have to continue it for the good of the child. When it is obvious that they cannot afford the cash burden these practices imply, they buy cheaper and cheaper goods of less and less nutritive value, or they dilute the expensive product with the polluted water which is at their disposal, completing the cycle leading to protein-calorie malnutrition.

Another unexpected result of the increase in artificial feeding is clearly explained by James. After age 3, the children get some cornmeal porridge, to which condensed milk is added. The amount of milk to be poured into the porridge is determined by the sweetness of the mixture. Since condensed milk is usually very sweet, the amount of milk added to the cornmeal is very small. Other weaning items include potato puree, vegetables, fish soup and tea. Unfortunately, the fish soup is strained for the baby who thus does not get the chunks of fish but only the water. Bananas are added later and are reputed by most of the mothers to be a superior food, better than calf's liver in iron content!

The FAO mission sent to study this problem (see page 95) suggested that: a) regional standards for the sale of imported infant foods be written into a law which all member governments of CARIFTA would pass; b) import duties on such products be lowered; c) low-priced weaning foods of established value such as INCAPARINA and others be promoted; d) government and private enterprise cooperate in promoting a regional industry which otherwise would have limited chances of success (see page 113); e) the existing methods used to handle distribution in food aid programs be improved; f) the production of protein-rich foods at home both for auto-consumption and for trade in urban areas be promoted; g) experimental plants for the processing of mixtures based on locally grown resources such as (in the case of Jamaica) coconuts and bananas, be established; h) educational programs and health and social services be promoted.

C. LEVELS OF NUTRITION [47]

Table No. 8 estimates, as stated, the average caloric intake at about 2,600, the protein intake at 66.7 grams and the fat intake at 64.4 grams. These are averages which are not available to all. On the basis of the figures given, the daily amount of cereals and wheat flour available to each Jamaican would amount to 276 grams a day. This would procure 28 grams of vegetable protein and about 2.7-3.3 grams of fat, depending upon the size of the corn contribution in the daily intake. Given the respective proportion of all foods indicated on the table, the calcium supplied would amount to about 500-600 milligrams, low but acceptable if totally absorbed.* The amount of iron at over 20 milligrams daily would be ample. Phosphorus would come to more than 1 gram a day, well within the normal range. The most important fat-soluble vitamin, namely vitamin A, would be found in three of the vegetables and fruits eaten: sweet potatoes (if the yellow variety is preferred to the pale one, which is not always the case) would provide 2,577 micrograms; spinach and other greens, especially in the quantity given, might bring 1,400 micrograms; and oranges would add a small but significant contribution. Such a diet as listed in the table might contain about 4,266 micrograms or 7,000 International Units of vitamin A, which is ample.

---

*The malabsorption problem has not yet been solved. Basically, the question is: do the large amounts of cereals and some of their by-products, such as phytates, prevent the absorption in the bowel of minerals like calcium, iron and others?

The water-soluble vitamins, such as thiamine, riboflavin and niacin, are adequately represented in this kind of diet. Ascorbic acid is overrepresented, as expected, given the high consumption of oranges mentioned in previous paragraphs. Three oranges per capita per day make 180 milligrams of ascorbic acid available. In view of these figures, the only conclusion that comes to mind is that while the diets as shown on the table should be sufficient to sustain health and growth, the distribution of these nutrients must be faulty since large pockets of malnutrition have been reported to exist.

IV. ADEQUACY OF FOOD RESOURCES [34] [29]

Tables 3 and 4 show that more food is imported than grown locally. When this happens in a developing country, the consequences are inescapable: a few have too much, many have too little. This has a tendency to create social unrest rather than to promote orderly economic development.

In the particular case of Jamaica, one is surprised to see the import list swollen by large orders of cereals and fish (salted cod) which are intended for the residential population and still larger ones of meat and dairy products, obviously for the tourist visitors whose impact on the economy is at the same time so profitable and so costly in terms of dietary consequences.

The dilemma is simple. The tourist trade demands foreign foods whose prices are prohibitive to the lower socioeconomic groups; yet without the income from tourists, the national budget could not finance the cost of development. Hence, the tourist is essential because of the money he leaves in the country, but he is costly because in spite of all efforts and laws, he causes the local production of food to be smothered by imports. The Government of Jamaica is well aware of this situation and is making heroic efforts to promote local food production, to stimulate the output of the small farms and to encourage the subsistence rural population to take part in the national economy. Definite progress has been made along those lines (witness the changes in food expenditures reported on page 120), but the weight of the traditional way of life is so heavy that progress cannot occur fast enough. Jamaica, like all the developing countries, is turning into a two-class society: a small upper class of merchants and technicians and a large rural mass trying to move to urban areas where it is reputed that "things happen"—unfortunately, not always good things.

The future could be favorable, given enough time. The climatic and soil conditions allow expansive and diversified agriculture wherever the ground is not eroded, which could provide a decent fare for all. The policies of the Five Year Independence Plan have guided planning and programming towards the goal of self-sufficiency. Since 1955 there have been three major programs aimed at promoting adequacy of food supplies: the 1955-1960 Farm Development Scheme which launched 22,500 farmers on the road to self-sufficiency; the

1961-1963 Agricultural Development Plan which helped another 20,600 farm families; and the 1963-1968 Farmers Production Program which was integrated into the Five Year Independence Plan and benefited 25,600 farmers. Under all these schemes, grants and loans intended to improve local food production were made. Farmers were invited to try new crops and were assisted with food aid during the transition periods. The Farmers Production Program has been replaced by a new agricultural program under the Second Five Year Plan (1968-1973) which emphasizes livestock production (see *Agricultural Policies*). Other development projects contributed significantly to the promotion of food adequacy. Prominent among those were support given to so-called "redundant sugar workers"—former employees of sugar estates who have established new farms on land granted by the estates. The support ended when it was felt that the new farmers were able to "go it alone."

There is no doubt that Jamaica is confronted by a transition period which may last a few years. During this time a generation of farmers eager to develop their land, to improve their food production and to do justice to their farms must be trained in modern techniques but must still grow the traditional sugar crop. Dependence upon the tourist trade, whose income cannot yet be dispensed with, should not be allowed to become an entrenched way of life.

V. NUTRITIONAL DISEASE PATTERNS [1] [3] [2] [4] [38]
[32] [22] [14] [17] [7]

Ashcroft and collaborators have made several studies of the heights and weights of Jamaican children at various ages and at various times. In a study of schoolchildren which took place in 1964, Ashcroft and Lovell found that male children of African origin ages 7 to 14 belonging to a low socioeconomic status were taller and heavier than those in a similar group investigated in the same schools in 1951. Girls also showed some increase in comparison to their predecessors, but to a much lesser degree than the boys. No explanation is given for this difference between sexes. The findings, however, can be considered evidence that standards of living have risen among certain population groups in the past 13 years. In another study of secondary schoolchildren 11 to 17 years old from middle- and upper-class families, Ashcroft, Heneage and Lovell found no significant difference between those of African, European and Chinese origin, except that the Chinese were of significantly shorter stature, but this may be ascribed to a genetic phenomenon—nature rather than nurture.

Comparing mean values for stature among children from three areas of Jamaica, Ashcroft and Lovell in another study found these values to lie between those obtaining for English children the same age in London at the beginning of the century and the figures found for a comparable group in 1959. Heights and weights of 363 men and 603 women from the city of Kingston and 766 men and 804 women from a neighboring hilly rural area were also compared by Ashcroft, Ling et al. The mean heights for men proved to be higher in towns than in the rural areas while the figures for women did not change. Moreover, the mean rural values were not different from British values obtained during World War II but were much less than those obtained in the United States in 1955. All these findings might be interpreted as a sign of improved standards of living which would bring this population to a better health level than the one enjoyed by Europeans at the turn of the century, but not as high as the one prevailing in the developed countries at present.

McKenzie and Lovell compared 204 Jamaican children who had died between the ages of 6 months and 3 years, pairing them with living children of the same ages. They were able to establish that 70 of the deaths had been caused by malnutrition and that malnutrition had been a contributory cause of death in 132 cases. The investigators established to their satisfaction that the standard of child care, as measured by attendance at antenatal and postnatal clinics, was lower among the mothers of those who died than among the mothers of the living children. They also determined that the children who died were breast-fed for shorter terms and received less protein food supplements than those who survived. W.P.T. James confirms that malnutrition is major cause of death among children during the first years of life in Jamaica. The significance of these various explorations seems to be that when a child survives the early dangers of malnutrition, he develops within normal limits but that there exist in Jamaica a number of areas where lack of education, restricted financial resources and the structure of society are conducive to serious levels of malnutrition.

Nutritional diseases are common among certain groups. Fox, Campbell and Morris found protein-calorie malnutrition (PCM) throughout the island among children between weaning age and 3 years due to energy intakes amounting to only 63 percent of requirements and protein intakes providing only 55 percent of the need. This confirms findings by other workers that malnutrition is more and more a problem of infants and that typical kwashiorkor is becoming rarer. Liver enlargement and loss of hair pigmentation were frequent, as were cases of dental caries. A. Fonoroff agrees that kwashiorkor and marasmus are the major nutritional problems among the population and she stresses the misconceptions and ignorance concerning the causes of these diseases. For instance, many women ascribe PCM to "bad blood" caused by the mother's own improper behavior, by the unsatisfactory burial of a close relative or by the mother's recent death.

The number of infants suffering from PCM is estimated by FAO to be between 35,000 and 50,000. Many youngsters weigh only 60-80 percent of the standard weight for their age, sex and ethnic groups, which places them in

Grades I and II of Gomez' classification of malnutrition.* Anemia is found throughout the Caribbean area, associated with iron or folic acid deficiency, particularly among preschool and young schoolchildren.

Infant mortality rates have declined in recent years from 37.4 per 1,000 in 1965 to 35.2 per 1,000 in 1968. Yet even at this level the role of malnutrition in causing death or contributing to early death through lessened resistance to infections or other disease, remains very important.

VI. CONCLUSIONS

Jamaica is bravely struggling to overcome many of the problems which usually beset developing countries and a few more that are typically Jamaican. The usual problems are climatic and social: erratic distribution of water and good soil; excessive population growth in relation to the carrying capacity of the land; disaffection of rural laborers needed to make the land productive and to fight erosion; unemployment in the crowded cities because of an excess of unskilled workers and a shortage of skilled ones; lack of investment capital to remedy the situation; and a system of education that has not been oriented towards the specific needs of the island.

In addition to these burdens common to all new nations, Jamaica has a few serious problems of its own: the ruggedness of the terrain makes inland communications difficult; the aftermath of slave emancipation has left a widespread number of undersized holdings at the periphery of large estates which cannot support the inhabitants without an infusion of cash wages from the outside or substantial government support; the local tradition sustains the right of all family members to partake in the meager fare provided by the farm whether they have actually helped produce it or not; the matriarchal structure of society encourages runaway population growth but further depresses the land's support of this very population; the emigration of skilled and educated people to the United Kingdom, the United States or Canada leaves only the unskilled and uneducated to fend for themselves as best they can; the importance of tourism to the economy makes it a resource that cannot be refused because of the $100 million a year it brings, but which cannot be enjoyed because it does not absorb the excess rural manpower and increases the bill of imported goods, especially food, which is priced beyond local family budgets. (The high quality of the imported food cuts both ways: it provides an example for local producers to imitate, but this example is so high as to discourage competition.) All these and

---

*GradeI = weight 10-24 percent below normal standard.
  Grade II = weight 25-39 percent below normal.
  Grade III = weight 40 percent or more below normal.

more are problems specific to Jamaica which are not going to be solved in the very near future.

Yet, there are solid assets to consider against this list of liabilities. First, the Government is aware of the existence of these problems and has taken many wise steps to steer a middle course between excessive dependence on tourism and excessive limitations against it. The ideal would be to promote local food production to the point where it would be attractive to tourists and priced sufficiently low for local budgets, but this is difficult and will take time. Second, nonagricultural resources such as the mineral wealth of the country (bauxite) have brought large chunks of developmental capital and will do so increasingly.

The change from an agricultural subsistence economy to an industrial economy of consumption is always dangerous and painful. It can only be hoped that wisdom will continue to prevail in the Government.

BIBLIOGRAPHY

1. Ashcroft, M.T. and Lovell, H.G. "Changes in Mean Size of Children in Some Jamaican Schools Between 1951 and 1964." *West Indian Medical Journal*, 1965, 14, 48-52.

2._____ , "Heights and Weights of Jamaican Primary Schoolchildren." *Journal of Tropical Pediatrics*, 1966, 12, 37-43.

3._____ , Heneage, P. and Lovell, H.G. "Heights and Weights of Jamaican Schoolchildren of Various Ethnic Groups." *American Journal of Physical Anthropology*, 1966, 24, 35-44.

4._____ , Ling, J., Lovell, H.G. and Miall, W.E. "Heights and Weights of Adults in Rural and Urban Areas of Jamaica." *British Journal of Preventive and Social Medicine*, 1966, 20, 22-26.

5. Ashworth, A. "An Investigation of Very Low Calorie Intakes Reported in Jamaica." *British Journal of Nutrition*, 1968, 22, 341-355.

5a. Barclay's Bank D.C.O. *Jamaica: An Economic Survey*. London, Barclay's Bank, 1970.

6. *Barclay's Overseas Review*, May 1971, 46-49.

7. Cook, R. "Nutrition and Mortality Under Five Years in the Caribbean Area." *Journal of Tropical Pediatrics*, 1969, 15, 109-117.

8. Crown Publishers, Inc. *Fact Book of the Countries of the World*. New York, Crown Publishers, Inc., 1970.

9. Dibbs, J.L. "Prospects of the Fishing Industry in the Caribbean." *Protein Foods for the Caribbean*. Jamaica, The Caribbean Food and Nutrition Institute, 1968, pp. 23-24.

10. Edwards, D.T. *An Economic Study of Small Farming in Jamaica*. Kingston, University of West Indies, 1965.

11. *Encyclopedia Britannica*. Chicago, William Benton, Publisher, 1970.

12. Evans, D.O.S. "Seeking Additional Markets for Traditional Foods: Jamaica." *Protein Foods for the Caribbean.* Jamaica, The Caribbean Food and Nutrition Institute, 1968, pp. 43-44.

13. Floyd, B. "Jamaica." *Focus,* 1968, XIX (2).

14. Fonaroff, A. "Differential Concepts of Protein-Calorie Malnutrition in Jamaica: An Exploratory Study of Information and Beliefs." *Journal of Tropical Pediatrics,* 1968, 14, Monograph No. 4, 81-105.

15. Fonaroff, L.S. "Settlement Typology and Infant Malnutrition in Jamaica." *Tropical and Geographical Medicine,* 1969, 21 (2), 177-185.

16. Food and Agriculture Organization of the United Nations. *Production Yearbook 1970.* Volume 24. Rome, FAO, 1971.

17. _____ . *Report to the Governments of Guyana, Jamaica and Trinidad and Tobago: Industrial Production of Protein Foods for Infants and Young Children in the Caribbean—A Feasibility Study.* Nutrition Consultants Reports Series 15. Rome, FAO, 1970.

18. _____ . *Trade Yearbook 1970.* Volume 24. Rome, FAO, 1971.

19. *Foreign Agriculture,* 1968, VI (31), 12-13.

20. _____ , 1969, VII (43), 9-10.

21. Fox, H.C., Campbell, V.S. and Elliot, J.A. "A Mixed Vegetable Protein Food for Child Feeding in Jamaica." *Information, Bulletin of the Scientific Research Council Jamaica,* 1968, 8, 52-67.

22. _____ , Campbell, V.S. and Morris, J.C. "The Dietary and Nutritional Status of Jamaican Infants and Toddlers." *Information, Bulletin of the Scientific Research Council Jamaica,* 1968, 8, 33-51.

23. Grantham-McGregor, S.M. and Back, E.H. "Breast Feeding in Kingston, Jamaica." *Archives of Disease in Childhood,* 1970, 45, 404-409.

24. Hopcraft, A. *Born to Hunger.* Boston, Houghton Mifflin Company, 1968.

25. Inter-American Development Bank. *Eleventh Annual Report 1970.* Washington, D.C., IDB, 1971.

26. _____ . *Socio-Economic Progress in Latin America.* Washington, D.C., IDB, 1971.

27. International Bank for Reconstruction and Development. *Statement of Loans—June 30, 1971.* Washington, D.C., IBRD, 1971.

28. Jamaica, Government of (Central Planning Unit). *Economic Survey—Jamaica 1969.* Kingston, The Government Printer, 1970.

29. _____ . *Five Year Independence Plan 1963-1968.* Kingston, The Government Printer, 1965.

30. _____ . (Ministry of Health), The Caribbean Food and Nutrition Institute and University of the West Indies. "Preliminary Results of the Jamaica Nutrition Survey Carried Out in March 1970." Kingston, Mimeographed, Undated.

31. James, P.E. *Latin America*. Fourth Edition. New York, The Odyssey Press, 1969.

32. James, W.P.T. "Patterns of Infant Feeding in Jamaica." *Cajanus* 1968, No. 2, 50-54.

33. Klaidman, S. "Indies' Sugar Blues." *The Washington Post*, July 11, 1971.

34. Knight, E.M. "Government's Outlook on Food Aid." *Protein Foods for the Caribbean*. Jamaica, The Caribbean Food and Nutrition Institute, 1968, pp. 116-118.

35. Knowles, W.H.C. "Diversification of Agriculture with Special Reference to Maize." *Protein Foods for the Caribbean*. Jamaica, The Caribbean Food and Nutrition Institute, 1968, pp. 52-54.

36. *Labor Developments Abroad*, 1968, 13 (9), 16-25.

37. Leung, W-T. Wu. *INCAP-ICNND Food Composition Table for Use in Latin America*. Washington, D.C., U.S. Government Printing Office, 1961.

38. McKenzie, H.I., Lovell, H.G., Standard, K.L. and Miall, W.E. "Child Mortality in Jamaica." *Milbank Memorial Fund Quarterly*, 1967, 45, 303-320.

39. McKigney, J.E. "Food Economics in Nutrition Policy and Planning." *Nutrition Newsletter*, 1969, 7 (4), 16-24.

40. Phillipsen, W.L. "CARIFTA and the Caribbean Market." *Foreign Agriculture*, 1969, VII (21), 10-11.

41. *Quarterly Economic Review: The West Indies, British Honduras, Bahamas, Bermuda, Guyana*, 1971 (1), 6.

42. United Nations (Department of Economic and Social Affairs). *Demographic Yearbook 1969*. New York, UN, 1970.

43. United Nations Children's Fund. *Digest of Projects Aided by UNICEF in the Americas*. New York, UNICEF, 1969.

44. United Nations Development Program. *Projects in the Special Fund Component As of 31 January 1971*. DP/SF/Reports Series B, No. 11. New York, UNDP, 1971.

45. U.S. Agency for International Development. *A.I.D. Economic Data Book— Latin America*. Washington, D.C., AID, 1970.

46. U.S. Department of Agriculture (Economic Research Service). *Agriculture and Trade of the Caribbean Region*. ERS-Foreign 309. Washington, D.C., U.S. Government Printing Office, 1971.

47. —————————. *Food Balances for 24 Countries of the Western Hemisphere—Projected 1970*. Washington, D.C., USDA, Undated.

48. —————————. *Indices of Agricultural Production for the Western Hemisphere Excluding the United States and Cuba—Revised 1961 through 1969, Preliminary 1970*. ERS-Foreign 264. Washington, D.C., U.S. Government Printing Office, 1971.

49. —————————. *Jamaica, Trinidad and Tobago, Leeward Islands, Windward Islands, Barbados, and British Guiana—Projected Levels of Demand,*

Supply, and Imports of Agricultural Products to 1975. ERS-Foreign 94. Jerusalem, Israel Program for Scientific Translations, 1963.

50. ————————. *Prospects for U.S. Agricultural Exports to Jamaica.* Foreign Agricultural Economic Report No. 56. Washington, D.C., U.S. Government Printing Office, 1969.

51. ————————. *Summary and Evaluation of Jamaica, Trinidad and Tobago, Leeward Islands, Windward Islands, Barbados, and British Guiana—Projected Levels of Demand, Supply, and Imports of Agricultural Products to 1975.* ERS-Foreign 148. Washington, D.C., U.S. Government Printing Office, 1966.

52. U.S. Department of Commerce (Bureau of International Commerce). "Basic Data on the Economy of Jamaica." *Overseas Business Reports.* OBR 67-38. Washington, D.C., U.S. Government Printing Office, 1967.

53. U.S. Department of Labor (Bureau of Labor Statistics). *Labor Conditions in Jamaica.* Labor Digest No. 51. Washington, D.C., USDL, 1964.

54. ————————. *Labor Law and Practice in Jamaica.* BLS Report No. 320. Washington, D.C., U.S. Government Printing Office, 1967.

55. West, R.C. and Augelli, J.P. *Middle America: Its Lands and Peoples.* Englewood Cliffs, Prentice-Hall, 1966.

56. Williams, E. *From Columbus to Castro: The History of the Caribbean 1492-1969.* New York, Harper & Row, Publishers, 1970.

LIST OF TABLES

LIST OF MAPS

TABLE NO. 1

Population by Parish — Jamaica, 1943-1970

Parish	1943	1960	1970*	Annual Rate of Increase
St. Andrews	128,146	296,013	520,973	7.6
Clarendon	123,505	163,950	195,091	1.9
St. Catherine	121,032	153,535	176,760	1.5
Kingston	110,083	123,403	130,807	.6
St. Elizabeth	100,182	116,706	133,412	1.0
St. Ann	96,193	114,360	126,933	1.1
Manchester	92,745	117,788	131,912	1.2
Westmoreland	90,109	109,606	122,758	1.2
St. Mary	90,902	94,233	96,117	.2
St. James	63,542	83,003	96,283	1.6
St. Thomas	60,693	68,725	74,221	.8
Portland	60,712	64,510	53,540	1.4
Trelawny	47,535	56,080	61,688	1.0
Hanover	51,684	53,902	54,980	.2
Total	1,237,063	1,615,814	1,995,475	Aver. 1.5

*Estimated

Source: After U.S. Department of Labor (Bureau of Labor Statistics), *Labor Law and Practice in Jamaica.*

TABLE NO. 2

Area Covered in Crops — Jamaica, 1948-1970
(in 1,000 hectares)

Crop	Annual Average 1948-1952	1964	1966	1968	1969	1970
Corn	17	4	4	4	4	4
Rice	3	2	1	1	1	1
Potatoes	1	1	1	1	2	2
Sweet potatoes and yams	16	40	41	42	45	n.a.
Manioc	5	3	4	4	4	n.a.
Cabbages	1	1	1	1	1	n.a.
Pulses	6	2	7	7	7	7
Sugarcane	46	60	60	60	55	55
Tobacco	1	1	1	1	5	5
Bananas	29	36	38	38	30	30

n.a.=data not available.

Source: Food and Agriculture Organization of the United Nations, *Production Yearbook 1970.*

TABLE NO. 3

Production of Crops – Jamaica, 1948-1970
(in 1,000 tons unless otherwise stated)

Crop	Annual Average 1948-1952	1964	1966	1968	1969	1970
Corn	13	4	4	4	4	4
Rice	6	3	1	1	2	2
Potatoes	1	11	13	13	13	13
Sweet potatoes and yams	64	215	216	207	210	n.a.
Manioc	17	8	10	10	10	11*
Cabbage	5	7	6	6	6	n.a.
Pulses	2	2	3	3	3	3
Sugarcane	2,663	4,793	4,400	3,800	4,000	n.a.
Centrifugal sugar	279	497	456	389	377	400
Oranges and tangerines	54	69	87	62	71	75
Grapefruit	19	30	19	21	21	22
Lemons and others	5	9	10	10	10	10
Bananas	131	290	330	210	210	145*
Pineapples	2	1	1	1	1	n.a.
Coconuts (million nuts)	74	120	125	120	115	n.a.
Copra	5.5	15.7	17.5	16.8	15.6	11.8
Coffee	2.5	1.4	1.0	1.0	1.2	1.2
Cocoa	2	2.2	1.7	1.8	1.9	2.2
Tobacco	1	1.3	4.6	4.8	4.9	4.9

n.a.=data not available.

Sources: Food and Agriculture Organization of the United Nations, *Production Yearbook 1970.*

*U.S. Department of Agriculture (Economic Research Service). *Indices of Agricultural Production for the Western Hemisphere.*

TABLE NO. 4

Food Imports — Jamaica, 1963-1969
(in 1,000 tons)

	1963	1964	1965	1966	1967	1968	1969
Meat (fresh, chilled, frozen)	5.6	4.7	7.0	8.6	8.8	10.4	26.3
Meat (dried, salted, smoked)	3.4	3.7	3.6	2.7	2.2	2.2	1.5
Dry milk and cream	5.4	6.3	6.5	5.7	7.7	9.1	7.5
Butter	2.8	3.9	3.1	3.4	4.3	4.5	4.2
Cheese and curd	1.3	1.6	1.3	2.0	2.0	2.4	2.4
Wheat and wheat flour	126	138	142	141	151	173	146
Rice	22	27	33	27	33	24	26
Corn	16	26	23	49	46	42	53
Oats	1	1	1	1	1	–	–
Potatoes	4.8	3.2	1.4	5.1	2.4	2.9	5.0
Legumes	3.0	4.1	3.0	1.3	1.7	2.2	3.7
Onions	3.5	3.8	4.1	4.1	4.3	4.4	4.8
Animal fats except lard and butter	3.2	3.6	3.8	3.2	5.3	3.8	3.8
Soybean oil	–	–	0.1	1.8	4.3	3.5	5.2

Source: Food and Agriculture Organization of the United Nations, *Trade Yearbook 1970.*

TABLE NO. 5

Food Exports — Jamaica, 1963-1969
(in 1,000 tons)

	1963	1964	1965	1966	1967	1968	1969
Oranges and tangerines	6.6	2.9	2.8	2.7	4.0	2.1	2.0
Other citrus	9.1	4.8	6.1	3.9	4.2	7.6	6.5
Bananas	116	177	203	203	193	155	153
Coconuts	0.1	0.2	1.3	1.7	0.1	0.2	–
Sugar (raw)	400	424	431	414	358	389	299
Cocoa beans	1.2	1.4	2.2	1.5	–	1.4	1.4
Pepper & pimento	2.5	2.3	1.3	2.4	1.9	2.3	3.2

Source: Food and Agriculture Organization of the United Nations, *Trade Yearbook 1970.*

TABLE NO. 6

Food Imports by Value – Jamaica, 1965-1969
(in $1,000)

Item	1965	1966	1967	1968	1969
Meat and meat preparations	6,482	7,562	6,744	8,658	9,058
Dairy products, eggs and honey	6,872	7,126	8,034	8,332	8,264
Fish and fish preparations	5,738	7,126	7,156	7,958	8,806
Cereals and cereal preparations	15,324	16,096	18,618	20,486	20,368
Fruits and vegetables	2,850	2,856	3,002	3,760	3,778
Sugar and sugar preparations	431	428	559	688	2,725
Animal feed	1,750	2,536	2,844	6,226	4,892
Beverages	1,536	1,670	1,682	2,354	2,740
Totals	40,983	45,400	48,639	58,462	60,631

Source: Government of Jamaica (Central Planning Unit), *Economic Survey – Jamaica 1969.*

TABLE NO. 7

Nutrient Availability Per Capita Per Day – Jamaica, 1964

	Q.p.d.[a] g	Calcium mg	Phosphorous mg	Iron mg	Vitamin A mcg	Thiamine mg	Riboflavin mg	Niacin mg	Vitamin C mg
Flour	175	28.0	150	1.4	0	.10	.08	1.5	0
Corn	25	1.5	72	.6	1.2	.10	.02	.5	0
Rice	41	3.6	42	.5	0	.03	.01	.6	0
Sugar	117	59.0	51	4.9	0	.03	.11	.3	2.0
Potatoes	21	1.2	8	.1	0	.02	neg.	.3	3.0
Sweet potatoes[b]	142	44.0	48.0	1.4	2,577.0	.12	.05	1.0	34.0
Manioc	13	4.6	5	.1	0	neg.	neg.	neg.	neg.
Legumes[c]	12	5.6	22	.3	neg.	neg.	neg.	neg.	neg.
Coconuts	49	6.4	141	.8	0	neg.	neg.	1.3	2.0
Vegetables[d]	136	80.0[e]	40	4.0	1,400.0	.08	.23	.8	60.0
Bananas	119	8.5	33	.6	78.0	.05	.05	.8	18.0
Other fruit (oranges)	548	187.0	110	3.6	210.0	.47	.16	1.0	300.0
Beef and veal (lean)	34	5.0	60	1.3	0	.02	.07	1.0	0
Other meat (pig)	26	1.5	50	.4	0	.20	.05	1.0	0
Fish (dried cod)	63	33.0	580	2.2	0	.06	.30	7.1	0
Vegetable oils	24	0	0	0	0	0	0	0	0
Other fats	10	0	0	0	0	0	0	0	0
Milk[f]	61	94.0	0	.3	(150)	.03	.31	.2	0

[a]Quantity per day
[b]Deep orange type
[c]P. vulgaris
[d]Spinach
[e]Due to oxalic acid, may not be fully utilized
[f]Whole and reconstituted

Sources: U.S. Department of Agriculture (Economic Research Service), Food Balances for 24 Countries of the Western Hemisphere – Projected 1970.

W-T. Wu Leung, Food Composition Table for Use in Latin America.

TABLE NO. 8

Food Balance Sheet – Jamaica, 1964 (Estimated)
(Population: 2,000,000 approximately)

Product	Supply — Production (1,000 m.tons)	Imports (1,000 m.tons)	Exports (1,000 m.tons)	Changes in stocks (1,000 m.tons)	Total supply (1,000 m.tons)	Nonfood use — Seed and waste (1,000 m.tons)	Feed (1,000 m.tons)	Industrial (1,000 m.tons)	Total (1,000 m.tons)	Utilization — Total gross (1,000 m.tons)	Extraction rate (Per cent)	Total (1,000 m.tons)	Supply for food — Net Per capita — Per year — Kilograms	Per day — Calories	Grams protein	Grams fat
Flour	–	121	–	–	121	–	–	–	–	121	–	121	64.0	638	22.3	1.9
Corn	4	18	–	–	22	–	4	–	4	18	95	17	9.2	91	2.3	1.0
Rice	4	45	–	–	49	1	–	–	1	48	60	29	15.2	150	2.8	.3
Other cereal prod.	–	5	–	–	5	–	–	–	–	5	–	5	2.5	26	.6	.1
Total cereals					197								90.9	905	28.0	3.3
Sugar: Raw	510	–	429	–	81	–	–	–	–	81	–	81	43.0	412	1.2	–
Potatoes	12	6	–	–	18	3	–	–	3	15	–	15	8.0	15	.4	–
Sweet potatoes	101	–	–	–	101	3	–	–	3	98	–	98	52.0	130	2.8	.3
Cassava	13	–	–	–	13	–	–	4	4	9	–	9	4.7	14	.1	–
Pulses	6	4	–	–	8	–	–	–	–	8	–	8	4.2	44	2.8	.3
Coconuts	17	–	–	–	77	–	–	43	43	34	–	34	18.0	70	.9	6.7
Other vegetables	104	–	–	–	104	5	–	5	10	94	–	94	49.8	40	1.6	.3
Bananas	271	–	171	–	100	12	–	–	12	82	–	82	43.5	81	1.1	.4
Other fruit	459	–	–	–	459	35	46	–	81	378	–	378	200.2	262	4.7	3.3
Cacao	2	–	–	–	2	–	–	–	–	2	88.5	2	1.3	13	.3	.9

Beef and veal	20	3	—	—		23	23	12.0	51	5.1	3.3
Other meat	18	—	—	—		18	18	9.5	67	3.2	6.0
Total meat								21.5	118	8.3	9.3
Fish	13	32	—	—		45	45	23.9	41	5.8	1.8
Vegetable oils	16	—	—	—		16	16	8.5	206	—	23.3
Slaughter fats	4	—	—	—		4	4	2.2	51	.1	5.6
Butter	4	3	—	—		3	3	1.5	29	—	3.3
Total fats								12.2	286	.1	32.2
Whole milk	75	—	16	38	56	17	17	9.2	15	.8	.8
Dried milk	—	7	—	2	2	5	5	2.8	28	2.8	.1
Canned milk	20	—	—	—	—	20	20	10.4	91	2.3	2.4
Cheese	—	1	—	—	—	1	1	.7	7	.7	.4
Total milk and cheese									141	6.6	3.7
Eggs	15	—	2	—	2	13	13	6.8	27	2.0	1.9
Total consumption									2559	66.7	64.4

Source: U.S. Department of Agriculture (Economic Research Service), *Food Balance Sheets for 24 Countries of the Western Hemisphere – Projected 1970.*

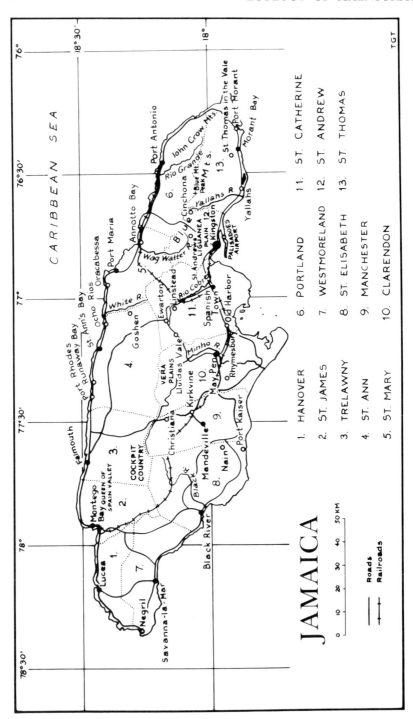

JAMAICA

Roads
Railroads

MAP NO. 1.

1. HANOVER   6. PORTLAND   11. ST. CATHERINE
2. ST. JAMES   7. WESTMORELAND   12. ST. ANDREW
3. TRELAWNY   8. ST. ELISABETH   13. ST. THOMAS
4. ST. ANN   9. MANCHESTER
5. ST. MARY   10. CLARENDON

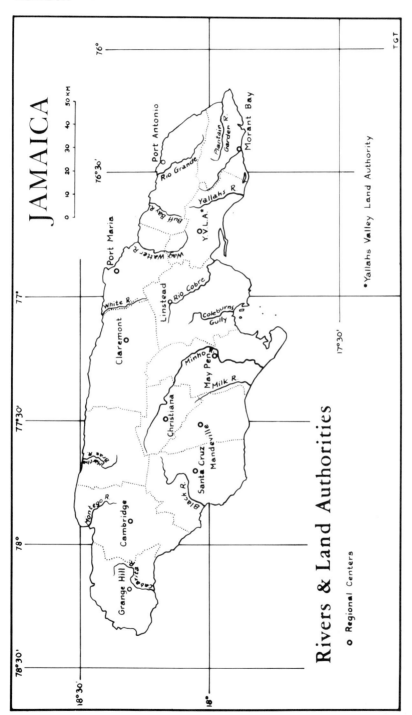

JAMAICA

Rivers & Land Authorities

o Regional Centers

*Yallahs Valley Land Authority

MAP NO. 2.

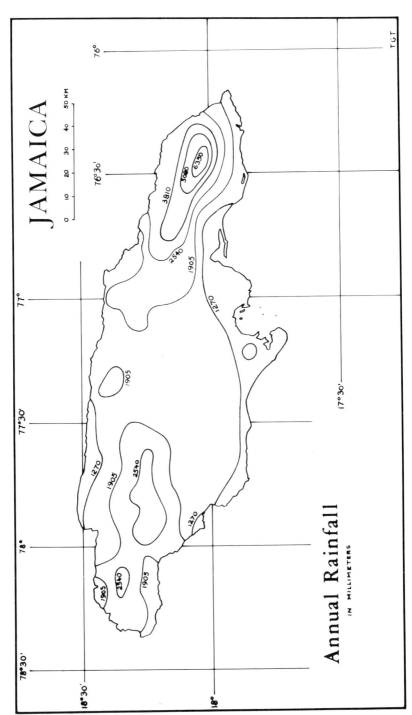

JAMAICA

Annual Rainfall

IN MILLIMETERS

MAP NO. 3.

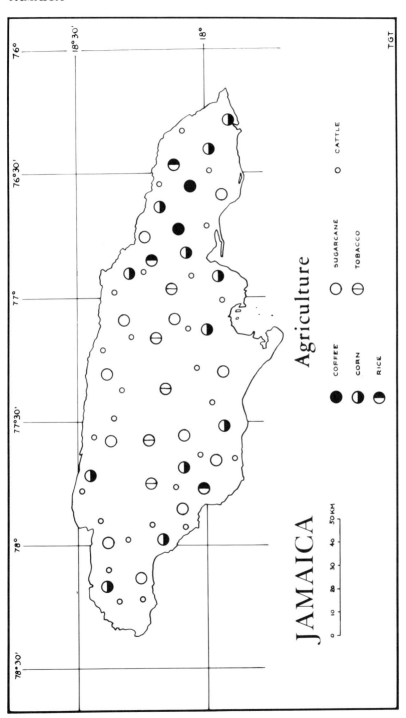

JAMAICA

Agriculture

COFFEE   SUGARCANE

CORN   TOBACCO

RICE   CATTLE

0 10 20 30 40 50 KM

MAP NO. 4.

THE ISLAND OF HISPANIOLA

In December 1492, Columbus discovered a 77,644-square-kilometer island lying between 17°36' and 20°04' north latitude and 63°20' and 74°29' west longitude. He named it La Isla Española (Spanish Island) and it eventually came to be known as Hispaniola. The island was inhabited by peaceful Arawak and Taino Indians who called their homeland *Hayti* or "the mountainous country." By the end of the 16th century most of the Indians had been killed by disease and maltreatment.

Hispaniola provided the Spaniards with a base for further expansion of the empire to Cuba, Mexico, Panama and South America. With the discovery of gold in the central part of the island, Spanish settlements multiplied rapidly, but the eastern part remained virtually untouched. In addition to the mining activities, plantations were established and with the disappearance of the Indian population, African slaves were imported to work the plantations and the mines.

In the mid-17th century, buccanneers from the island of Tortuga established settlements on the practically uninhabited western end of the island. These settlements were taken over by the French West India Company in 1664 and in 1697, according to the Treaty of Ryswick, Spain ceded the western part of the island to France. Thus, before the beginning of the 18th century, the island became divided culturally and linguistically and the foundations for the present countries of Haiti and the Dominican Republic were laid.

" HISTORICAL EXTERNAL ORIENT

THE REPUBLIC OF HAITI

TABLE OF CONTENTS

THE REPUBLIC OF HAITI

I. BACKGROUND INFORMATION

A. PHYSICAL SETTING [6] [44] [11] [5] [17]

The Republic of Haiti encompasses 27,770 square kilometers at the western end of the island of Hispaniola which it shares with the Dominican Republic. It comprises two peninsulas connected by a land mass. Over 40 percent of the land area is above 500 meters in altitude. The northern part of the country is dominated by the Massif du Nord, which is a continuation of the Cordillera Centrale that runs across the island in a southeasterly direction. These mountains have been described by West and Augelli as "a tangled maze of peaks and ridges with, here and there, a flat-bottomed intermontane valley." There is an area of coastal lowland around Anse Rouge. The Massif gives way briefly to the Plaine du Nord (see Map No. 1), an extension of the lengthy Cibao Lowlands of the Dominican Republic. Cap Haïtien, one of the best farming areas in the country, is located in this region. The Cap is a small patch of coastal lowland with fertile alluvial soil and a relatively humid climate. To the south of the Massif du Nord, leading to the southern peninsula, are five parallel configurations of alternating lowlands and ranges: the Plaine Centrale to the east, the Montagnes Noires, the Artibonite Valley, the Chaine des Mateux and the Cul-de-Sac Depression. Due to the rain shadow effect of the mountains, the lowlands are arid and require irrigation. Parts of the Cul-de-Sac Depression are below sea level and covered by extensive salt lakes, the largest of which are the Etang Saumâtre and Lac Enriquillo. Coffee is cultivated on the rainy windward slopes of the mountain chains, while sugar and rice are grown on the irrigated lowlands (see Map No. 3). Cotton is cultivated on the semiarid plateaus and plains. Subsistence food crops are grown everywhere possible, even on steep mountain slopes which the peasants cultivate, using ropes to support themselves.

Most of the southern part of Haiti is a long peninsula jutting into the sea. This region is composed primarily of highlands (Massif de la Selle to the east and Massif de la Hotte to the west) with small patches of coastal plains located between Aquin and a point just beyond Chardonnières, and around Corail. The highest point in the country is the Mont de la Selle (2,680 meters) in the Massif de la Selle. The island of Gonâve lies in the bay off Port-au-Prince and resembles the southern highlands in topography.

The major river of importance in Haiti is the Artibonite, which is 280 kilometers long. The second largest is the Trois Rivières (102 kilometers). The other rivers are short and irregular, often receding to a trickle during the dry season and turning into raging torrents following the heavy rains.

Vegetation is extremely varied. The Cul-de-Sac Depression, which is the most arid zone, is desert-like with cacti, thornbush and dry scrub the primary cover. The Artibonite Valley, classified as subhumid, supports savanna with scattered palms. In the few coastal swamps which are found in the country, mangroves thrive. Although much of Haiti, especially the north and northeast, apparently was once covered with tropical rainforests, stands of trees (mostly pine) are now limited to the upper slopes of the mountains and represent only secondary growth. Almost all virgin forest has been cut, mainly for fuel, and the Government's efforts at reforestation to fight erosion have been thwarted by the peasants who cut the newly-planted young trees for firewood.

The soils of Haiti are varied. In the sierras a dense, rocky red soil is spread over a limestone base and is subject to erosion because of deforestation. The Artibonite Valley, except in its lower reaches, has alkaline soils unfavorable to agriculture. As already mentioned, the best land is found in the Cap Haïtien area where fertile alluvial soils are ideal for farming. Other areas especially favorable to agriculture are the coastal plains above Les Cayes and the Asile Valley, both of which are characterized by alluvium. Actually, the whole area extending from the western Cul-de-Sac through Port-au-Prince on the southwest peninsula is the site of intensive farming. The peasants do not make use of fertilizer and many fail to practice crop rotation or fallowing which would restore the soil's fertility. Moreover, even though outlawed, the slash-and-burn method of farming is often practiced to the subsequent detriment of the soil, since burning destroys the humus and promotes erosion.

B. CLIMATE [44] [6] [17]

Temperatures vary with altitude and exposure to trade winds and range from the *tierra caliente* to the *tierra fría* type.* In the lowlands, annual temperatures average about 25.5°C, except in sheltered spots like Gonaives, Port-au-Prince and

---

Tierra caliente means "hot land" and generally refers to the climate found at sea level to 833 meters elevation, where the daytime temperature ranges from 29.5°C to 32°C and the nighttime reading drops to 24° or even 21°C. *Tierra fría* means "cold land" and is used to describe the climate at elevations above 1,830 meters where daytime temperatures are a pleasant 24-27°C and nights are cold at 10-8°C.

the Cul-de-Sac Depression where the average exceeds 27°C (see Table No. 1). In the mountains, winter temperatures frequently fall below the freezing mark. Precipitation patterns are equally varied although, in general, rainfall decreases from northeast to southwest and is heavier in the highlands than in the lowlands. Windward areas receive more rain than leeward ones. Irrigation is a necessity in the Artibonite Valley, the Plaine du Nord, the Cul-de-Sac and other lowland areas. The driest zone is in the Cul-de-Sac Depression.

C. POPULATION [14] [35] [1] [6] [44]

In 1971 the population of Haiti was estimated to total about 5.2 million, but no accurate census has ever been taken. The rate of natural increase is thought to be around 2.5 percent a year. Life expectancy at birth is estimated by the Government to be about 50 years, although other sources estimate a shorter life span. The infant mortality rate is very high at 146.5 per 1,000 live births. These figures reflect the poor health and poor nutritional status of the population and the lack of adequate public health facilities. The density is about 179 persons per square kilometer when figured on an overall basis, but on arable land it is probably nearer 400 per square kilometer. The population is about 85 percent rural. There are only two towns with more than 20,000 inhabitants: the capital city of Port-au-Prince (about 280,000) and the town of Cap Haïtien (33,000).

Except for a miniscule community of Caucasian families engaged in commerce at Port-au-Prince, the population of Haiti is about 95 percent Negro *(brun)* and 5 percent mulatto *(jaune)*. The latter form the elite of the upper class and are descendants of unions between French men and African women during the 18th century. The mulattoes live in the principal towns, enter commerce, the professions and government service. They speak French, adhere to Roman Catholicism and take pride in their cultural heritage. Their position in society is based on skin color, family history and money. With the exception of a small elite, the blacks are peasant farmers in the rural areas or workmen and household servants in the towns. Most are illiterate and speak only a local patois which is an admixture primarily of French, Spanish and English, with a few remnants of African and Indian words. It is estimated that about 89.5 percent of the population over 15 years of age is illiterate. This is the highest rate in the western hemisphere. The peasants are nominally Catholic but *voudun* (voodoo-ism), a belief in spirits and spells carried over from the original African culture, is widely practiced.

A few black families with money, whose members have been educated abroad, have joined the ranks of the elite. There is no viable middle class in Haiti, but a few people, such as artisans, skilled laborers, minor civil servants and some of the more advanced peasant farmers, have begun to occupy a place on the ladder between the masses and the upper class.

The Haitian peasants are the most impoverished in the Americas. Most live in small one- or two-room huts called *cailles-pailles*, which average no more than 3.5 x 4.0 meters, with an adjacent pen for chickens and pigs. The hut's floor is made of beaten earth, the walls of bamboo or like plant material plastered with mud and lime, and the roof of thatched straw or palm leaves. Some *cailles-pailles* are dispersed, some grouped into tiny villages of four to 10 huts. A small village is lucky if it can boast a community privy. There is not even a primitive stove in the *caille-paille*: a metal brazier for cooking is kept outside the house. Furniture is minimal and rarely includes beds; hammocks or straw mats are used for sleeping. The huts are quite stuffy at night because the windows and doors are kept tightly closed to protect against the night air and against ghosts. These dwellings are wet during the rainy season and are usually infested with vermin the year round. Landless families called *sans maman* (motherless ones) may have even poorer accommodations than the ones described while a peasant with larger than average holdings (called a *gros habitant*) may be able to afford a wooden frame house with corrugated iron roof. Because of the widespread deforestation, construction materials are costly and even an ordinary *caille-paille* may cost the equivalent of $80 or more.

Regional variations in housing reflect the local availability of materials and the climatic conditions of the area. In the high elevations of the Plaine Centrale, for instance, unfinished palm boards are used for the walls while on the Plaine du Nord the frame is plastered with a mixture of clay and brick fragments. In the cold mountain zone of the *tierra fría*, the huts are broader and sturdier than in the lowlands and a heavier thatch is used for the roofs.

D. HISTORY AND GOVERNMENT (6) (1) (44) (43)

Haiti's history as a distinct national entity began in 1697 when Spain ceded to France the western third of the island of Hispaniola. The colony was then called Saint Domingue and it became one of France's richest possessions. During the 18th century, the plantations of Saint Domingue were exporting sugar, coffee and other tropical crops produced by the thousands of African slaves who had been brought to the colony by the French landowners. By 1789, out of a total population of 520,000 there were about 27,500 mulattoes (freedmen of mixed ancestry) and about 450,000 black slaves. While many of the mulattoes owned plantations and held slaves themselves, effective power was in the hands of the white French planters.

The upheaval of the French Revolution of 1789 was felt in Saint Domingue, bringing unrest and disorders which culminated in an overall slave revolt in 1791. Plantations were burned and the white ruling class was massacred. Spain and Britain tried to invade the island during this period of turmoil and were repelled by the first of Haiti's black leaders. General Pierre Toussaint l'Ouverture, who restored order in the country. In 1793, the French Government abolished slavery in Saint Domingue and guaranteed to all the colony's inhabitants the Rights of Man proclaimed by the French Revolution. Toussaint l'Ouverture was designated Governor General. In 1803, Napoleon sent his brother-in-law, General Leclerc, to Saint Domingue with 70 warships, 45,000 men and orders to seize Toussaint and restore slavery in the colony. During the war which ensued Toussaint was tricked into capture, shipped to France and imprisoned.

At this point, three of Toussaint's leading generals, Henri Christophe, Jean Jacques Dessalines and Alexandre Pétion, resumed the war against the French. In 1803 the French, decimated by yellow fever and with their military commander dead from the disease, capitulated and the victors proclaimed their independence, adopting the original Arawak name of the country, *Hayti*. Dessalines proclaimed himself emperor of the newly-independent country but he was soon assassinated (1806). A republic was then proclaimed and Henri Christophe was named its first president. However, Christophe was opposed by the southern mulatto elite who feared black domination. A civil war soon developed and Christophe withdrew to the north where he proclaimed himself King of the North, the Northwest and the Artibonite and began surrounding himself with a newly-created black nobility. The southwestern part of the country became a mulatto stronghold under the leadership of Pétion. Christophe committed suicide in 1820 and the country was reunited, only to experience the rise and fall of governments with relative anarchy prevailing. In 1915, the United States Government stepped in, partly to keep other foreign interventionists out, partly to have a base from which to protect the Panama Canal from attack by German U-boats during the First World War. The American occupation lasted until 1934. During this time roads were built, sanitation was improved, public health services were established and the country's financial situation was stabilized. Soon after the American withdrawal the economy and the nation's infrastructure began to deteriorate once again.

The current Government of Haiti is based on the Constitution of 1964. That document gave then President Dr. Francois Duvalier tenure for life. Duvalier died in 1971, naming his son as his successor. Legislative authority is in the hands of a unicameral legislature composed of 58 deputies elected for a term of 6 years.

Administration of the country is highly centralized. The nation is divided into five departments—North, Northwest, Artibonite, West and South—each under the authority of a military commandant who reports to the President at Port-au-Prince. The departments are subdivided into circumscriptions called "rural sections," each one headed by a section chief who receives orders from the military commandant of the department to which his section belongs. The cities have councils and ruling magistrates (mayors) but the magistrates have little decision-making initiative; real power is focused in the President at Port-au-Prince.

E. AGRICULTURAL AND NUTRITION POLICIES [14] [1] [39] [40]

1. Agricultural Policies

Haiti is highly dependent on the agricultural sector which gives jobs to 80-87 percent of the employed population, provides 50 percent of the gross domestic product and accounts for 50-60 percent of exports by value. Yet productivity is low, capital investment in agriculture is limited, supporting services are inadequate and the systems of storage and transportation are poor.

In 1963 the Government established a National Development and Planning Council (CONADEP) to draw up and administer the country's development plans. CONADEP is attached directly to the presidency. Under the most recent plan, highest priority has been given to developing the economic infrastructure of the nation: power, transportation and telecommunications. Since inadequate transportation is one of the most serious problems facing agriculture, impeding food distribution and making many communities inaccessible to agricultural extension (and health) services, this priority should benefit the agricultural as well as the industrial sector. Projects related to agriculture under the plan have included construction of irrigation facilities, promotion of export crops (especially coffee) and food import substitution.*

There are two government agencies operating in the field of rural development: the Ministry of Agriculture, Natural Resources and Rural Development, and the Institute of Agricultural and Industrial Development. Under the Ministry are an Office of Agricultural Credit, a Rural Development Service and a Cooperative Service. The Office of Agricultural Credit serves low-income farmers and promotes cultivation of staple crops such as rice, beans, corn, yams and potatoes. Small farmers are encouraged to establish their own rural credit societies and in 1970 there were 66 such societies with about 1,000 members. The intention is good, but credit resources are very limited. In 1970 the Office authorized credit totaling only about $202,300. The Rural Development Service provides extension services to small farmers but its operations are hampered by the shortage of trained personnel. In 1970 the Service staff included 143 field technicians who provided assistance to 4,063 farmers, a small achievement considering that there are an estimated 250,000 small farms throughout the country. The Cooperative Service, as its name implies, encourages the creation of agricultural cooperatives. In 1970 there were three coffee cooperatives with 474 members and 40 other agricultural cooperatives with 3,250 members.

The Institute of Agricultural and Industrial Development (IDAI) was estab-

---

*In the past, some attention has been given to increasing the use of fertilizers and insecticides, ameliorating pastures, improving the quality of cattle and establishing small-scale processing industries.

lished in 1961 to stimulate economic growth through provision of direct loans to business and agriculture. The IDAI has sponsored a short-term supervised credit program for small farmers and has authorized loans for the establishment or improvement of agricultural enterprises. The Institute has also promoted cotton cultivation since 1962. Through a subsidiary, the National Equipment Society, IDAI has invested in facilities needed for agricultural development, such as agricultural storage centers (the largest of which is at Gonaives), small irrigation works, a dairy and slaughterhouse at Les Cayes and a cottonseed oil refinery at Gonaives.

Agricultural education is being promoted by the Government, with the financial assistance of the Inter-American Development Bank. Since 1967 the Government has supported a program at the University of Haiti to improve instruction in agriculture and to establish a program of veterinary medicine. On the intermediate level, the Government is promoting rural teacher training and rural vocational education.

The work of the Government in providing technical assistance to farmers is hampered by the uneven distribution of trained personnel within the bureaucracy, by the emigration of numerous technicians to the United States and to the United Nations agencies, by shortage of funds and by inadequate means of transportation.

2. Nutrition Policies [9] [23] [1]

In 1962 a Nutrition Bureau was formed within the Ministry of Public Health which works in close cooperation with a like office in the Ministry of Agriculture. The principal functions of the Bureau are: a) to define the nutritional problems of Haiti; b) to propose solutions; c) to develop nutritional norms and standards; d) to give technical advice to the ministries of Health and Agriculture; e) to train personnel; and f) to coordinate nutrition programs. In addition, the Bureau operates a program of research and demonstration which at the moment is aimed primarily at combating protein-calorie malnutrition. To this end, the Bureau has initiated two projects: the establishment of nutrition rehabilitation centers (mother-craft centers); and the development of a weaning food based on local resources.

A network of nutrition rehabilitation centers has been set up throughout the countryside. At last count, there were 26 such centers. The malnourished children in a village are identified, using the Gomez classification,* and are admitted to the center for about 4 months, which is generally the time needed

---

*Grade I malnutrition = weight 10-24 percent below normal standard.
  Grade II = weight 25-39 percent below normal.
  Grade III = weight 40 percent or more below normal.

for recuperation. Concurrent with the treatment of their children, the mothers are required to participate in a nutrition education and child care program conducted at the center. Six days a week, rotating teams of mothers prepare the meals for the children, learning about the value of the foods being cooked and the relationship of these foods to the health of their infants. There is a followup program for discharged children, and mothers who have attended the centers are encouraged to share with their neighbors the information they have obtained, giving a multiplier effect to the program.

The Nutrition Bureau has worked on the development of a protein-rich weaning food called AK-1000, based on a mixture of cereals (corn, sorghum or rice) and beans, of which there is a variety in Haiti including *Phaseolus vulgaris* (red, black or white kidney beans), *Phaseolus lunatus* (lima beans) and *Cajanus indicus* (pigeon peas).

There are numerous school feeding programs in Haiti but their effectiveness is uneven. Provisions are not always supplied on a regular basis and the menu is not well-balanced from a nutritional point of view, especially considering the fact that for many children the lunch they receive at school is their only meal for the day.

The Department of Agriculture's Nutrition Bureau is part of the Department's Extension Service. At Guerin this Bureau has promoted the cultivation of sweet potatoes (rich is vitamin A), selected beans, hybrid corn and legumes and has encouraged rabbit-raising. At Fond-Parisien the Bureau has succeeded in expanding the cultivation of tomatoes, legumes, sorghum and fruit trees. In addition, the Department of Agriculture's Home Economic Service has for many years conducted nutrition education programs for rural women.

F. FOREIGN AID

1. Bilateral Aid [6] [38]

The United States has been Haiti's main source of bilateral aid but assistance has been drastically curtailed since 1962, due to disputes over the way in which the work was carried out and questions about the diversion of funds for improper uses. Total U.S. economic assistance between 1946 and 1968 amounted to $111.4 million, of which $77.5 million were in the form of technical assistance grants for the improvement of health services and agriculture, including the Artibonite Valley irrigation project. About $3.5 million were for emergency relief under Title II of the Public Law 480 (Food for Freedom) progam and $13.0 million were in the form of food donations distributed through voluntary agencies, such as CARE, Catholic Relief Services and Church World Services; $28 million in long-term loans were made available through the Export-Import Bank.

2. Multilateral Aid (13) (14) (37) (36) (34) (15) (16)

Haiti receives assistance from a number of multilateral agencies. Since 1961 the Inter-American Development Bank (IDB) has approved loans to Haiti in the amount of $12,260,000. In 1970, the IDB made a $5.1 million long-term, low-interest loan to Haiti for the improvement and expansion of the Port-au-Prince water system. This is the second stage of a project begun in 1964 with a $2.4 million loan from the IDB. In 1971 the Bank authorized a $3.2 million loan for agricultural and industrial development. The United Nations Development Program Special Fund has provided Haiti with a total of almost $4.1 million for agricultural projects, including an animal husbandry demonstration project in the Plaine des Cayes region, land and water surveys in the Gonaives Plain and the Department of the Northwest, agricultural surveys and demonstrations in southern Haiti, and engineering and feasibility studies of the Port-au-Prince–Les Cayes–Jérémie road. All but the last of these projects have been carried out with the technical assistance of the Food and Agricultural Organization of the United Nations. The United Nations Children's Fund has supported projects totaling $2.4 million, including a program to strengthen the health services, a malaria eradication program in cooperation with the World Health Organization, a training program for rural teachers in cooperation with the United Nations Educational, Scientific and Cultural Organization and a prevocational training program for rural boys and girls in cooperation with the International Labor Organization. The World Bank has made a $2.6 million loan to Haiti for road construction, and its affiliate, the International Development Association, has provided credit in the amount of $350,000 for a highway project. The expansion of the road system should help to improve the distribution of food crops.

II. FOOD RESOURCES

A. GENERAL (33) (44) (1) (14) (21)

According to the Food and Agriculture Organization of the United Nations (FAO), the total land area of Haiti encompasses 2.7 million hectares, of which 370,000 hectares were arable or under permanent crops at the time of the 1950 agricultural census, 500,000 hectares were in prairies and pastures and 700,000 hectares were wooded. In 1958, Sebrell, Smith et al. computed the land under permanent crops to total 1,254,000 hectares, a figure somewhat lower than that given by the Haitian Department of Agriculture in 1965 of 1.4 million hectares. This relatively small discrepancy may be explained by the fact that the former source gives the amount of land actually sown in specific crops while the latter includes 250,000 hectares of semiarid mountainous land. Sixty percent of the cultivated acreage is located in the Plaine des Cayes (around the city of Les Cayes), the Plaine du Nord, the Artibonite Valley and the Cul-de-Sac Depression. The Artibonite is fertile only where irrigation is available and the Cul-de-Sac Depression is of low fertility. The rest of the land under crops is scattered through several cordilleras.

According to the Sebrell, Smith et al. computation, about 45.1 percent of the land is used for food production. There seems to be a consensus of opinion that further extension of arable acreage will be costly and difficult. The most valuable land is already thickly settled and the other potentially usable land is either mountainous and difficult to reach, or dry and requiring irrigation, or poor and demanding fertilization. Four hundred thousand hectares are either semiproductive or semiarid and 1,170,000 more hectares are unusable. Hence, the hope for increased food production rests with the adoption of improved technology.

However, there are many obstacles to the modernization of agriculture in Haiti, including lack of funds, lack of education and lack of transportation facilities for both goods and people. The lack of funds is due to the very narrow base of the Haitian economy which relies almost exclusively on agriculture, with coffee representing about 60 percent of all money-earning exports. The lack of education is the result of many circumstances, most important of which is the fact that 84.9 percent of the peasantry speaks almost only Creole. This causes instruction to remain verbal and elemental. There are not enough instructors and even if there were, they would be hampered by the scarcity of good roads in a mountainous country where mules and donkeys remain the major means of transportation (see *Transportation*). Instruction by radio has limited effectiveness due to the extreme poverty of the peasants. Moreover, the rate of growth of the population at 2.5 percent a year erodes whatever progress can be made in spite of all difficulties.

Behgin et al.* have made a list of the major food crops contributing to the Haitian diet (see Table No. 2). Corn and millet, in true African tradition, are the most popular cereals. Sorghum is not identified separately from millet and its consumption is considered to be lower than that of millet. Rice and wheat, the latter imported, are the next favored grains. The plantain is the most widely consumed fruit, while manioc, sweet potatoes and yams are the preferred tubers. The cocoyam or *malanga* is commonly used. Legumes, such as dry beans and the ubiquitous pigeon pea, complete the list of the foods most typically found in the diet. In addition, a large variety of vegetables and tropical fruits are available.

The resources of the sea, as well as those of Haiti's rivers, lakes and ponds, contribute modestly to the food supply. The amount of fish landed is very small,

---

*Throughout this section *(Food Resources)*, "Beghin et al." refers to Beghin, Fougère and King, *L'Alimentation et la Nutrition en Haiti.*

amounting to only 4,000 tons a year of seafood and 500 tons of freshwater fish. This catch does not meet the local demand and another 3,000 tons of fish are imported, representing 41.3 percent of all protein food purchased abroad. This additional fish could be obtained locally if Haiti would follow the example of the Dominican Republic or Jamaica and expand the fishing industry.

With this background, it is easy to see that the food resources are limited and that the majority of the population must feed itself on a very narrow budget. In 1968, it was computed that the gross domestic product (GDP) allowed an annual per capita income of no more than $74. The rate of growth of the population is estimated at over 2.5 percent a year, while the rate of growth of the GDP is only about 1.5 percent, hence the average income of each Haitian must be diminishing. According to Beghin et al., the population of Haiti can be divided into the five following income groups:

Distribution of Population by Income – Haiti, 1962			
Category	Average Annual Income	Percent of Total Income	Percent of Total Population
Comfortable	$800	13	1
Rural middle class	300	24	5
Urban middle class	280	9	2
Poor rural farmers	32	43	83
Poor urban residents	72	11	9

Source: After I.D. Beghin, W. Fougère and K.W. King, L'Alimentation et La Nutrition en Haiti.

If the picture conveyed by the table above is correct, we can expect to find considerable malnutrition in Haiti. King, Dominique, et al. made a survey of the food expenditures per capita in a poor region of Haiti in 1964 and 1965. They found that the daily food cost per person ranged from a minimum of 7.8¢ at Fond-Parisien to a maximum of 11.4¢ at Les Cayes. In 1968, Dominique et al. (cited in Beghin, et al.) made another survey and reported that the daily food expenditure per capita per day in Haiti was found to be between 8¢ and 8.5.

B. MEANS OF PRODUCTION [5] [1] [12]

The means of production are limited in every sense, which leads to an economy characterized by a restrictive subsistence sector combined with a localized domestic money sector. According to Herskovits, de Young, Beghin and others, the production from individual farms is intended for the local market as well as home consumption. The market is within walking or donkey-riding distance from the farm. This is, of course, the case in most developing lands, except that in Haiti the commercial part of the output of food crops is larger than it is in most developing countries. Therefore, researchers point out, it is inaccurate to apply the term "subsistence" in its true sense to Haitian peasant farming. While no figures and percentages are given, de Young, supported by

Beghin et al., remarks that the small plot is extremely diversified in its crops and that eggs, chickens and pork are usually sold for cash at the nearest market while vegetables, roots and sugarcane are more frequently consumed at home. Such a pattern reproduces on a tiny scale the one which existed in Eastern Europe just after the Second World War when valuable protein-rich foods were sold and starchy carbohydrates were retained on the farm to provide the basis of the diet.

1. Agricultural Labor Force [42] [1] [21] [5] [12]

In 1960, the labor force included about 56 percent of the population. On the basis of 1971 estimates, this would mean about 3 million people. Eighty-seven percent of the work force is believed to be employed in agriculture, 3.6 percent in services (including government), 2.9 percent in commerce, 2.7 percent in manufacturing, and 3.8 percent in diverse activities. It is estimated that a very large percentage—as much as 80 percent—is unpaid and self-employed. In agriculture, this percentage rises to 93, reflecting the family farming of small plots which does not require the help of hired farmhands. In 1964 it was reported that only one out of nine persons received a salary and that over half of the country's workers were unemployed or underemployed. Women, of course, are an important part of the labor force, sowing, planting and harvesting whenever the case demands it. They also act as saleswomen, going to the nearby market to sell the most valuable items of their plots' output. In the home, they select and prepare the family's food and take care of the children. The paid labor force is often composed of migrant workers who settle down with their families in huts located at the periphery of the larger sugarcane, sisal and banana estates. They work part-time on the plot around the hut, which they may have rented for as long as there is work to do on the estate, and when the plantation crop needs their help they work in the owner's field.

Wages are low: the overall minimum wage rate in Haiti is 70¢ a day for an 8-hour day but this does not necessarily apply to farmhands, who are paid on the basis of a personal agreement with the plantation owner or his foreman. The 48-hour work week schedule is not enforced. The Labor Code allows up to 60 hours with time and a half after 48 hours. Labor organizations exist on paper but are unstable. Many have come and disappeared.

The productivity of the labor force under these conditions is very low. One reason could be the fact that the Haitian carries out several activities at the same time, on his own account and as a member of a cooperative work system, such as a *coumbite*. The *coumbite* represents a tradition of mutual self-help which can be found almost everywhere in Africa. The occasion of a *coumbite* involves not only strenuous physical labor but also recreation and enjoyment. It may include only a few men helping to work a small field for a few hours or it can consist of a large party gathered to accomplish a specific task to the rhythm of a drumbeat and ending the day with a "feast" accompanied by rum drinking, singing and dancing. *Coumbites* may not be called on Sundays (for religious reasons) nor on Tuesdays, when each man is supposed to be free to work on his own fields. A *coumbite* is well-organized with a director and a number of team leaders. Loafers are identified and ridiculed; often they are penalized by being given a contemptuously small portion of food.

(2) The lack of stamina which is the result of undernutrition may also be responsible for the low level of productivity. This lack of stamina may explain to a large degree what Beghin et al. call the "plasticity" of the Haitian villager's attitude, offering no resistance to pressure from outside but refraining from throwing his weight behind reforms and programs intended to improve his lot.

(3) Lack of education and the high level of illiteracy are also responsible for the low productivity, since they prevent the training of semiskilled workers who could use and maintain mechanical equipment. (Other reasons also militate against the use of such machines in Haiti—see *Mechanical Equipment.*)

2. Farms ^{(40) (33) (1) (12) (44)}

Land holdings in Haiti are of three major types: the small family plot, the estate and the government domain. The first category is the most numerous, resulting in extreme fragmentation of the arable land. Sharecropping *(métayage)* is widespread, reflecting the population pressure on the land and the fragmentation of holdings. Families who have inherited miniscule plots must sharecrop additional land in order to survive, while some peasants are forced to let part of their holdings out to *métayage* because their inheritance is in the form of scattered parcels, all of which they cannot reach.

a. Small Family Plots

There are approximately 560,000 farms in Haiti, about one-half of which are actually owned by the families living on them, according to most estimates. Few of the landowners have title to their property and the inheritance customs complicate the problem. The average family farm covers only two-thirds of a hectare. About 40 percent of the farm families have holdings estimated at less than 1.29 hectares (1 *carreau* in local language), 70 percent have less than 2.58 hectares (2 *carreaux*), 94 percent have less than 6.45 hectares (5 *carreaux*) and only 6 percent have over 6.45 hectares. (Better-off farmers who live on their own property are known as *gros habitants.*) Sebrell, Smith et al. point out that in the fertile Artibonite Valley, which encompasses 33,000 hectares, a few families have "substantial" holdings of up to 400 hectares, while the rest of the 33,000 resident farm families share the remainder of the land among them. The fact that these very small holdings have to provide both dietary needs and pocket money implies considerable diversification on small acreages and, given the backward techniques used, very low effeciency for each crop.

b. Estates

There are probably 1,000 estates of 100 hectares or more belonging to absentee landlords who live in towns on the income their managers *(géreurs)* procure for them. Some of these large holdings belong to foreign companies and individuals who operate them for profit using hired manpower.

c. Government Domain

The public domain held by the Government is generally located in the less fertile areas of the country or in the mountains. Nevertheless, the Government finds tenants for some small plots and charges a rent that varies with the size of the holding and the productivity of the soil.

In the fertile valleys the houses are clustered together, reaching very high densities which threaten human survival. Some of the oldest settlements show a certain degree of structuralization: a central market place, better buildings around it, huts at the periphery. Others are just houses or huts put together haphazardly in places of difficult access, creating various problems for extension services and nutrition education efforts.

These different aspects of land use are not conducive to efficient development. In addition, agricultural practices are primitive and often influenced by the African cultural heritage, e.g., the multiple planting of compatible crops like corn, beans and root crops. There is no crop rotation. Diminishing returns of the same crop on the same field tell the farmer that it is time for a change: first a change of crop, then a change of field. Slash-and-burn techniques are used to clear the new land. This practice of shifting cultivation is less and less acceptable because on the one hand unused land is becoming scarce, while on the other the population is expanding. The Government opposes the system by law with little success so far.

3. Fertilizers [7] [24]

Fertilizers are used in very limited quantities because the people are not convinced of their advantage and because farmers do not have enough cash to buy them and the amount of credit for such purposes is limited. Teaching the Haitian farmer to fertilize his crop and enabling him to purchase fertilizers could increase food output in just one year's time. Thus far, however, small amounts of fertilizers are used only on estates. In 1969, 600 tons of nitrogenous fertilizers and 700 tons of phosphatic mixtures were used, a 33 percent increase over 1965. In the same year 1,500 tons of potassic fertilizers were spread, an amount almost twice as great as that used in 1965. Animal manure is available in small amounts only in the pastoral areas of the Plaine des Cayes, and around Port-au-Prince, Gonaives and the Cul-de-Sac Depression where cattle are found in substantial quantities.

4. Mechanical Equipment [33] [7] [14] [44]

The number of tractors in use is unknown. This means that practically all food cultivation is carried out with hoe and machete. Very few of the simplest tools for agriculture and even for gardening are available. A few spades or watering jugs are found on most Haitian farms. Plows, which were introduced long ago, are not part of the agricultural arsenal, probably because most of the terrain is unsuitable due to gradients and shallowness of the soil. Moreover, the cost of plows is relatively high and animal power is not available on the small hilly farms where they would be needed. Finally, the continued physical exertion required to use even a small wooden plow is too much for the underfed Haitian. The most widely used hand tools are the hoe, machete, billhook, dibble and knife.

C. PRODUCTION [12] [33]

It is almost impossible to have an accurate estimate of agricultural production in Haiti. Cash crops are also food crops since most farmers, even smallholders, plant a little sugarcane, tend some coffee bushes and cultivate a few banana trees to provide products for both home consumption and for sale at the nearest market. The data on production is thus approximate. Returns could be better than they are if a small amount of fertilizer were available to each small farmer and if pests could be efficiently controlled. Birds and rats play havoc with the crops and Sebrell, Smith et al. reported a probably loss of 5,000 tons of rice to rats in 1957 even though about half a million of the rodents were killed.

A typical timetable for planting and harvesting on Haitian farms would look something like this:

Planting and Harvesting Seasons – Haiti

Crop	Planting Season	Harvesting Season
Corn	March-April	July-August
Pigeon peas	March-April	July-August
Rice	May-August	September-December
Millet	July-September	January-March
Tubers	October-December	Next dry season
Bananas	April-September	March-July
Red beans (lowlands)	January-February	June-September
Red beans (mountains)	August-September	January-February
Sugarcane	May-July	May-July following year

Source: After M.J. Herskovits, *Life in a Haitian Valley.*

The Haitian has a strong feeling for the unconquerable forces of nature. Thus no crops are planted during the first quarter of the moon and crop reversals are thought to be due to the intervention of ghosts and spirits which are everywhere and which can be propitiated by specialists.

1. Food Crops [7] [33] [1] [27]

a. Cereals

As indicated in Table No. 2, the most important cereal is corn. The area sown has fluctuated in the last 20 years between 270,000 and 320,000 hectares. Most of the crop comes from the fertile Artibonite Valley (34 percent), followed by the departments of the West (31 Percent), the South (21 percent), the North (11 percent) and the Northwest (3 percent). These figures are admittedly approximate and various researchers have made their own slightly different estimates. Corn is so popular that it is sown practically everywhere. Hence, yields and production are both poor and uneven, oscillating between a recorded 200,000 and 240,000 a year. Yields are better in the Department of the West which results in the crop sometimes being more abundant there than in the more extensively sown Artibonite Valley.

Millet and sorghum, indiscriminately referred to as *petit mil,* together cover around 240,000 hectares, mostly in the Department of the West, followed by the departments of the Artibonite and the South. Sebrell, Smith et al. report on the special nutritional value attributed to the *mil chandelle* which is grown mostly in the Gonaives area. Beghin et al. state that millet is less commercialized than corn and is mostly consumed at home. Production varies from 150,000 to 190,000 tons a year, but yields are better the the Department of the Artibonite than in the Department of the West.

Rice, the preferred cereal but also the most expensive, is grown mostly in the Artibonite valley where nearly half of the whole paddy acreage is located. According to FAO, rice covered 25,000 hectares in 1968, but Sebrell, Smith et al. gave a 1958 figure of 63,000 hectares. Two factors can explain this discrepancy: first, the extensive small plots belonging to individual farmers may not have been included in the 1968 statistics; and second, some newly irrigated areas in the Artibonite Valley had not yet reached their full yield in 1968 while older areas were temporarily infertile, although undergoing improvement. The amount of rice produced is uncertain and estimates vary fourfold, depending upon the year and the reference consulted. The amount seems to be adequate to meet the domestic needs, however, since no rice appears to have been imported since 1963.

b. Roots and Tubers

As shown by Table No. 2, Haitians eat large amounts of tubers, and manioc most of all. Amounts recorded are certainly below the true levels. Moreover, only a small fraction of these roots is sold on the market. Manioc is sown on at least 25,000-30,000 hectares and the production is variously estimated at 80,000-120,000 tons. Forty-eight percent is grown in the Department of the South, 21 percent in the North, 14 percent in the West, 10 percent in the

Artibonite and 7 percent in the Northwest. Other well-liked tubers are *malanga* or cocoyam *(Xanthosoma terviride)* and taro *(Colocasia esculenta)*. Potatoes are also eaten in small quantities in the cities.

c. Legumes and Nuts

Legumes provide a substantial amount of protein and consist of beans, either the usual kidney bean *(Phaseolus vulgaris)* or the pigeon pea *(Cajanus indicus)* so common in the Caribbean area, or even the groundnut *(Arachis hypogea)*. Many other varieties exist which permit the farmer to harvest some beans at any time of the year. FAO gives an area sown of 25,000-27,000 hectares while Sebrell, Smith et al. in 1958 had reason to estimate the acreage at a higher figure. The crop is reported to vary narrowly from 17,000 to 19,000 tons a year, but in 1968 FAO reported a sudden drop to 10,000 tons, probably due to hurricane damage. The Department of the West produces an estimated 39 percent of the crop, the Artibonite 30 percent, the South 18 percent, the North 11 percent and the Northwest 2 percent. The groundnut is sown on approximately 12,000 hectares, most of it in the Department of the South, but also in substantial quantities in the West and in the Artibonite. The crop is small, reportedly about 2,000-2,500 tons a year but, of course, a substantial portion is not recorded. Among the nuts eaten are coconuts and cashews.

d. Vegetables and Fruits

Wild and cultivated vegetables or green leaves are eaten at most of the main meals. Sebrell, Smith et al. have recorded a number of green leaves, some of which are domestically commercialized. They mention watercress, wild spinach, the leaves of bean bushes, pumpkins and chayote *(Sechium edule)*. Others, such as tomatoes, onions, eggplants, carrots, beets, cucumbers and cabbages, are also found in many markets and are, in fact, domestic cash crops.

Fruits are consumed in great quantities. The plantain *(Musa paradisiaca)* is especially popular and, as in other Caribbean countries, is boiled or fried but not exported. Sebrell, Smith et al. gave a 1959 figure of 130,000 hectares planted, providing 45,000 tons of plantains, mostly in the departments of the South, West and the Artibonite, but also in smaller quantities in the other departments. Beghin et al. stress that the export banana *(Musa sapientum)* is no longer commercialized. FAO, however, reports a small 500-ton export in 1968. The most important wild fruit, both in quantity and quality (because of its carotene content), is the mango *(Mangifera indica)*. Sebrell, Smith et al. estimate the number of mangoes eaten by humans during the season at 2 billion. Given a 150-day season, this would mean approximately two mangoes a day per person or 1,260-1,890 micrograms of carotene per capita per day. Citrus fruit and pineapples are also cultivated in Haiti. FAO indicates a yearly crop of 6,000 tons of oranges and tangerines and 15,000 tons of other citrus fruits. No figures are given for pineapples. All this output is sold in local markets or consumed at home. Other fruits currently popular, mostly as snacks, are papayas, peaches, custard apples, avocadoes, sapodilla and breadfruit, all contributing minerals and vitamins in uncertain amounts.

Sugarcane *(Saccharum officinarum)*, which is both a food and a cash crop, is planted on 90,000 hectares according to FAO, a little less according to Sebrell, Smith et al. The production of cane averages about 4 million tons, occasionally reaching 4.6 million tons as it did between 1952 and 1957. Beghin et al. believe that this estimate is perhaps too high. Raw sugar amounts to about 60,000 tons, some of which (18 percent) is refined into white sugar. The rest of the crop becomes a brown type of sugar called *sucre populaire.* La Gra, writing in *Foreign Agriculture,* estimates the yearly average production of sugarcane at 2.5 million tons, of which less than 20 percent is grown on farms larger than 3 hectares, which reduces to 12,000 hectares the total acreage of sugarcane plantations in Haiti. Whatever the size of the cane crop, part of it is consumed at home as cane or as processed sugar, part of it is processed into an exportable product, more or less refined. Some molasses is produced (about 3.5 million gallons per year) but almost all of it is exported. The home portion of the cane crop is eaten in five different forms: raw cane which is munched by all children and grownups; various types of refined or semi-refined sugar; sugarcane juice or syrup; *rapadou* (sticks of crystallized sugarcane syrup made from unrefined dark brown sugar and reputed to be rich in iron); and *clairin* (light rum).

e. Fats

The production of vegetable and animal fats is based on cottonseed, palm oil, coconut oil and lard or pig fat. A few plants and a large number of presses produce the oil, which is sold in neighborhood markets. The lard is rendered in abbatoirs or after home slaughtering in unknown quantities. No production figures are available for fats, but Beghin et al. estimate the average daily consumption of all kinds at 37 grams per capita. Hence, based on a population of 5.2 million people, the total availability of fats per year must reach 64,532 tons. If the import of all kinds of edible fats reaches 12,000 tons (see *Trade*), the local production must then be about 52,000 tons. Beghin et al. report that 100 grams of Haitian palm oil brought on the local market contain 44,000 international units of vitamin A. If all the oil used were of that kind, there could be no vitamin A deficiency in Haiti (see *Nutritional Disease Patterns*).

2. Cash Crops [33] [1] [44] [30] [5] [7] [27]

The cash crops of Haiti are limited almost entirely to coffee, cocoa, sisal and sugar. In addition, some essential oils or small items of manufacture contribute to the GNP. As stated previously, this does not mean that the Haitian farmer does not make money with other crops. We have already indicated the importance of the domestic garden markets in large villages and towns, but the earnings from sales at such markets provide only small amounts of money for the purchase of daily food items not produced on the farm, clothing, oil, coal and household utensils. The cash crops are too limited to really support the development of the country.

Coffee is planted wherever soil, light and humidity permit. This has made coffee a pocket-money crop rather than a significant cash crop for most of the population. In 1958, Sebrell, Smith et al. estimated the area sown in coffee at 145,000 hectares, the largest part of which (46 percent) was in the Department of the South, 28 percent in the West, 15 percent in the North and the rest in the Northwest and the Artibonite. This last is a valley of food crops and is not used much for coffee, a major shift from the colonial period when coffee was grown almost exclusively on large plantations around Cap Haïtien. The coffee center is now in the southwestern peninsula. The shift is the outcome of the civil strife and insecurity which led to the opposition between north and south following independence (see *History and Government*) and resulted in more orderly and organized life in the peninsula than in the quarrelsome north.

Coffee production has become a daily gathering activity more than a plantation enterprise for many of the Haitian farmers. Following the destruction of the French estates around 1800, the trees ceased to be tended and the berries fell on the ground where rats gnawed at the shells and scattered the seed. The plants grew wild and spread on the mountain slopes. Even today these wild-growing thickets supply much of the peasants' coffee crop. The problems of erosion and deforestation threaten the future of coffee in Haiti. The coffee bush needs shade, but the indiscriminate cutting of trees for fuel and other purposes is steadily depriving the coffee plants of protection from the sun.

No recent figures on coffee acreage are available. FAO has not reported any since 1956 when an average of 147,000 hectares (close to the 1958 estimate of Sebrell, Smith et al.) was given for the period 1952-1956. Production figures are available, however, and according to FAO, the amount produced has steadily declined over the last 20 years. About 34,000 tons were harvested in the early 1950's and only about 28,000 tons were produced in 1968. The productivity of the plants is constantly diminishing because the peasant farmers take no real care of the wild-growing trees, seldom pruning or topping them to stimulate the growth of berry-bearing branches.

Sugar, which we have already discussed as a food crop, is also the second most important cash crop. About half the output is exported (see *Trade*). Plantation sugar is the consequence of the American occupation from 1915 to 1934, which resulted in the establishment of the Haïtian-American Sugar Company. This company owns 10,000-11,000 hectares of land in Haiti. The main areas of sugar production are the irrigated plains of Cul-de-Sac, the coastal region around Les

Cayes, the Plaine du Nord near Cap Haitien and the Plaine de Léogane near Port-au-Prince. The domestic sale of cane and *rapadou*, although in small quantities, also justifies the outlooks of de Young and Beghin et al., who stress the commercial facet of the subsistence economy. There are three types of sugarcane production, according to Moral: the largest plantations, whose output goes to a major refining plant; medium-sized plantations producing syrup, *rapadou* and *clairin* for the domestic market, using small open-air presses *(guildives)*; and very small plots of cane producing for family consumption.

Cocoa is grown on about 9,000 hectares. The year Sebrell, Smith et al. made their excellent survey (1958) most of the plantings were in the south and west. FAO has no figures on present-day sowings. Production, however, has increased considerably from 1,900 tons two decades ago to 3,500 tons in 1969, although the harvest fluctuates markedly from year to year. In 1968 it was reported that 500 tons were sold abroad, compared to only 110 tons in 1965.

Sisal is planted on variable acreages, oscillating between 30,000 and 50,000 hectares. Since 1959 it has been the country's only plantation crop, in the true sense of the word.

3. Animal Husbandry [7] [1] [33]

As is the case for all other food items, considerable uncertainties exist with regard to data concerning livestock and poultry in Haiti. FAO gives the numerical facts as best known from 1948 to 1968.

Livestock – Haiti, 1948-1968
(in 1,000 head)

Livestock	Annual Average 1948-1952	Annual Average 1951-1956	1964	1965	1966	1967	1968
Cattle	582	614	690	694	699	769	845
Pigs	1,137	1,137	1,301	1,334	1,367	1,504	1,654
Sheep	52	53	59	61	62	69	76
Goats	854	868	1,019	1,045	1,070	1,177	1,295
Chickens and other poultry	3,903	3,720	3,200	2,960	3,256	3,581	3,600

Source: Food and Agriculture Organization of the United Nations, *Production Yearbook 1969.*

A cattle increase of 45 percent in 20 years compares poorly with the Dominican Republic where the herd was augmented by 54 percent during the same period, or St. Lucia (100 percent) or Cuba (65 percent). It is true that other countries have fared worse, however. Thirty percent of the Haitian cattle graze in the south, in the Plaine des Cayes where 38 percent of the sheep, 28 percent of the goats and 28 percent of the poultry are also found. Pigs are found practically everywhere, but the greatest numbers are in the Artibonite Valley.

b. Meat, Milk and Eggs

The amount of meat available to the Haitian has been thoroughly studied and discussed by a number of competent investigators. Beghin et al. and Sebrell, Smith et al. estimate the amount of meat available each year at 27,000 and 32,000 tons, respectively. In 1960, an FAO expert placed it at 31,500 tons. Latest FAO reports estimate the total amount of meat provided by indigenous animals at a conservative 20,000 tons, of which 12,000 tons were beef, 2,000 tons mutton and 6,000 tons pork. The gain over the last 20 years is small, amounting to only 3,000 tons. These totals do not include poultry which Beghin et al., based on the report of an FAO expert, place at 22,000 tons a year. To these amounts a number of private slaughterings must be added, the weight of which cannot be accurately known. Some meat is imported but it is doubtful whether it is accessible to the inhabitants of the rural areas. More likely it remains in the cities. FAO statistics do not show any imports, probably because they are too small for the record. Neither do they show any exports which, however, do take place by air to other Caribbean islands. Beghin et al. estimate these exports at 1,600-2,000 tons a year and understandably deplore this exodus of valuable proteins.

There is no doubt that the number of animals slaughtered officially seems to be on the decrease. Between 1952 and 1956, FAO reported the average annual slaughter of 184,000 animals—69,000 cattle, 36,000 goats and 79,000 pigs. Beghin et al., quoting the Haitian Department of Agriculture, give a total of almost 152,000 animals slaughtered in 1962, about 148,000 in 1963 and around 92,000 in 1964. No doubt there is a slowdown in the slaughtering of cattle, and the availability of meat is probably lower than earlier surveys showed. On the basis of the figures presently at our disposal, the annual availability of meat should not exceed 4.5 kilograms per capita per year, a sizable drop from the 7 or 8.5 kilograms variously estimated by investigators researching this question some 10 or 12 years ago.

The information on the cow's or goat's milk available for home consumption or trade is, like the rest, difficult to interpret. FAO gives an estimate of 19,000 metric tons of cow's milk a year consumed in Haiti. This would give about 4 kilograms per capita per year, to which goat's milk and imported milk must be added, which probably would allow a total of at least 8 or 9 kilograms, an estimate consistent with the amount suggested by Beghin et al. The amount imported is figured in tons of condensed or dried milk and would amount to over 2,000 tons which, diluted in an equal amount of water, would provide another 4,000 tons of fluid milk or slightly over 1 liter per capita per year. The amount must also vary considerably with the season. On the basis of individual consumption verified in nutrition surveys, Beghin et al. conclude that a figure of 11 kilograms of milk per capita per year is reasonably near the truth. This would give an availability of about 30 grams of milk per capita per day, a believable figure. Yet, this gives no indication of the way the milk is distributed. The most likely guess is that most of it is sold in the cities, some of it distributed to hospitals, orphanages and mothercraft centers and that the population of the rural areas either does without or drinks the milk of its own animals when available. Some butter is produced in Haiti at the rate of 30-40 tons a year, but this is probably for the urban trade. Butter imports amounted to 49 tons in 1967. Figures are published by FAO irregularly: 71 tons were imported in 1965 and 53 tons in 1964.

Egg production is difficult to estimate. The 1969 FAO *Production Yearbook* gives a 1968 figure of 340 million units weighing 9,500 tons. If this estimate is correct, it reflects a static situation, since 344 million were already available yearly between 1948 and 1952. The weight of each egg must have increased, as the same report gives a bulk weight of 7,300 tons in 1948. Beghin et al. report that another FAO source estimated the 1960 egg production to be 82 million eggs weighing 3,718 tons or 45 grams per egg. This estimate would provide 20 eggs per capita per year, whereas the 340 million estimate would provide 68 eggs per capita per year. It is entirely possible that production has increased faster than population during the last 10 years, since a modern chicken farm was created with the help of FAO during the decade. However, the total seems high. An unknown percent of this production must be broken, hatched or lost and the actual number consumed must be far below the 68 per capita estimated above. Moreover, we know that the Haitian farmwoman will not eat her own eggs because they are part of the minicommercial economy which drains the products from the countryside to the cities.

4. Fisheries [1] [9]

There is no real fishing tradition in Haiti, despite the fact that the country enjoys a long coastline. Beghin et al. have estimated that the annual production of fish between 1960 and 1965 amounted to 4,500 tons, of which only 500 tons represented freshwater fish. In 1952, the Haitian Institute of Statistics (cited by Beghin et al.) reported that 8,293 tons of salted or smoked fish were imported, mostly from Canada. During the following 12 years these imports declined regularly, until in 1964 they amounted to only 2,616 tons. The per capita availability of domestic and imported fish would then have been 7,000 tons, or roughly 1.4 kilograms in 1964. Fougère et al. report that in 1968 the per capita fish intake actually rose to 5.7 kilograms. They did not indicate the source of the increase (domestic production or imports) but credited the population with having made a good choice in increasing the consumption of fish in a hurricane year when most other foods were in short supply. This seems to indicate that fish can be made available in larger quantities when needed. While the exact consumption of fish per capita per year in Haiti is a matter for controversy, it may be safely concluded from all statistical and other sources consulted that it is now probably between 2 and 4 kilograms per capita per year. The 5.7 kilos

(16.62 grams) per day quoted by Fougère in 1968 (see Table No. 6) was probably exceptional since people relied more heavily on fish than usual that year due to the shortage of other food supplies.

D. FOOD INDUSTRIES [1] [31]

The Haitian food industry, although in its infancy, still represents a sizable portion of total industrial production. The figure of 42 percent given in 1960 is probably still accurate. These enterprises process sugar, cereals, coffee, meat, oilseeds and other fats, fruits, vegetables, milk and other dairy products, cocoa, fish and beverages. The major activity is sugar refining, which is carried out primarily under the aegis of the American-owned Haïtian-American Sugar Company (HASCO). HASCO operates a 65,000-ton capacity plant at Port-au-Prince, the Centrale Dessalines owns a 30,000-ton capacity plant at Les Cayes and the Usine Larue operates at 1,000-ton capacity in Cap Haitien. There are about 600 small traditional sugar plants called *guildives* producing syrup, *rapadou* and *clairin*. Two-thirds of the *guildives* are located in the central plateau region. The name, and often the equipment used, dates back to the colonial period. Beghin et al. have given a good description of the *guildive*, which is comprised of an open-air cane mill and the equipment needed to cook the cane juice, ferment the syrup and distill the fermented syrup. The cane stalks are pressed between two steel cylinders moved either by oxen or horses or, more rarely, by a water wheel. The raw juice is then cooked in steel vats until it becomes a thick syrup while the discarded fiber *(bagasse)* is used as fuel. Some of the syrup is marketed as is, some is crystallized into *rapadou* and some is distilled into *clairin*. In addition to the *guildives*, there are more than 5,000 portable hand presses in use throughout the country. These are used to extract the sugar juice needed by the family for its daily requirements.

Coffee production is another major industry, employing an unknown number of women who sort the grains, and giving work to over 23 decortication plants. Cereals, such as wheat, rice and corn, play a major role in Haitian food industries. Wheat imported from Canada and the United States is processed at a mill owned by Caribbean Mills Incorporated, located at Port-au-Prince. The mill has a capacity of 52,000 tons of flour annually, most of which is re-exported to other islands and some of which is used locally. The mill is thoroughly mechanized, thus providing little employment. Strangely enough, Beghin et al. report that the flour for export is enriched with minerals and vitamins in conformity with United States practice, while the flour intended for domestic consumption is not. Bakeries produce various kinds of bread, especially a 28-gram roll which is very popular and finds its way through itinerant vendors into the remotest villages of the country. It is estimated that the consumption of this bread amounts to 14 grams per capita per day. Rice is processed in the mills of the IDVA Company *(Office de Développement de la Vallée de l'Artibonite)*. Other mills exist at Des Chapelles and Grande Rivière du Nord. Much rice is milled at home. Corn is also processed on a large scale by industrial mills as well as by hand machines for home consumption. However, the grain is of low prestige and is the food given to prisoners. Corn is also the base for a popular Haitian broth called *acassan.* *

Meat processing is an important component of the food industry. There is a large abattoir owned and operated by the Haitian-American Meat and Provision Company (HAMPCO) near Port-au-Prince. This factory is modern and owns adequate freezing/storage space. HAMPCO sells to other islands in the Caribbean. Meat for domestic consumption is provided by home slaughterings made in very unsanitary conditions. Beghin et al. remark that since the state collects a tax on each animal reported slaughtered, much clandestine slaughtering takes place which may mean that more meat is available than is officially believed to exist. Meat is preserved by various methods. The most famous is *boucanage* (smoking and drying), the term from which the name "buccaneer" was derived to designate the French pirates based on Haiti in the days of the Spanish Main (probably because they prepared their meat in this manner). Another method used is to marinate slices of meat in orange or lime juice, then dry them in the sun.

Beverages, especially rum, are manufactured in Haiti. Beghin et al. praise one brand of Haitian rum (Barbancourt) as the best in the world. It is prepared with great care according to ancient recipes, using oak casks which do not allow more than 120,000 gallons (5,000 hectoliters) to be produced a year, only 500 of which are exported. The manufacturing technique is elaborate as befits a regal product. Lesser beverages brewed from fermented cane juice include *tafia* and *clairin*, the latter containing 25-35 percent alcohol. *Clairin* is produced at the rate of about 7.4 liters per capita per year. There are two large ice-making plants which also prepare carbonated beverages.

Cottonseed oil is manufactured by the *Huilerie Nationale* at Port-au-Prince and another refinery at Mantèque which has branches at Gonaives and Petit Goâve. Other oils, such as coconut and palm, are produced on an artisanal basis. A few small plants preserve fruits and vegetables, especially tomato paste.

Fish is preserved by drying and salting but the salt, say Beghin et al., is too rich in magnesium, calcium and copper to permit its extensive use in fish processing. With the help of FAO, dairying has been developed in the last 10 years. Although the industry is still small, several plants have freezing and pasteurizing facilities. One of these plants is located at Les Cayes and utilizes the cream and butter of the regional livestock industry. Small quantities of cheese are also being manufactured.

Acassan is a corn broth, usually spiced, sweetened and sometimes diluted with milk. It is very similar to Mexican *atole* and is a very popular drink, consumed mostly as a snack and more often in the morning.

THE REPUBLIC OF HAITI

E. TRADE

1. Domestic Trade [12] [44]

As already stated, domestic trade is important in Haiti, both economically and psychologically. From the point of view of the internal economy, domestic trade provides the majority of the population with the indispensable pocket money needed to round out the diet and to buy the simple necessities of everyday life that cannot be conveniently manufactured. From the psychological standpoint, the smallest sale brings the seller a sense of achievement. Markets are held at regular intervals. Saturday is the main market day; lesser markets are held on other days. However, road stands and squatting women selling produce or cooked foods can be seen at all times in village streets or along country roads. In a given region, markets are staggered in such a way that almost every day some village holds one. Women pay a fee for the stalls they occupy and usually keep the same location for years. Prices are set according to what the traffic will bear, but it is a slight on a woman's reputation as a competent trader if she is not sold out at the end of the day, regardless of the price she obtains in the last hours.

In the African tradition, women will walk tens of kilometers to attend a village market where they know that the eggs or sticks of sugarcane or even the tomatoes and vegetables which have been grown at home will find a purchaser. Women will go alone or with a donkey or in groups, carrying their wares from one village to another, and the miniscule amount of cash they bring back home will permit the purchase of oil or bottled gas or a machete or even a dress from another market on another day. As in Africa, the market is also a club where women gather news and gossip. In addition to this petty trading, larger amounts of coffee, sugarcane or cocoa are sold to intermediaries who eventually resell them to others until the product reaches the exporter.

2. Foreign Trade [27] [40] [1] [38] [8]

Haitian foreign trade has been in general decline in recent years. In 1963 exports brought an income of over $26 million, but had dropped to $19.4 million by 1968. Because of drought and loss of productivity through erosion and hurricane damage, the country has not filled its international coffee or sugar quotas in recent years, mostly because low earnings have discouraged new plantings. Table No. 4 shows that sugar exports during the 1963-1968 period decreased from 35,900 tons in 1963 to 22,600 tons in 1964, rose to 33,600 tons in 1966 but fell back to 24,400 tons in 1968. Exports of coffee, the most profitable crop, fell from 26,000 tons in 1963 to 18,000 tons in 1967 and 1968. Sisal, whose future is doomed anyway, declined from 32,000 tons in 1951-1958 to 14,702 tons in 1968 and the area sown from 24,000 to 9,000 hectares. Bananas have ceased to be a moneymaking crop for several years now. Essential oils, for which a good market exists, represent a small but positive factor, as do bauxite and copper resources, which so far have not been extensively developed,

On the import side of the ledger, foodstuffs account for about 16 percent of all imports. Most striking is the size of the wheat, fats and milk or milk products purchased, which represent practically all the incoming food trade (see Table No. 3). While imports of milk and milk products have increased since 1963, cereal imports have fallen, possibly because of increased domestic production of rice and corn. About 31,100 tons of wheat were imported in 1968. Wheat is used mostly for making bread and is primarily for urban consumption, although the rural people who have contacts with the cities soon come to like it. It is, nevertheless, the least consumed cereal of all. Beghin et al., adopting the figures of the U.S. Department of Agriculture, estimate Haitian wheat use at 6 kilos per capita per year. If the figure given in the 1969 FAO *Trade Yearbook* is correct, this estimate is near the truth. However, given the urban/rural ratio, the consumption must be more like 500 or 600 grams a week for the urbanite and an occasional loaf or roll for the most progressive farmer.

The sustained need to import fats is a drain on the narrow economy of the country. The nearly 12,000 tons of imported fats of all kinds provided 6.4 grams of fat per capita per day in 1968, which is consistent with the findings of Beghin et al. Imported fats added to visible and invisible local fats provided by domestic foods and the oil processing industry yield an approximate national average of 37 grams per capita per day (see Table No. 2).

Total income from exports has varied little between $39 million in 1958 and $36 million in 1968. Total imports cost $43 million in 1958 but had dropped to $38 million in 1968, bringing the trade deficit down from $4 million to $2 million. Using the figures available, which admittedly are only partial but refer to some of the most vital items, the cost of these food imports was about $6.9 million in 1968. The contribution of trade to the diet is, therefore, very important, mostly because of fats and cereals. It is very doubtful whether the rural masses who comprise 85 percent of the population, derive any benefit from the milk imported except insofar as they patronize the mothercraft centers where some of the nonfat dry milk or evaporated milk is distributed.

F. FOOD SUPPLY

The food supply of Haiti is very small, as could be expected in a country where the population has managed to survive on a day-to-day, hand-to-mouth basis.

1. Storage [33] [1]

There is no need for food to be stored between harvest and market, except in small quantities. Grain is dried in the sun by spreading it over the hot earth and any surplus is kept in small ratproof granaries built of mud and covered with straw. Most often, these granaries are raised on pillars of concrete or earth. Some farmers improvise granaries, using jerrycans or oil drums elevated above the ground. Corn is collected in bundles and hung from the roof of the hut or from nearby trees. Wheat, which is imported rather than grown and therefore needs to be stored before being distributed, is adequately handled in modern silos at Port-au-Prince. The capacity of these is not reported but must be small given the limited amount (less than 50,000 tons) imported each year. Rodents, parasites and moles destroy a substantial portion of all crops. The Government is aware of this situation and through the Institute of Development is pursuing experiments aimed at designing storage space that would respond to the Haitian climate as well as to the requirements of the various crops.

2. Transportation [12] [43] [44]

Lack of adequate transportation is one of the great problems of Haiti. Until independence, the country had quite a number of roads and bridges but the war with the French and the following unrest and strife not only destroyed what existed but prevented rebuilding a network of roads that would provide remote producers with outlets for their salable agricultural products. Present roads are not numerous and are unasphalted except for some short stretches in and around the major cities. There are three main trunk roads: a northern one from Môle St. Nicolas to Cap Haitien and thence to the Dominican Republic; a central road from St. Marc to Mirebalais and Elias Pina in the Dominican Republic; and a third, southern road joining Dame Marie, Les Cayes, Mirâgoane and Port-au-Prince, continuing to St. Marc along the coast. In addition, there is a north-south road linking Cap Haïtien to Port-au-Prince. Several branches spread out from this network, making it possible to drive from the southernmost to the northernmost point in the country. The successive valleys have paths and mountain trails passable on foot or with mules and donkeys. This causes a segmented population pattern and a lack of exchange beyond one's region. There is a short coastal railroad north and west of Port-au-Prince belonging to the sugar and sisal companies. Domestic air transportation serves the major part of the country. No information exists on the use made of these air facilities for the transport of food. Most of the food commerce takes place by bus, donkey or on the heads of the lady merchants who do not hesitate to walk several days to carry a basket of their homegrown vegetables to the market at distances of 30-40 kilometers.

III. DIETS

A. GENERAL [1] [21]

Given the narrow production base described earlier, the diets of Haiti must be monotonous, poor in quality and inadequate in quantity. Beghin et al.* have

---

L'Alimentation et la Nutrition en Haïti.

made a masterful analysis of the role of food and nutrition in the 300-year-old Haitian culture. They stress its heterogeneous origin—Caribbean, African and French—and the rugged environmental background in which it has developed.

The Western man, accustomed to basking in his chromium-laden, mechanized environment and measuring its success in terms of gross national product and degrees of pollution, may be disappointed by the primitive culture of the Haitian. Yet, the Haitian has survived so far, although he has shown no more respect for his habitat than has Western man. He has hampered his survival not by spewing tons of carbon monoxide into his air or phosphates into his water, but rather by destroying his soil cover for fuel and in doing so, bringing about a frightful degree of erosion.

Basically, the Haïtian diet rests on the tripod of corn, sugar and manioc. There are, of course, substitutes and additions. Millet may supplement corn; wheat and rice are luxuries. Malanga, sweet potatoes and yams replace manioc. Legumes, especially the kidney bean and the pigeon pea, strengthen the poor basic menu with their kind of protein. Animal proteins are scarce and come in the form of dried, smoked fish and sometimes pork or beef. Fats come mainly from cotton-seed, coconut and palm oil, and lard is present at each meal because, like his West African cousin, the Haitian believes that fat equals health, although one does not meet in Port-au-Prince the obese women so frequently seen in the streets of Dakar and Accra. Meals are prepared outside the house over braziers where charcoal is used as fuel, a paradoxical fuel that is cheap because it burns for a long time but costly because it represents the destruction of forest resources and consequent erosion of the soil. Foods are usually boiled and served with a variety of spices, especially red peppers.

There are at least two and sometimes three meals in the day, the most substantial of which is taken in the evening in most areas of the country. On that occasion, the family is gathered together and the company sometimes includes relatives and friends. Breakfast is light: highly sweetened coffee, manioc bread, a fruit or a roll, and often a glass of rum. A snack lunch is taken in the field around 9:00 or 10:00 a.m. and is brought to the man by his wife. The snack is usually spartan, consisting of a piece of corn or a plantain porridge or smoked fish with manioc, washed down with *acassan*. Supper is served to the man of the household around 6:00 p.m., the wife and children having eaten earlier.* It is based on a diet of roots, malanga, manioc, sweet potatoes, plantains or roasted corn with greens and a main dish of rice and beans, if the family can afford rice. If not, a corn porridge may be served, and occasionally meat or dried or fresh fish is added, especially if the family lives near the coast or has access to a river.

---

*The Haitian family used to be quite large as a result of polygamy. The present form is known as *plaçage*, which gives status to a concubine. The extended family forms a clan *(lakou)*.

Obviously, there are many variations according to circumstances, such as season, occasion, social status, urban or rural location. As expected, the urban people and the *gros habitants* eat less manioc and corn, and more bread, rice, meat, eggs, milk and fresh fish,

Many studies have been made to try to estimate the quantities consumed of each major staple; enormous discrepancies exist among the data of investigators operating in different places and at different times. King, Dominique et al. documented significant differences in dietary intakes depending upon the location and the time of year. Rice was found to be the major cereal in Port Margot and corn the major one in Guérin. The cereal base of the diet amounted to only 33 kilograms per capita per year in Port Margot while it was 116 kilograms in Guérin. On the other hand, the diet seemed to be based on roots in Port Margot (91 kilograms per capita per year) and on cereals in Guérin. Beghin et al. suggest an average corn intake for the whole nation of 29 kilograms per capita per year. Sebrell, Smith et al. estimated 22 kilograms. In fact, only orders of magnitude can be given in this discussion and the time of year, as King, Dominique et al. demonstrate, must be taken into consideration.

Sugar consumption is higher in Port Margot and Ganthier than it is in Fond-Parisien and Guérin. Dried beans are more abundant at Ganthier and Fond-Parisien, less so at Guérin and Port Margot and the same observations can be repeated for other staples. While considerable variations can thus be elicited, the national average of food intake is low and the presumption exists of large areas of serious malnutrition. Beghin et al. have made a review, compilation and critique of all previous surveys and, adding considerations of their own, have come up with the estimates of food intake shown in Table No. 2. They calculate an average caloric consumption for the country as a whole of 1,700 calories per capita per day. This average tells much about the lowest levels. The protein intake averages 41 grams and the fat 37 grams. These figures are probably as near the truth as can be reached. Carbohydrates, especially sugar, account for 77 percent of all calories (300 calories from raw sugar can be considered empty of nutrients), fats for 15 percent and proteins for 8 percent.

B. INFANT DIETS [1]

In rural areas, practically all mothers breast feed their babies for at least 6 months. This is not the case in cities, where more sophistication causes more bottle feeding and hence more diarrheas. According to Beghin et al., a number of taboos for the mother and the child are still observed. White beans, tomatoes and fish are generally taboo for nursing mothers and in certain places lard, eggplants, pork and fruit are also forbidden. Infants are not allowed any kind of beans, meat or eggs and, as in most developing countries, they are weaned on a light porridge of cornmeal and sweet water, and later receive a bread soup which may contain some fresh or reconstituted milk.

C. VERY POOR DIETS [1] [9] [4] [21] [3]

A remarkable effort was started in 1964 by the bureau of Nutrition of the Haitian Department of Health to restore to health the much-ailing preschool children of Haiti. Nutrition rehabilitation centers, later to be called mothercraft centers, were planned as early as 1955. They came into being in 1965 and consist of simple Haitian-type houses where a responsible monitor, specially trained, using complete Haitian methods and foods, educates mothers in the preparation of a proper diet for their children. These monitors have 9 years of regular schooling and 2 years of special training at the Institute of Social and Family Education. They assist women at the center for a duration of 4 months, after which the mothers are on their own but are followed up by the monitor and are urged to convince other mothers from their own villages of the benefits of the center's approaches.

The studies made in connection with this rehabilitation effort give us an idea of what a diet can be in a very poor environment, as in the village of Fond-Parisien. The irrigation system in this village was totally destroyed by hurricane Hazel in 1954 and the fertile areas were covered with silt brought down from higher regions by the torrential rains. Only basic crops—millet, roots, beans, a few vegetables and a little rice—were grown after the hurricane. Caloric intake under those circumstances did not exceed 1,269 calories per person per day in 1964. Proteins were limited to 32 grams, of which only 3.36 grams were of animal origin. Tables 5 and 6 illustrate the type of diet and the levels of nutrition which resulted. These are among the poorest diets imaginable that are compatible with survival. Except for the consumption of iron and ascorbic acid, none of the nutrients approaches the minimum level required. While some improvement was observable in the years 1965 and 1966, possibly due to the opening of a mothercraft center in 1964, a severe drought slapped ascending curves down again in 1968.

D. LEVELS OF NUTRITION [1] [21] [28]

The levels of nutrition are low in almost all areas considered. In their book *L'Alimentation et la Nutrition en Haiti*, Beghin et al. have summarized surveys conducted prior to 1965. In 1964-1965 King, Dominique et al. conducted additional surveys which are especially useful because they are the only ones providing information collected by the same investigators at two different times of the year. They stress the widespread caloric deficit (which in 1964 reached a low of 1,360 calories at Fond-Parisien and 1,500-1,600 calories in many other places), as well as the important seasonal variations. Protein nutrition is not as bad as one could expect and not as seasonally dominated as that of other nutrients. The role of dry beans in providing proteins is certainly important. As is the case almost everywhere in the developing world, riboflavin deficiency dominates the picture of vitamin shortages. Calcium intake is always low. However, the minimum desirable requirement of this mineral varies with age, time of day and activity and, in fact, is not clearly known. Iron seems to be adequately provided for by most diets but anemias are common, leading to a number of hypotheses as to how to explain the nature of those anemias. Intestinal parasitism depletes the organism of its hemoglobin faster than iron replacements can be ingested. Some anemias observed may have causes other than nutrition, the most important of which could be that part of the iron ingested is not absorbed. Adequacy in vitamin A almost all year round (see *Nutritional Disease Patterns*) may be explained by the high level of consumption of mangoes and by the usage of palm oil in many, although not all, areas.

IV. ADEQUACY OF FOOD RESOURCES [7] [1] [23]

The food resources of Haiti, given the present state of affairs, are obviously inadequate and the previous section shows to what extent, in terms of calories and nutrients. Haiti has to purchase at least $7 million worth of food every year, amounting to about one-fifth of its total import bill. Most of the food bought abroad is wheat, wheat flour, milk, milk products and fats. One may wonder whether wheat is really necessary in a country which grows rice and whether domestic production of milk and fats could be expanded.

Estimating the inadequacies of the food resources of Haiti is difficult because of the uncertainties as to the source of information. Hence, the following computation is only approximate, using official FAO figures.

Approximate Production of Basic Crops — Haiti, 1948 and 1968

| | 1948-1952 | | 1968 | | | |
| | Area | Production | Area | Production | Change in % | |
Crop	(1,000 ha)	(1,000 tons)	(1,000 ha)	(1,000 tons)	Area	Production
Corn	270	203	320	240	+18.5	+18.2
Millet	242	171	230	150	−4.9	−12.2
Rice	28	28	25	20	−10.7	−28.5
Manioc	30	104	25	80	−16.6	−23.0
Sweet potatoes and yams	20	100	22	110	+10.0	+10.0
Dry beans	26	17	25	10	−3.8	−31.0
Bananas	20	247	18	220	−10.0	−10.9

Source: Food and Agriculture Organization of the United Nations, *Production Yearbook 1969.*

The preceding table, if near the truth, is alarming. While the population has grown by an estimated 2.4 percent a year, the production of corn has increased by only 0.9 percent a year, the production of sweet potatoes and yams by 0.5 percent a year and the production of all other basic foods has decreased in actual quantities. Moreover, according to a calculation by the U.S. Agency for International Development, the per capita production index in 1968 was evaluated at 64 from a base of 91 in 1958. Production is going down and, given the importance of food in aggregate total output, the spiral is to be taken seriously.

The Government of Haiti has taken it seriously. It has created a Bureau of Nutrition which is charged with six basic functions (see page 151). Given its limited resources, the Bureau has done well in creating two programs which have been successful: the mothercraft centers and the weaning food based on local cereals and beans (AK-1000). It may be appropriate to mention that the problem of coordinating governmental efforts to ensure adequacy of food resources and to combat malnutrition has been a concern of all organizations and authorities interested in international health in the past decade. The last three conferences on nutrition and child feeding in Africa held between 1967 and 1970 under the auspices of the U.S. Agency for International Development, stressed that in establishing an institute or bureau of nutrition, it is essential that it be given an adequate budget for carrying out operational programs and that it be placed high enough on the administrative ladder to have its recommendations heeded. It is not clear at this time if the Bureau of Nutrition in Haiti meets these two criteria.

V. NUTRITIONAL DISEASE PATTERNS [3] [4] [33] [22] [26] [18] [19] [10] [2] [1]

Infant mortality is very high and stands at 146.5 deaths per 1,000 live births. Malnutrition is deemed by many authors to be one of the first three causes of admissions and deaths of infants in the hospitals. Only infants with diarrhea and tetanus (through the umbilical cord) are as numerous.

There is considerable evidence that the nutritional health of Haiti is not satisfactory. Prior to the establishment of the mothercraft centers at Fond-Parisien, a thorough clinical investigation of the population was undertaken which revealed the seriousness of the problem. Three hundred sixty-six children were examined* who represented 11 percent of the total population of the village and almost all the child population from 4 months up to 6 years. These included 166 boys and 200 girls. The height of these children was found to average 10 percent lower than American standards for children of the same age. Weights were 20 percent lower than the American standards. It was also found that the gap between norms and findings increased with age. While 75 percent of the children

---

*See Beghin, Fougère and King, "Enquête Clinique sur l'Etat de Nutrition des Enfants Préscolaires de Fond-Parisien et de Ganthier (Haïti): Juin 1964."

aged 9-5 months were within normal range for weight, only 50 percent of the children from 6-11 months, 16 percent of those 12-17 months old and 7 percent of all 5-year-olds were normal, giving an average of 20 percent for the whole group. According to the well-accepted Gomez classification (see page 151), 46 percent of the children suffered from first degree malnutrition, 23 percent from second degree and 11 percent from third degree malnutrition. As to be expected, the 1-4 year group was the most seriously affected.

In Ganthier, another village, findings were comparable to those at Fond-Parisien, except that the general level of food consumption was slightly higher: caloric intake averaged 1,547 instead of 1,359 and protein intake 36 grams instead of 32 grams. In this village, only 2 percent of the children 1-4 years of age showed third degree malnutrition instead 12 percent and 23 percent were in the normal range instead of only 16 percent at Fond-Parisien.

Jelliffe and Jelliffe, using Jamaican rather than United States anthropometric standards, reported in 1960 that 7 percent of the 1-3-year-old children in Haiti suffer from protein-calorie malnutrition. Clinical examination of children is no less revealing. Girls seem to present symptoms of malnutrition twice as frequently as boys. Hair fragility and depigmentation, a sign of protein-calorie malnutrition and incipient kwashiorkor, was found in 6.8 percent of the boys and 15 percent of the girls. The children examined showed angular cheilosis, active or in the form of scars, indicating faulty riboflavin nutrition. This finding was in agreement with those of other investigators. In 1958, Sebrell, Smith et al. examined a total of 3,113 children and adults in 12 different villages and observed active cheilosis in 0-47 percent of the cases seen and scar cheilosis in 3-55 percent, nasolabial seborrhea in 0-34 percent and glossitis in 1-55 percent, depending upon the location. In all, 51.5 percent of all people seen presented evidence of existing or past riboflavin deficiency. Fougère, King and Bernadotte found high frequencies in the south of Haiti in 1959. In one locality, Civadier, 78 percent of the boys aged 7-10 years showed the same symptoms while the investigators found 25.7 percent in the northwest peninsula.

Jelliffe and Jelliffe report a frequent association of ariboflavinosis symptoms and kwashiorkor. Other investigators also confirm the ubiquitous presence of riboflavin deficiency at different rates of prevalence which, understandably, seem to change with the season. Age seems a factor, if not per se then because of diet and other circumstances correlated with age. The 6-15-year-olds seem to suffer most, at least in the northwest and along the south coast, where rates above 40 percent are found. Sebrell, Smith et al. discovered ariboflavinosis to be more common in the rural than in the urban areas. Since mangoes and avocados are the best source of riboflavin in Haiti, it is not surprising to observe most cases of ariboflavinosis during the off-season of these fruits. Other foods are rich in riboflavin but, unfortunately, they are either too expensive (e.g., meat) or too scarce (e.g., milk).

As we have seen, vitamin A is abundant in the foods of Haiti, especially in mangoes, avocados and palm oil. While at least one investigator* believes that vitamin A deficiency could be the cause of some cases of blindness among Haitian children, other researchers have failed to find significant symptoms of avitaminosis A. Again, the time of year at which surveys are made is important. In 1958 Sebrell, Smith et al. found the daily intake of vitamin A to reach over 13,000 IU per day while Dominique at Fond-Parisien measured a low of 342 IU and Beghin et al. in 1952 a low of 1,092 IU. These variations in findings may be due to seasonal differences. King et al. observed temporary shortages in November, January and March. Given the fact that vitamin A is stored in the liver when consumed in large amounts, reserves are built up during the fruit season on which the individual draws during the lean months. The dispensation of vitamin A in the blood and tissues is controlled by at least two factors: 1) the balance sheet of outgo against reserves; and 2) the genetic factors which control the rhythm and speed at which the reserves are delivered to the tissues in usable form, a process about which very little is known.

The question is: are there many signs of vitamin A deficiency among the Haitian people? Sebrell, Smith et al. noted Bitot spots in 0.3-13.9 percent and follicular hyperkeratosis in 10-31.6 percent of the subject examined, but the latter sign is at least controversial. Moreover, the same investigators found low levels of vitamin A in the serum, but high levels of serum carotene, suggesting a possible problem at the point were carotene is converted into vitamin A. Most other investigators concede that findings of minor symptoms of vitamin A deficiency are uncommon in Haiti. As for major symptoms, Beghin et al. support Escapini and estimate at 12 percent the number of very malnourished children who will eventually suffer the severe form of vitamin A deficiency. The absolute number of such children may not be very high, but the consequence (blindness) is so cruel and the prevention so simple that the problem should be in the forefront of the preoccupations of health personnel in Haiti.

Sebrell, Smith et al. found anemia to be relatively common among various samples of population: 12.6 percent of 356 people had less than 12 grams of hemoglobin per 100 milliliters of serum and 7 percent had less than 11 milliliters. Pregnant women, as usual, showed higher percentages of hemoglobin shortage, reaching 33 percent. These findings were confirmed by Jelliffe and Jelliffe, especially among children between 1 and 3 years. As usual, the respective roles of malaria and intestinal parasitism in the causation of anemia are difficult to ascertain, but there is a likelihood that, as elsewhere, marginal consumption of iron (which in this case was below 11 milligrams per capita per day in most of the places investigated), combined with defective absorption,

*Escapini, a World Health Organization expert whose 1963 study is reported in Beghin et al., *L'Alimentation et la Nutrition en Haïti.*

may be responsible for at least a large proportion of the prevalent anemia. Klipstein has also indicated a possible role for folic acid deficiency in some of the Haitian anemias.

Sebrell, Smith et al. reported a high level of prevalence of thyroid enlargement, mostly in females. Rates vary from 17.5 percent to 39 percent among the females and between 1.4 and 16 percent among the males, depending upon the group considered. A program of salt iodization would certainly be in order, but Haitian salt would have to be submitted to a serious overhaul to eliminate impurities in order to support such a campaign to eradicate goiter.

In spite of a low consumption of niacin, pellagra is very uncommon. Ascorbic acid needs seem to be adequately covered, and no true scurvy has been reported in recent years. Rickets is uncommon, although Jelliffe and Jelliffe and Beghin et al. have spotted a few cases among young children.

VI. CONCLUSIONS

It is not easy to draw any optimistic conclusions after viewing the situation in Haiti. The land is poor, eroded and overpopulated for its carrying capacity. As a consequence, the country is the home of too many malnourished children and adults. The usual consequences of malnutrition are, therefore, present/high rates of mortality among infants and children and low productivity among the adults. The uncertain climate is probably responsible in large part for this situation. Haiti is in the path of cyclones and hurricanes which flood the crops, carry away the topsoil, destroy the fruit and kill the livestock. The frequency of these catastrophic events, which occur to some extent almost every 2 or 3 years, is depressing. The people carry on an ever-recurring struggle to restore soil fertility, repair crop damage and rebuild houses. Severe droughts occur periodically everywhere, but especially in the northwest. These droughts eventually kill the trees, suppress the shade and ruin the prospects for coffee plants. Droughts also dwarf the food crops and, if repeated for several consecutive years, may create a vacuum difficult to fill. Finally, a combination of hurricanes and droughts, if occurring consecutively, can at any time assume the proportions of a terrible disaster.

Obviously, the country is not equipped to fight these circumstances on its own. One is hard put to suggest a practical solution to these ills. The population should be brought down to a level which the soil and the financial resources of the country can carry, but what is such a level? It is difficult to say, because it would depend very much upon the people themselves. What standard of living are they willing to accept to live in Haiti? What would be the consumption level that would be at the same time worth living for, attainable through the restoration and development of local resources, and purchasable with the income of the land aided by a modest indebtedness? The questions are unanswerable. The task is enormous and the difficulties awe-inspiring because most of them are part of the makeup of man.

BIBLIOGRAPHY

1. Beghin, I.D., Fougère, W. and King, K.W. *L'Alimentation et la Nutrition en Haiti.* Paris, Presses Universitaires de France, 1970.

2. _____, Fougère, W. and King, K.W. "L'Ariboflavinose en Haiti." *Archivos Latinoamericanos de Nutrición,* 1967, XVII (2), 95-107.

3. _____, Fougère, W. and King, K.W. "Enquête Clinique sur l'Etat de Nutrition des Enfants Préscolaires de Fond-Parisien et de Ganthier (Haite): Juin 1964." *Annales de la Société Belge de Médicine Tropicale,* 1965, 45 (5), 577-602.

4. _____, King, K.W., Fougère, W., Foucauld, J. and Dominique, G. "Le Centre de Récupération pour Enfants Malnourris de Fond-Parisien (Haiti). Rapport Préliminaire sur le Fonctionnement de Centre et Resultats de Quatre Premier Mois d'Activités." *Annales de la Société Belge de Médecine Tropicale,* 1965, 45 (5), 557-576.

5. de Young, M. *Man and Land in the Haitian Economy.* Latin American Monograph No. 3. University of Florida Press, Gainesville, 1958.

6. *Encyclopedia Britannica.* Chicago, William Benton Publisher, 1970.

7. Food and Agriculture Organization of the United Nations. *Production Yearbook 1969.* Volume 23. Rome, FAO, 1970.

8. _____. *Trade Yearbook 1969.* Volume 23. Rome, FAO, 1970.

9. Fougère, W., Dominique, G. and Gonzales, L. *Report from Haiti on Mothercraft Centers.* Bogota, Working Conference on Nutrition Rehabilitation Centers, Undated.

10. _____, King, K.W. and Bernadotte, J. Unpublished data, 1959. Cited in (3) above, p. 588.

11. Gildea, R.Y., Jr. "Haiti." *Focus,* 1967, XVII (9).

12. Herskovits, M.J. *Life in a Haitian Valley.* Garden City, Doubleday and Company, Inc., 1971.

13. Inter-American Development Bank. *Eleventh Annual Report.* Washington, D.C., IDB, 1970.

14. _____. *Socio-Economic Progress in Latin America.* Social Progress Trust Fund Tenth Annual Report. Washington, D.C., IDB, 1970.

15. International Bank for Reconstruction and Development. *Statement of Loans.* Washington, D.C., IBRD, 1971.

16. International Development Association. *Statement of Development Credits.* Washington, D.C., IDA, 1971.

17. James, P.E. *Latin America.* Fourth Edition. New York, The Odyssey Press, 1969.

18. Jelliffe, D.B. and Jelliffe, E.F.P. "The Nutritional Status of Haitian Children." *Acta Tropica,* 1961. 18, 1-45.

19. _____. "Prevalence of Protein-Calorie Malnutrition in Haitian Preschool Children." *American Journal of Public Health,* 1960, L (9), 1355-1366.

20. King, K.W. "Development of All-plant Food Mixture Using Crops Indigenous to Haiti: Amino Acid Composition and Protein Quality." *Economic Botany,* 1964, 18 (6).

21. _____, Dominique, G., Uriodain, G., Fougère, W. and Beghin, I.D. "Food Patterns from Dietary Surveys in Rural Haiti." *Journal of the American Dietetic Association,* 1968, 53 (2), 114-118.

22. _____, Foucauld, J., Fougère, W. and Severinghaus, E.L. "Height and Weight of Haitian Children." *American Journal of Clinical Nutrition,* 1963, 13 (2), 106-109.

23. _____, Fougère, W. and Beghin, I.D. "Un Mélange de Protéines Végétales (AK-1000) pour les Enfants Haitiens." *Annales de la Société Belge de Médecine Tropicale,* 1966, 46 (6), 741-754.

24. _____ and Price, N.O. "Nutritional Value of Haitian Forages." *Archivos Latinoamericanos de Nutrición,* 1966, XVI (2), 221-226.

25. _____ and Price, N.O. "Mineral Composition of Cereals and Legumes Indigenous to Haiti." *Archivos Latinoamericanos de Nutrición,* 1966, XVI (2), 213-219.

26. Klipstein, F.A. "Folate Deficiency Secondary to Disease of the Intestinal Tract." *Bulletin of the New York Academy of Medicine,* 1966, 42 (8), 653-683.

27. LaGra, J. "Haitian Sisal Plantations on the Wane." *Foreign Agriculture,* 1971, IX (2), 10.

28. Leung, W-T. Wu. *INCAP-ICNND Food Composition Tables for Use in Latin America.* Washington, D.C., U.S. Government Printing Office, 1961.

29. *Monthly Bulletin of Agricultural Economics and Statistics* (FAO), 1971, 20 (2).

30. Moral, P. *Le Paysan Haitien.* Paris, Maisonneuse et Larose, 1961.

31. Olcott, H.S. and Nicolas, G. "Food Technology in Haiti." *Food Technology,* 1969, XIII (9), 10-18.

32. Sebrell, W.H. and King, K.W. "The Role of Community Mothercraft Centers in Combating Malnutrition." *Malnutrition is a Problem of Ecology.* Bibliotheca Nutritio Dieta No. 14. Basel, S. Karger, 1970.

33. _____, Smith, S.C. et al. "Appraisal of Nutrition in Haiti." *The American Journal of Clinical Nutrition,* 1959, 7 (5), 1-48.

34. *Time Magazine,* October 11, 1971, p. 54.

35. United Nations (Department of Economic and Social Affairs). *Demographic Yearbook 1969.* New York, UN, 1970.

36. United Nations Children's Fund. *Digest of Projects Aided by UNICEF in the Americas.* New York, UNICEF, 1969.

37. United Nations Development Program. *Projects in the Special Fund Component as of 30 June 1971.* DP/SF/Reports, Series B, No. 12. New York, UNDP, 1971.

38. U.S. Agency for International Development. *A.I.D. Economic Data Book-Latin America.* Washington, D.C., AID, 1970.

39. U.S. Department of Agriculture (Economic Research Service). *Agricultural Policies in the Western Hemisphere.* FAER No. 36. Washington, D.C., U.S. Government Printing Office, 1967.

40. _____ . *Agriculture and Trade of the Caribbean Region.* ERS-Foreign 309. Washington, D.C., U.S. Government Printing Office, 1971.

41. _____ . *Food Balances for 24 Countries of the Western Hemisphere 1959-1961.* ERS-Foreign 86, Washington, D.C., U.S. Government Printing Office, 1964.

42. U.S. Department of Labor (Bureau of Labor Statistics). *Labor Conditions in Haiti.* Labor Digest No. 49. Washington, D.C., USDL, 1964.

43. U.S. Department of State. "Republic of Haiti." *Background Notes.* Washington, D.C., U.S. Government Printing Office, 1968.

44. West, R.C. and Augelli, J.P. *Middle America: Its Lands and Peoples.* Englewood Cliffs, Prentice Hall, 1966.

LIST OF TABLES

LIST OF MAPS

TABLE NO. 1

Annual Average Temperature – Haiti
(in degrees centigrade)

Station	Altitude (meters)	Annual Average
Port-au-Prince	40	27.3
Cap Haitien	10	26.1
Les Cayes	5	28.2
Gonaives	5	28.2
Port-de-Paix	10	25.9
Jérémie	30	26.1
Jacmel	20	25.4
Mirebalais	120	25.6
Kenscoff	1,350	17.1
Pétionville	400	25.9
Fond-Parisien	50	25.8

Source: I. Beghin, W. Fougère and K.W. King, *L'Alimentation et la Nutrition en Háiti.*

TABLE NO. 2

Yearly and Daily Intakes and Nutritive Values of Foods – Haiti, 1970

Food	Annual Intake (kg)	Daily Calories	Daily Proteins (g)	Daily Fats (g)
Cereals and products	63.0	617	16.9	5.6
Wheat	6.0	60	1.9	0.2
Corn	29.0	289	7.6	3.4
Rice	9.0	89	2.0	0.3
Millet	19.0	179	5.4	1.7
Roots and tubers	69.4	191	1.5	0.4
Potatoes	0.2	1	0.0	0.0
Sweet potatoes	21.9	54	0.6	0.2
Manioc	39.0	116	0.6	0.2
Yams	5.0	11	0.2	0.1
Others	3.3	9	0.1	0.1
Sugars	66.8	300	0.0	0.0
Sugar	11.7	124	0.0	0.0
Rapadou	14.6	133	0.0	0.0
Sugarcane	40.5	43	0.0	0.0
Legumes, nuts	25.6	116	11.3	3.6
Beans	19.0	79	10.6	0.2
Groundnuts	0.6	6	0.3	0.5
Coconuts	6.0	31	0.4	2.9
Vegetables	43.0	35	1.3	0.0

TABLE NO. 2 (continued)

Yearly and Daily Intakes and Nutritive Values of Foods – Haiti, 1970

Food	Annual Intake (kg)	Daily Calories	Daily Proteins (g)	Daily Fats (g)
Fruits	145.5	184	1.9	2.9
Bananas	9.0	16	0.2	0.0
Plantains	36.5	75	0.6	0.2
Mangoes	60	48	0.4	0.2
Avocados	15	28	0.4	2.5
Citrus	15	10	0.2	0.0
Others	10	7	0.1	0.0
Meats	8.0	50	3.7	3.8
Beef	2.7	18	1.4	1.3
Pork	4.6	27	2.0	2.1
Chicken	0.7	5	0.3	0.4
Eggs	0.9	3	0.3	0.2
Fish	1.8	9	1.9	0.3
Fresh	1.1	3	0.5	0.1
Dry	0.7	6	1.4	0.2
Milk and products	11.2	20	1.2	1.0
Milk	11.0	18	1.1	0.9
Cheese	0.2	2	0.1	0.1
Fats	6.6	155	0.0	17.7
Cottonseed oil	5.1	125	0.0	14.0
Others	1.5	30	0.0	3.7
Miscellaneous	10.6	20	1.0	1.5
Clairin	7.5	–	–	–
Rum	0.1	–	–	–
Cocoa	0.5	5	0.1	0.5
Coffee	2.5	15	0.9	1.0
Total	452.4	1,700	41.0	37.0

Source: I. Beghin, W. Fougère and K.W. King, *L'Alimentation et la Nutrition en Haiti.*

TABLE NO. 3

Major Food Imports – Haiti, 1963-1968

	Quantity in Tons						Value in $1,000					
	1963	1964	1965	1966	1967	1968	1963	1964	1965	1966	1967	1968
Milk	1,170	2,110	2,990	1,750	2,190	2,820	872	447	1,060	693	958	1,225
Butter	8	53	71	–	49	–	6	46	84	–	48	–
Cheese	80	33	115	14	151	–	70	29	119	18	136	–
Wheat and flour	48,500	47,300	61,700	32,300	36,100	31,100	3,550	3,290	3,960	2,200	2,880	2,560
Rice	2,000	n.a.	1,000	–	–	–	320	10	30	n.a.	–	–
Onions	45	88	–	–	–	–	4	8	–	–	–	–
All animal fat*	7,208	8,698	7,168	7,657	5,202	5,877	1,408	1,878	2,043	1,849	1,444	1,470
All vegetable fats	5,178	4,566	5,900	6,357	5,466	5,938	1,376	1,201	1,659	1,886	1,990	1,645

*Pig, poultry, all other kinds.

Source: Food and Agriculture Organization of the United Nations, *Trade Yearbook 1969.*

TABLE NO. 4

Major Agricultural Exports – Haiti, 1963-1968

	Quantity in Tons						Value in $1,000					
	1963	1964	1965	1966	1967	1968	1963	1964	1965	1966	1967	1968
Bananas	3,990	110	400	500	390	500	241	9	33	50	22	40
Sugar**	35,900	22,600	23,100	33,600	30,700	24,400	4,760	2,500	2,420	3,100	3,770	3,070
Coffee	26,390	22,780	22,650	24,350	18,660	18,940	16,790	19,400	19,320	20,720	14,260	14,610
Cocoa	1,150	460	110	40	360	500	544	270	45	167	105	150
Sisal	18,613	17,453	13,754	17,700	12,080	14,702	3,820	3,840	2,759	2,784	1,448	1,615

**Raw and refined in raw equivalent

Source: Food and Agriculture Organization of the United Nations, *Trade Yearbook 1969.*

TABLE NO. 5

Nutrient Intakes in a Poor Village – Haiti, 1964-1968

(per capita per day)

Calories and Nutrients	Unit	1964	1965	1966	1968
Calories		1,269	1,608	1,633	1,350
Total proteins	g	30	43.1	47.3	39.1
Animal proteins	g	3.36	6.05	6.78	7.18
Carbohydrates	g	207.7	286.1	291.3	230.2
Fat	g	42.6	36.2	37.9	33.6
Calcium	mg	148	239	221	212
Iron	mg	10.8	16.1	16.3	13
Vitamin A	IU	1,111	1,154	724	1,766
Niacin	mg	6.96	11.57	10.82	8.52
Thiamine	mg	0.94	1.32	1.38	1.06
Riboflavin	mg	0.42	0.67	0.62	0.52
Ascorbic acid	mg	32.5	38.2	48	40.8

Source: After W. Fougère, G. Dominique and L.D. Gonzales, *Report from Haiti on Mothercraft Centers.*

TABLE NO. 6

Food Consumption According to Dietary Surveys in a Poor Village – Haiti, 1964-1968
(grams per person per day)

Foods	1964	1965	1966	1968
Meats	13.89	13.0	11.05	11.50
Eggs	–	–	–	.04
Fish	2.81	8.38	12.68	15.62
Milk	23.26	58.31	36.43	44.28
Fats and oils	29.46	21.68	24.35	22.79
Native beans	47.31	59.03	73.02	59.67
Green beans	3.06	11.56	4.48	9.01
Rice and rice products	45.82	41.55	48.87	39.78
Corn and corn products	77.74	82.26	102.81	135.68
Millet and millet products	55.88	109.37	92.89	15.40
Sweet potatoes (yellow)	8.83	–	–	.39
Sweet potatoes (white)	35.58	44.90	97.24	11.24
Plantains	20.85	5.86	15.57	4.35
Avocados	17.50	8.75	7.84	3.00
Mangoes	4.12	16.52	5.82	49.37
Sugar	14.52	21.02	19.10	24.41

Source: After W. Fougère, G. Dominique and L.D. Gonzales, *Report from Haiti on Mothercraft Centers.*

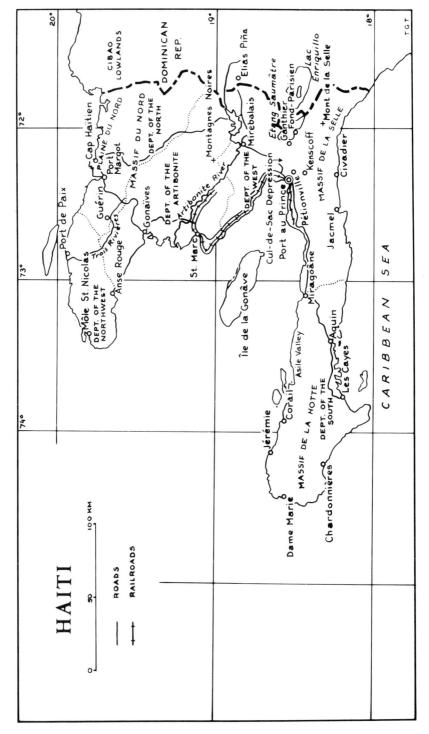

MAP NO. 1.

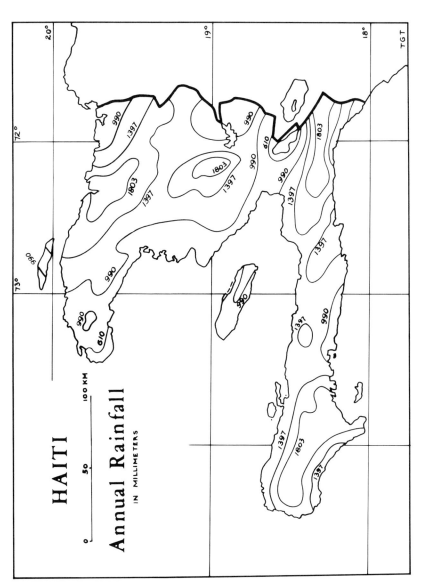

HAITI

Annual Rainfall

IN MILLIMETERS

0   50   100 KM

MAP NO. 2.

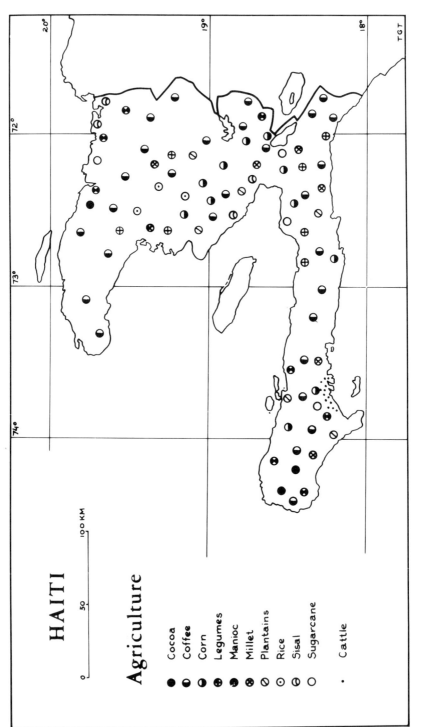

MAP NO. 3.

HAITI

Agriculture

Cocoa
Coffee
Corn
Legumes
Manioc
Millet
Plantains
Rice
Sisal
Sugarcane

Cattle

THE DOMINICAN REPUBLIC

TABLE OF CONTENTS

THE DOMINICAN REPUBLIC

I. BACKGROUND INFORMATION

A. PHYSICAL SETTING [7] [1] [23] [34] [17]

The Dominican Republic occupies the eastern two-thirds of the island of Hispaniola and is bounded on the west by the Republic of Haiti along a 358-kilometer border extending from Pedernales on the southern Caribbean coast along a meandering line to Pepillo Salcedo on the northern Atlantic coast. On all other sides, the country is bounded by the sea: the Atlantic Ocean to the north, the Caribbean Sea to the south. The coastline measures 1,392 kilometers.

About two-thirds of the country's territory consists of highlands, primarily in the west, although there is also an upland area in the northeast. The remaining third is gently rolling lowland. As in Haiti, the highlands comprise a series of parallel mountain ranges: the Cordillera Septentrional in the north (500-1,000 meters), the Cordillera Central in the west-central part of the country (1,660-3,400 meters), the Sierra de Neiba and the Sierra de Bahoruco in the southwest (both 1,000-2,000 meters) and the Cordillera Oriental in the northeast (350-660 meters). The highest point in the country, Pico Duarte (3,471 meters), lies in the Cordillera Central and is the tallest peak in the West Indies. The western highlands are rugged, forest covered and sparsely inhabited. Many streams originate in these mountains, forming the basis of the country's drainage system. The Cordillera Oriental is lower and less rugged than the western ranges. Like the other highlands, it is forested, cut by many streams, and largely uninhabited.

The lowlands include the southeastern plain, the three large valleys which separate the western mountain ranges (Cibao, Azua-San Juan and Neiba), and the narrow coastal bands found in both the north and the south. The southeastern plain extends for about 160 kilometers from the foot of the Cordillera Central near Santo Domingo, eastward to the Mona Passage (see Map No. 1) and is limited on the north by the Cordillera Oriental. The land is flat or gently undulating and is well-drained by numerous rivers which originate in the cordilleras and empty into the Caribbean, including the Rio Jaina, the Rio Ozama and the Rio Macoris. Animal husbandry and sugarcane cultivation are the primary agricultural activities. About one-third of the country's populace lives in the plain, but the capital city of Santo Domingo is the only large urban center. However, there are scattered towns servicing the surrounding rural areas, and along the coast there are a few port cities.

The Cibao Valley or Lowlands (which become the Plaine du Nord in Haiti) separates the Cordillera Septentrional from the central range. This region is the largest and most important flatland in the country. Its fertile, rich soil is drained by the Rio Yaque del Norte and by the Rio Yuna-Río Camu systems. This lowland is intensely cultivated and is the site of the country's second largest city, Santiago de los Caballeros, which lies in the middle of the valley. Many food crops (including dryland rice, corn, beans, vegetables, groundnuts and yams) are grown in the humid eastern section of the valley known as the Vega Real, and the primary cash crop in this area is cocoa. Tobacco is the crop of the upper Yaque Plain, and rice is grown on the flood plain of the river and in the irrigated semiarid lower plains. Bananas are cultivated in the western end of the Cibao.

The Azua-San Juan Valley, running between the Cordillera Central and the Sierra de Neiba, is the next most important lowland. Rural life predominates in this area, although there are numerous villages along the north-south axis of the valley. Most of the cultivated land is in the eastern half of the corridor and on the edge of the western half, which is largely uncleared scrub forest. A number of streams flow through the valley. The Río Macosia, a tributary of the Artibonite, drains the western part of the valley. The San Juan Valley has always been of strategic importance as the easiest route between eastern and western Hispaniola.

The Neiba Valley, which lies between the Sierra de Neiba and the Sierra de Bahoruco, is the lowest and driest region of the Dominican Republic. The western half of the valley is a deep depression (called the Cul-de-Sac in Haiti) occupied by large, saline Lake Enriquillo which lies about 47 meters below sea level. Except for the city of Neiba, the depression is relatively uninhabited. The eastern part of the Neiba Valley, however, is irrigated farmland, watered by the Río Yaque del Sur.

Northern coastal crops include sugarcane, bananas, tobacco, manioc, coconuts and miscellaneous food crops. Animal husbandry is also practiced. The southern coastal lowlands are devoted primarily to sugarcane, although there are some pastures to the extreme east and small areas scattered along the coast where food crops are cultivated.

B. CLIMATE [7] [1] [34]

In spite of the country's location in the tropics, the Dominican Republic enjoys a mild climate due to the tempering influence of the highland elevations and prevailing trade winds. readings above 32°C or below 0°C are unusual. The average annual temperature in the lowlands (as typified by Santo Domingo) is about 26.5°C; in the highlands (as represented by Constanza) it is about 19.5°C; and in the nation as a whole it is 25°C.

Humidity is high since the northeast rain-bearing trade winds blow all year long. Rainfall is heaviest in the northeast (averaging 1,500 millimeters a year) and lightest along the Haitian border (1,000 millimeters average). Map No. 2 shows the pattern of precipitation. There is a period of lesser rainfall between November and April. The island of Hispaniola lies within the hurricane belt and on the average, about one hurricane every 2 years causes serious damage.

C. POPULATION [1] [7] [23] [34] [25]

The 1970 population of the Dominican Republic was estimated at 4.0 million. The annual rate of increase is thought to be around 3.6 percent. The overall density is 86 persons per square kilometer, one of the highest rates in Latin America. In the heavily populated Cibao Lowlands and in the northern coastal region the density rises to 560 per square kilometer. This figure is still not as high as in Haiti, however, and the Dominican Republic has for years felt the mounting population pressure of its neighbor. The largest city is Santo Domingo with about 655,000 inhabitants. The only other city in excess of 100,000 people is Santiago de los Caballeros (104,000). Table No. 1 shows the population distribution by province in 1967. The infant mortality rate was about 72.6 per 1,000 live births in 1968 (compared to 22 per 1,000 in the United States). Life expectancy is 57 years for males and 58.6 years for women.

The original inhabitants of Hispaniola were Taino Indians who were pressed into forced labor gangs by the Spanish to work the mines and plantations. Harsh treatment and disease almost completely annihilated the Indian population by the middle of the 15th century, resulting in the importation of Negro slaves from Africa around 1503. The present population is predominantly mixed. There are about 2,000 Chinese in the country, settled mainly in the cities where most are engaged in the restaurant business. A few hundred Japanese have established agricultural communities in the countryside.

As in most developing nations, there is an increasing trend toward rural-urban migration in the Dominican Republic, but so far the country has retained its rural character. Nevertheless, the population growth rate is higher in the cities than in the countryside. Many factors are cited as contributing to this internal migration pattern: the hardship of subsistence farming; the difficulty of obtaining clear title to land; the static rural social structure; the improvement in communications and transportation between rural and urban areas; the "excitement" of city life and the attraction of urban amenities; and the hope of finding remunerative employment in the cities, As usual, however, the unskilled rural immigrants find it difficult to obtain jobs, and housing and other facilities are inadequate to accommodate the influx. The problem of internal migration has increased since the 1961 overthrow of General Trujillo, who controlled population movement during his dictatorship. The cityward trend has increased the demand for food imports since domestic production has not yet increased sufficiently to meet the needs of the urban centers.

Spanish is the official language of the country and is spoken by about 98 percent of the people. About 1.2 percent speak Haitian patois, 0.6 percent English, and 0.2 percent a variety of other languages.

Social stratification is based on ancestry, wealth and political power. The elite, who comprise less than 5 percent of the population, owe their status mainly to family heritage and consider themselves to be pure-blooded Spanish noblemen. Wealth alone will not buy entry into this class and some members of the elite are no longer rich but retain their position due to family name. Most live in urban centers and are engaged in business, industry, politics or the professions. The boundaries of this class are unbreachable. The so-called new rich who form the stratum just below the elite have gained their position through the acquisition of political and economic power rather than the inheritance of family name. During the Trujillo period, this class included many military officers. Like the elite, the new rich live in the urban centers. Since wealth and power are the entrees to this class, the boundaries are easily crossed—in both directions.

There is a significant middle class in the Dominican Republic, due largely to Trujillo's expansion of the government bureaucracy and his maintenance of stability which led to the growth of industry and commerce. The middle class is found in rural areas and small towns as well as in the cities. At the bottom of the scale is the lower class—laborers, itinerant vendors, craftsmen, tenant farmers, etc. At the very lowest rung of the social ladder is the canecutter.

The Dominicans are predominantly Roman Catholic. About 95 percent profess the Catholic religion, about 2 percent are Protestants and some 1,000 are Jewish.

D. HISTORY AND GOVERNMENT [7] [1] [17] [34] [23]

The island of Hispaniola was discovered by Columbus in 1492 and in 1496 his brother Bartolomé founded the city of Santo Domingo, now the capital of the Dominican Republic. The island served as the base for Spanish exploration of the rest of the hemisphere. Gold was discovered early and the Spanish were soon engaged in mining and plantation agriculture (primarily sugarcane), using the indigenous Taino Indians as slave labor. Spanish settlements came to be concentrated east of the Artibonite River; the western end of the island was later settled by the French and was ceded to France in 1697, eventually becoming the Republic of Haiti.

As mentioned previously, the disappearance of the Indian labor force led to the importation of Negro slaves from Africa and by 1520 Negro laborers dominated in the population. About this time, the gold deposits of Hispaniola became exhausted and many Spaniards began leaving Santo Domingo for the more promising colonies of Mexico and Peru. For the next 250 years, the economy stagnated.

In 1795, having been forced out of Santo Domingo by French forces, the Spanish ceded the colony to France. The black Haitian Toussaint l'Ouverture was made Governor and the slaves were freed. This resulted in a second major exodus of Spanish settlers. In 1809, however, the Spanish retrieved control of Santo Domingo with the help of the British. In 1822 the Haitians, who had achieved their independence from France in 1804, again seized the entire island of Hispaniola and ruled it as an entity until 1844 when the Dominicans revolted, drove the Haitians back into the western end of the island, and declared their independence. The Haitians made repeated incursions into the Dominican Republic until 1855. Fear of reconquest by Haiti led Dominican leaders to request at various times annexation to Spain, France, England and the United States. Finally, in 1861 Spain resumed colonial administration of the territory but the occupation was short-lived and independence was restored in 1865. The fear of Haitian domination which led to this series of events has persisted to the present day. (One manifestation of this fear is the strict limitation maintained by the Government on the entry of Haitians to work as temporary field hands on the sugar plantations.)

The succeeding years brought alternating periods of political turmoil and dictatorship to the Dominican Republic. Economic conditions were so bad by 1905 that the United States Government established a receivership over the Dominican customs houses to protect the interests of U.S. and other foreign investors. Further difficulties, including the threat of European intervention, led to U.S. military occupation of the Republic from 1916 until 1924 when democratic self-government was restored.

In 1930, political power was seized by General Leonidas Trujillo who, through a repressive dictatorship, initiated a 31-year period of economic and political stability in the Republic. With his assassination in 1961, a new period of political turmoil began which culminated in a second U.S. occupation in April 1965. United States forces were merged with an Inter-American Peace Force of the Organization of American States in May and in September a provisional government was established. Elections were held in June 1966 and a democratic government has been in office since.

A new constitution was adopted in 1966 which vests executive power in a President elected by direct vote for a 4-year term. The President is assisted by a Vice-President, also elected for 4 years, and by a Cabinet of 12 secretaries of state, a judicial adviser and two ministers without portfolio. Legislative power is exercised by a bicameral Congress. The 27 members of the Senate and the 74 members of the House of Deputies are elected for terms of 4 years. The country is divided into the National District (Santo Domingo) and 26 provinces (see Map No. 1).

E. AGRICULTURAL POLICIES [24] [15] [2] [1] [3]

The 1968-1975 Economic and Social Development Policy Plan* gives high priority to the agricultural sector and calls for an annual increment in nonsugar crop output of 5.5 percent between 1970 and 1974. In 1968 it was reported that over $9.3 million were allocated to various government agencies involved in agriculture, including the Ministry of Agriculture, the Irrigation Institute, the Cooperative Institute and the Agrarian Institute.

The Government's agricultural policies are two-pronged: the first goal is self-sufficiency in food crops; the second is diversification and upgrading of agricultural exports. Special emphasis has been given to improving production of rice, one of the staples of the Dominican diet. The Government has supported the price of this cereal at a level about 33 percent above the prevailing world market rate, and the Agricultural Bank has granted production credit to rice farmers with the crop as security. Through successful research efforts, varieties which can more than double the yield of native rice have been developed, tested and distributed to producers. The overall program has been so successful that recently there has been an oversupply of rice, in spite of increased domestic consumption.

Land reform has been one of the Government's major programs. In 1962 an Agrarian Reform Law was enacted and the Dominican Agrarian Institute (*Instituto de Agrario Dominicana*—IAD) was established under the Secretariat of Agriculture. The Institute's mandate included distributing publicly-owned land, consolidating inefficient small farms into economically viable units and providing credit and technical assistance to small farmers. Following the termination of the Trujillo regime in 1961 when thousands of hectares of land previously held by Trujillo, his family and friends were confiscated, the Government became the country's major landholder. In 1964 about 37,000 hectares were turned over to the IAD for land settlement and distribution. An additional 121,000 hectares were transferred from the General Land Settlement Administration in the same year. Most of this land had already been settled by homesteaders under earlier government programs. In 1970 the Dominican Congress passed legislation transferring another 1,800 hectares to the IAD for agrarian reform purposes. Further land acquisitions are planned. Between 1963 and 1970 the IAD had granted provisional property deeds to 10,500 families and had initiated projects expected to benefit 3,000 more. The IAD has supported the agrarian reform effort

---

*Transformed in 1970 into the 1970-1974 National Development Plan.

with a program of infrastructure works (irrigation, drainage, road construction and repair, etc.) and technical assistance to farmers through the services of 46 field technicians.

Agricultural credit is provided by the Agricultural Bank of the Dominican Republic. Supervised credit programs are administered by the Secretariat of Agriculture, the IAD and the Institute for Cooperative Credit (*Instituto de Desarollo y Credito Cooperative*–IDECOOP). During 1970 the Agricultural Bank made loans totaling more than $22.4 million through these agencies which benefited over 20,650 farmers, including at least 2,328 participants in the agrarian reform projects. It is reported that over 90 percent of the production loans administered by the IAD are allocated to rice farmers, and growers interested in other commodities find it difficult to obtain adequate credit. The Secretariat of Agriculture sponsors loans aimed primarily at rehabilitating cocoa plantations. IDECOOP loans are limited and have generally been made for diversification and rehabilitation of coffee plantations. Commercial agricultural enterprises are able to obtain financing from the Fund for Economic Development Investments (*Fondo de Inversiones para el Desarollo Economico*–FIDE) which was created in 1966 with the assistance of the U.S. Agency for International Development and the Inter-American Development Bank (IDB). About half of the jobs created as a result of FIDE loans have been in the agro-industrial sector.

The Cooperative Credit Institute promotes various types of agricultural cooperatives, but the movement has not received very wide support among small farmers. Nevertheless, about 25,000 farmers are reported to belong to 250 cooperatives devoted to coffee, rice, cocoa and banana cultivation. One of the most successful organizations is a rice production enterprise at Yuma. Rural housing, school construction, road building, well construction and other such projects are promoted by the Office of Community Development with emphasis on self-help.

An Institute of Price Stabilization was established in 1969 to regulate the output of crops and livestock products through pricing policies. Rice, which has been in oversupply recently, has been the Institute's major concern, but price stabilization programs have also been initiated for corn, sorghum and beans.

Irrigation has received major attention since 1964 under the auspices of the National Institute for Water Resources. Although the country has had an irrigation program since 1932 and by 1961 some 80 canals had been constructed to water 162,000 hectares, many irrigation ditches had not been properly maintained and as a result had silted up. The United States has provided over $1 million for the repair and expansion of the irrigation system. In addition, the Government has obtained loans from international credit institutions to build a $22 million dam at Valdesia on the Nizao River which will irrigate some 32,000 hectares of farmland besides providing electric power and potable water for rural communities. Another irrigation scheme is included in the Tavera Project on the

Río Yaque del Norte (see Map No. 1). Scheduled for completion in 1972, this project will provide irrigation for 400,000 hectares of land and will generate 152 million kilowatts of electric power per year. Financing was provided by AID, the IDB and by public subscription.

An Agricultural Extension Service was established in 1962 as part of the Secretariat of Agriculture but its effectiveness is hampered by the scarcity of trained agronomists and veterinarians. Teachers from Puerto Rico's Extension Service and U.S. Peace Corps volunteers have helped to fill the gap while training Dominican counterparts. There are about 12 experimental stations in the country which are engaged in trying to determine what crops are best adapted for the regions in which they are located.

Many experts have pointed out that one of the major weaknesses of the Government's programs affecting agriculture is the lack of coordination among the various agencies involved. The result is often duplication and fragmentation of efforts. There appears to be a real need for an integrated national policy on agricultural development and effective administrative machinery for coordinating the work of all government agencies engaged in activities related to agriculture.

F. FOREIGN AID

1. Bilateral Aid [28]

The United States has been the Dominican Republic's primary source of bilateral aid. Between 1946 and 1968, U.S. economic assistance totaled $235.4 million in loans and $178.6 million in grants. These funds have been used for agricultural education, irrigation, community self-help and many other purposes. A Peace Corps contingent assigned to the Dominican Republic has been primarily concerned with agricultural extension and rural community development activities.

2. Multilateral Aid [26] [16] [14] [27]

The Dominican Republic receives multilateral assistance from the United Nations Children's Fund (UNICEF), the World Bank, the International Development Association (IDA), the Inter-American Development Bank (IDB) and the United Nations Development Program (UNDP). Aid to improve the country's food resources and the population's nutritional status has included: the creation of a model health center with UNICEF assistance where pre- and post-natal services as well as helath and nutrition education are offered; the provision of IDA development credits in the amount of $5 million for a livestock development project; the granting of almost $1.3 million by the UNDP Special Fund for animal production and veterinary training in cooperation with the Food and

Agriculture Organization of the United Nations (FAO); the approval of a $2.8 million UNDP Special Fund grant for multipurpose development surveys of the Yaque del Norte and Yaque del Sur river basins (carried out by the World Bank); and the provision by the UNDP of $2.1 million for crop diversification and increased production in the Cibao Valley, with the technical assistance of FAO. Earlier loans from the IDB have enabled the Republic to expand its rural water supply system.

II. FOOD RESOURCES

A. GENERAL [1] [34] [27]

The total land area of the Dominican Republic covers 4,873,000 hectares. Only 1,067,000 hectares or less than 22 percent of this acreage is under crops and another 17 percent (828,000 hectares) consists of pastures. Vast forests cover 2,225,000 hectares or 45 percent of the country; the remaining area is idle or covered with brush. Until the present day there has been no shortage of land and no pressure brought to bear on the farmers to emigrate. On the contrary, the Trujillo era was marked by an intensive land occupation program, settlement of the western reaches and an effort to relocate slumdwellers from the cities to the rural areas.

Although, as we shall see, malnutrition is a major health problem, it is not caused by an actual scarcity of food, but rather by lack of education as to what constitutes a proper diet and lack of effort to grow the right foods and distribute them to the right people. Few Dominican peasants are ever really hungry. The farmers' ignorance and apathy is probably encouraged by the fertility of much of the land, which rewards small efforts handsomely. The fertility could be exploited for more impressive returns, especially in the Cibao Valley (called "the food basket of the Republic") and in the Vega Real Plain east of Santiago.

Most of the rice is grown on the flood plain of the Río Yaque del Norte. Coconuts, manioc and groundnuts come from the northern plains. The eastern half of the country is fully exploited: pastures are maintained at the tip, while sugarcane grows in much of the remaining area. The western half of the Republic includes most of the undeveloped brush and forestland and many of the irrigated estates (20 percent of the last are along the Haitian border). There, irrigation projects created after 1930 have brought some prosperity to the semiarid regions of the western Cibao lowlands, the San Juan Valley and the Lake Enriquillo area. In very recent years, as a result of agricultural credit programs, the Government has been able to stimulate increased planting of cocoa and expanded cultivation of fruits and vegetables as well as the production of beef and poultry.

The southern valley of the Neiba is also in need of irrigation and wherever it is available sugar and rice are produced. The southwestern Pedernales area is rather poor but some coffee and food crops can be grown. Unfortunately, the irrigation services are said to be handicapped by lack of funds and equipment and some of the ditches have been left to fill up with silt (see *Agricultural Policies*). Both the World Bank and the United Nations Development Program have provided assistance for rehabilitation of the network of canals which, when completed, may enable several hundred thousand new hectares of farmland to be brought under production.

B. MEANS OF PRODUCTION

1. Agricultural Labor Force [33] [1] [2]

As stated previously, the population of the Dominican Republic increases at a rate which is one of the highest in the world, estimated at 3.6 percent a year, creating a constantly growing demand for jobs. About 47 percent of the population is under 15 years old with 3 percent aged 65 or over. This leaves 50 percent of the population or about 2.2 million people (1970) in the economically active bracket. The slow motion of the economy, however, has discouraged many young people from looking for jobs and in 1966 the work force numbered only around 807,000. It is now estimated at over 1 million and believed to be increasing at the rate of 30,000 new workers each year. The following table shows the distribution of the labor force among the different sectors of the economy in 1966. It is doubtful that the percentages have changed much since.

Distribution of Labor Force by Economic Sector –
Dominican Republic, 1966

Economic Activity	Number	Percent of Total
Agriculture, forestry, hunting and fishing	471,000	58
Manufacturing	88,000	11
Construction	26,000	3
Services	222,000	28
Total	807,000	100

Source: R.H. Bateman, "Basic Data on the Economy of the Dominican Republic."

Women in the work force represent only 10 percent of the total number of people seeking employment. More than 60 percent of these women are in domestic services and 10 percent are in agriculture.

About 60 percent of the agricultural workers operate farms of less than 2 hectares with the help of unpaid family members; another 25 percent probably work as paid employees on farms varying in size up to 35 hectares, while the rest (15 percent) are migrant farmhands seeking seasonal employment on the 8,000 estates which exceed 35 hectares in size. Two-thirds of all agricultural workers are employed in the sugar industry. Agricultural employment is offered in the sugarcane fields from December to June or July and on coffee and cocoa plantations from October to March. During August and September no employment is available. Sugarcane cutting is unpopular in the Dominican Republic as elsewhere in the Caribbean, resulting in labor shortages. Canecutters sometimes have to be imported from Haiti in spite of the high unemployment and underemployment rates among Dominicans. About three-fourths of the workers in the manufacturing sector are engaged in sugar processing.

Wages are low, not exceeding $50 or $60 a month for more than half of the labor force and less than $200 for 75 percent of all salaried persons. The U.S. Department of Labor estimates that one-third of the total labor force was unemployed in 1968. Moreover, 40 percent of the fieldhands work only 8 months a year and 20 percent of the whole force is underemployed all the time. It is no wonder that the applications for enlistment in the National Service System, which includes the Army, Navy and National Police, are high. A Vocational School of the Armed Forces and Police has been created to train young recruits in various practical skills. These trainees form a valuable crops of civilian semiskilled workers when they leave the services.

The labor force is more stable than in other countries of the Caribbean area and seasonal migrations are at a minimum. On the sugarcane plantations most workers remain in shacks or in dwellings provided by the employers and grow some food on their own plots. Some become squatters if there is vacant land in the vicinity.

2. Farms [34] [1] [24] [3] [2]

The overall number of people living on farms is not known with certainty. The 1960 census revealed that 70 percent of the population was rural and 30 percent urban. Since that time there has been a constant stream of farmers, especially young ones, from the fields to the cities, although in lesser numbers than in other countries. Preliminary results of the 1970 census place the present rural share of the population at 60 percent.

The number of farms is believed to be over 450,000 although this is not certain due to the enormous complexity of the Dominican cadastral system. Not only were many original titles lost during the period of Haitian domination, but the practice of common holding allows anyone showing a fraction of a title to land through inheritance to cultivate a portion of that land, providing it does not interfere with the activity of another owner. Moreover, large estates from the days of Trujillo and his partisans have reverted to the state for redistribution, an almost impossible task given the multiple claims and counterclaims confronting the Government. Thus, while the following table may give an idea of the sizes of farms, it certainly does not represent the true distribution of ownership or reflect the actual number of farming establishments.

Estimated Number of Farms by Size – Dominican Republic, 1950 and 1960

| Size | 1950 | | 1960 | |
| | Number of | | Number of | |
(hectares)	Farms	Percent	Farms	Percent
Less than 10	244,399	88.3	422,654	93.9
10–100	30,316	11.0	26,050	5.8
100–1,000	1,948	.7	1,518	0.3
1,000–2,500	124	<0.1	85	<0.1
More than 2,500	61	<0.1	28	<0.1
Total	276,848	100.0	450,335	100.0

Source: Adapted from American University, *Area Handbook for the Dominican Republic.*

The table shows the enormous difference between the large number of small farms and the large size of a few farms, as well as the changes that occurred over the 10-year period 1950-1960. The trend in the same direction has continued since 1960 and has, in fact, accelerated but recent figures are not yet available. The table also shows that in 1950 about 55 percent of the cropland was occupied by 61 large estates while the rest was shared by 276,787 farms. In 1960 the situation had improved: the number of farms had almost doubled while the bigger units were less numerous and the area covered by the largest units had been reduced by about one-half. This trend no doubt continued between 1960 and 1970.

Of the 450,335 farms existing in 1960, it was indicated that 262,979 were owned by the farmers exploiting them and the area covered was said to be 1.66 million hectares or an average of a little over 6.4 hectares per holding. It is probable, however, that this is an overly optimistic estimate. While many *campesinos* may have a kind of title to a piece of land or to a share of a piece of land, they do not really enjoy the prerogatives of "landowners" in the usual sense of the word. Others may be tolerated on a plot near a large estate where they work part of the year, while still others may be landless and work wherever they find employment. The 1960 distribution of farms by types of tenure was as follows:

Since 1962 an effort has been made to facilitate land ownership. *Campesinos* have been settled on state-owned land and given facilities for term payments as well as credits for seeds and fertilizers. Between 1930 and 1960 new land was brought under cultivation without a parallel increase in the reported number of farms, while later the registered number of farms increased faster than the acreage cultivated, probably because government bookkeeping efforts began to catch up with reality. The trend towards larger estates was interrupted by the 1962 land reform, which endeavored to divide these holdings and to discourage the establishment of large companies and commercial farms. While wisdom dictates that industrialization of agriculture in developing countries should be undertaken very cautiously, there is no dearth of people who deplore the lack of economic efficiency that the persistence of small holdings entails.

Number and Size of Farms According to Land Tenure –
Dominican Republic, 1960

| Type of Tenure | Farms | | Farmland | |
	Units	Percent of Total	Area (1,000 ha)	Percent of Total
Owner-operators	262,979	58.8	1,512.4	73.1
Renter-operators	137,865	30.8	427.2	20.6
(Sharecroppers)	(30,782)	(6.9)	(86.6)	(4.2)
Concessional operators[a]	35,596	8.9	109.3	5.3
Other arrangements	6,658	1.5	20.3	1.0
Total	443,098	100.0	2,069.2[b]	100.0

[a]Operators without land titles, excluding renters and sharecroppers.
[b]Does not include approximately 189,000 hectares suitable for sugarcane.

Source: Dominican Republic (Oficina Nacional de Estadística), *República Dominicana en Cifras, 1969* as cited by W.F. Buck in *Agriculture and Trade of the Dominican Republic.*

Efforts are being made to encourage cooperative farming. This is viewed as the only way to reconcile the principle of private ownership of land, in however small amounts, with the efficient introduction of modern technology. Cooperatives would also facilitate the extension of agricultural credit (which is at present woefully inadequate) to small farmers. The spirit of cooperative farming is promoted by the Institute for Cooperative Credit but response to date has been limited. As stated earlier, 250 cooperative farms are said to exist with a membership of 25,000 people. Education in cooperatives is provided by the *Confederación Autónoma de Sindicatos Cristianos.*

3. Fertilizers and Irrigation [1] [2] [9] [14]

The use of fertilizers is limited in amount and in location in spite of the fact that since June 1956 the law has required that under certain circumstances some fertilizers be spread on some acreage. However, the law is not enforced and the improvements it brought about were only temporary. The Dominican Republic has a small fertilizer industry that produces about 30 tons of chemical fertilizers every year. The following table shows the average quantities and kinds used over the 20-year period 1948-1969.

Use of Fertilizers – Dominican Republic, 1948-1969
(in tons)

Kind of Fertilizer	Annual Average 1948-1953	1964	1965	1966	1967	1968	1969
Nitrogenous	1,300	8,500	10,000	14,300	15,000	13,000	20,000
Phosphatic	900	1,100	1,000	700	800	1,000	1,500
Potassic	400	1,800	1,000	900	2,000	2,500	3,000

Source: Food and Agriculture Organization of the United Nations, *Production Yearbook 1970.*

These amounts are mostly applied on rice, sugarcane and tobacco fields. Even owners of large farms do not always know how to use the fertilizers to best advantage. Most of the imported product is not within the reach of the small farmer. Crops are not usually rotated and, as in Haiti, farmers still practice some slash-and-burn agriculture.

Although the country as a whole receives an adequate amount of rain, there are dry regions in the west where productivity is entirely dependent upon irrigation. An irrigation system was created in 1932 and now waters an estimated 172,000 hectares through 3,000 kilometers of canals. As mentioned earlier, substantial sections of this network need rehabilitation, and new construction has begun on the Tavera and Valdesia projects (see *Agricultural Policies*). Moreover, wells are being drilled and play an important role in the area of the Río Yaque del Sur in collecting water that otherwise would be lost in the permeable soils.

4. Mechanical Equipment [1] [21]

An agricultural machine service was created in 1949, but for many reasons only a few farms or estates are mechanized. In 1950 only about 6 percent of the agricultural enterprises used machines and the proportion has increased only slightly since, judging by the scant data available. One of the reasons for the low level of mechanization is the fear that too many tractors would increase unemployment. Moreover, the cost of the machines is high and cheap labor is available. In 1969, according to FAO, 4,400 tractors were in use, most of them on rice and sugarcane fields. Small farmers utilize mostly hand tools and plows powered by oxen, mules or donkeys. It is reported that a number of machine stations have been established which lend their equipment to farmers and that the trend is to increase the use of these facilities.

C. PRODUCTION [9] [23] [8] [29]

The production of agricultural crops is remarkable for two reasons: the favor given to cash crops over food crops in terms of land use; and the decline in both total agricultural production and food output on a per capita basis over the period 1956-1969, as shown in the following table.

Indices of Per Capita Total Agricultural Production and Per Capita
Food Production – Dominican Republic, 1952-1969
(Index 1952-1956 = 100)

	1952-56	1958	1960	1962	1964	1966	1968	1969
Total agricultural production	100	103	115	98	93	82	77	83
Food production	100	103	116	97	91	82	77	84

Source: Food and Agriculture Organization of the United Nations, *Production Yearbook 1970.*

The relationship between land devoted to basic food crops and land devoted to cash crops is shown hereunder.

Comparison of Land Use Between Food Crops and Cash Crops
Dominican Republic, 1948-1968
(in 1,000 hectares)

Kind of Crop	1948-52	1964	1965	1966	1967	1968
Food crops	218	216	237	242	239	249
Cash crops	338	364	368	389	366	377

Sources: Food and Agriculture Organization of the United Nations, *Production Yearbook 1969.*

Food and Agriculture Organization of the United Nations, *Monthly Bulletin,* 1969, 11, 24.

Statesman's Yearbook 1970-1971.

It is apparent that the area devoted to basic food crops has constantly remained below that allocated to cash crops. This series of volumes on the ecology of malnutrition contains many examples of this practice in developing countries, which is always and understandably accompanied by serious nutritional health problems. The income derived from the sale of cash crops does not trickle down to the small producer, who is paid only a fraction of what the exporter receives. Thus the smallholder is unable to buy high-priced imported foods. The Government is well aware of this situation and is trying to increase food production. Yet, although self-sufficiency in food is the stated goal of the Government, the economy is still cash-crop dominated and mostly dependent upon the United States market.

1. Food Crops [14] [1] [24] [9] [6] [3] [11] [12]

As stated, the basic food crops are rice, manioc, corn and beans.

a. Cereals

Rice is the main cereal and is the only basic food that has made spectacular progress since 1952. The area sown has more or less doubled and production has almost tripled (see Tables 2 and 3). This is undoubtedly the result of irrigation and fertilization which have both been applied preferentially to rice. The best area of production is in the western part of the Cibao Valley, Santiago and La Vega provinces, and the reclaimed swamps surrounding the Río Yuna estuary. The method of cultivation is similar to the replanting practiced in Viet Nam where nursery seedlings are moved after 3 or 4 weeks to be replanted in waterlogged fields. Rice cultivation is supported by an experimental station in La Vega Province. As a result of Government promotion and price support programs, no rice has had to be imported since 1967. The new "miracle seed" is beginning to be used and some consumer resistance to the taste and appearance of the grain has already been observed.

Corn, the second most important cereal, is grown on almost all farms. The area sown has declined from a yearly average of 40,000 hectares in the 1948-1952 period to 31,000 hectares in 1970. Production, however, has remained about the same, increasing slightly in 1970, thanks to better techniques. Corn is the cereal of low income people. It is estimated that 76 percent of the crop is used for human consumption, 15 percent for fodder and the rest for seed. Government efforts to boost the production of corn for animal feed have met with little success.

b. Roots, Tubers and Vegetables

Manioc, sweet potatoes, yams, taro and other tubers are also found in the basic diet. The area planted in these roots has remained almost constant, increasing slightly for sweet potatoes and yams, decreasing somewhat for manioc. Production of manioc, however, has increased by more than 10 percent, although the figures in Tables 2 and 3 indicate only orders of magnitude since this root is planted throughout the country in many small plots which defy statistical notation. Most of the crop is eaten where produced; a little is sold in nearby markets. White potatoes have begun to gain favor and have shown a fivefold increase in production since the 1948-1952 period. They are usually grown on the periphery of the cities for the urban market. Potato farming is forming the basis of a truck garden industry which could be developed to include more green and red vegetables. Tomatoes and plantains, hot peppers and chilies are planted on most farms. Tomatoes are particularly successful; production reached 76,000 tons in 1969, up from 6,000 tons in 1964. Production of plantains for domestic consumption has increased by more than one-third during the last few years.

c. Legumes

Legumes are essential to the nutrition of the population of the Dominican Republic because of their high protein content. The pigeon pea, the red kidney bean and the groundnut all contribute in different ways to the daily fare. The pigeon pea, found on almost all farms, is planted on 27,000 hectares and has produced a rather constant crop of 21,000-22,000 tons. The area sown in dry beans has practically tripled since 1964, but the harvest fluctuates widely, between 27,000 and 37,000 tons. Groundnuts have been the object of special attention from the Government, in hope that the country will become self-sufficient in vegetable oils. The area sown more than tripled between 1952 and 1970 and production increased almost fivefold. Although the entire crop is used for oil, vegetable oil imports are still necessary (primarily soybean oil from the United States). Areas of production are spread over the Cibao Valley, along the eastern coast and in the mountains around Elias Piña. Two crops are raised annually: a summer crop from April to September and a winter crop from November to April, the latter being by far the smaller of the two.

2. Cash Crops (21) (1) (6) (3) (11) (12)

The cash crops are essentially sugarcane, coffee, cocoa, bananas and tobacco. Sugar was introduced into Hispaniola as early as 1492 by Christopher Columbus himself, who had obtained the seedlings in Madeira, but it was not until 1950 that the economic value of the crop began to rise. This induced the Government to divert land from production of other crops or from pasturage to sugar production. Dominican cane is reputed to have a higher sugar content than other varieties in the Caribbean but this advantage is somewhat undercut by inefficient production methods which rely mostly (and probably wisely, from a social standpoint) on hand labor, and result in a lower output per land unit than elsewhere. As shown in Table No. 2, the area in sugarcane continued to increase after the 1950 decade by 52 percent and the production of cane increased by almost 70 percent. Sixteen major estates share the acreage, two of which—Río Haina and La Romana—both claim to be the largest sugarcane estates in the world.

In 1969, the processing of cane into raw sugar had more than doubled over the 1952 level. Twelve of the most important estates and mills are the property of the Government and operated by the State Sugar Council *(Consejo Estatal de Azúcar)*. In 1970 these government mills produced an estimated 604,700 tons of raw sugar. The crop grows in 18 months, is cut by machete and transported by oxcart to the mills. Large estates keep their own oxen and maintain pastures to feed them. As elsewhere in the Caribbean area, the profession of canecutter is looked down upon by the younger generation. The Government would like to restructure the industry but is waiting for a more auspicious time to undertake the considerable social and economic transformation which would be required to move production to selected fields better suited for sugar cultivation, relocate thousands of workers, increase the efficiency of transportation from plantation to sea outlets, modernize the factories, etc.

Coffee has been a pillar of the Dominican economy since 1715. Data on the area covered are not reported every year but between 1948 and 1952 a yearly average of 76,000 hectares was indicated and in 1968 the acreage was estimated to have risen to 148,000 hectares (see Table No. 2). Production rose by almost two-thirds during the same period (see Table No. 3). The coffee area encompasses the provinces of La Vega, Salcedo, Santiago and Duarte with more coffee groves in the mountains south of Barahona. The lower levels are harvested first and the migrant workers move from low to higher altitudes in pursuit of the later maturing bushes. The harvesting season starts in November or December. A Coffee and Cocoa Administration was established in 1961 which concerns itself with expanding the cultivation of the crop.

The area planted in cocoa is not known with exactitude, but it was estimated at 134,000 hectares in 1965. Like coffee, cocoa is cultivated on small farms and like coffee it grows best in the Cibao Valley. The major cocoa area is located between Moca and San Pedro de Macoris. Yearly production is around 28,000-30,000 tons but is strongly influenced by the international market which has sustained heavy losses during certain years when production was too abundant.

The area sown in tobacco has grown slowly in the past decade, fluctuating between 18,000 and 20,000 hectares, producing from 16,000 to 25,000 tons. The Tobacco Institute, established in 1962, aims at doubling the number of people dependent upon tobacco for their livelihood. This is being accomplished through a variety of support programs for tobacco farm families. Most of the tobacco acreage is found in Santiago Province.

The Dominican Republic grows bananas for export and plantains for home consumption. The export banana is grown on large plantations around Monte-cristi which cover about 13,000 hectares and produce around 250,000 tons of fruit. Sigatoka and Panama disease, the two fungoid enemies of the plant, are not as severe in the Dominican Republic as they are in other parts of the Caribbean, but they are, nevertheless, responsible for the drop in production in certain years. The future of the industry is in doubt as the most important plantations are gradually shifting to production of other crops. The plantain is grown everywhere possible by individual farmers and is, as elsewhere in the region, an important dietary staple. Plantain production was estimated at 1.4 million tons in 1966.

3. Animal Husbandry (1) (6) (9) (31) (14) (13) (3) (12)

a. Livestock and Poultry

The climatic conditions and the geography of the Dominican Republic lend themselves well to the development of a prosperous animal husbandry industry. Not only is abundant pastureland available, especially in the southeast, but some land diverted to sugarcane in earlier years could be returned to pasture. The area in grazing land is variously estimated by different sources. The Food and Agriculture Organization gives a total of 867,000 hectares, some of which is managed and some not. Both guinea grass and Pangola grass are found, the latter being the most advantageous and hence under expansion. The livestock industry receives substantial support from the National Government and from the Inter-American Development Bank. The IDB loaned the Government $6 million in 1963 and has since indirectly supported the industry through various rural development projects. Table No. 4 shows the growth of the livestock and poultry industry since the 1948-52 period.

Cattle herds now number about 1.1 million head, representing a steady development since 1948. The cattle are a mixed lot: depending upon the herd, crossbreeds between local types and Brahmans are found, together with Swiss and German steers of good quality. The farmer does not differentiate much between milk and meat strains but the quality seems to be slowly improving, as judged by the increasing weight of slaughtered animals. A livestock program was inaugurated in 1962, which included importing breeding animals and initiating veterinary measures to combat the endemic levels of brucellosis and tuberculosis. Beef cattle are found primarily in the eastern Cibao Valley, in the eastern provinces of El Seibo, San Cristóbal, San Pedro de Macoris and La Altagracia, and along the northern coast.

Pigs are found everywhere but are more numerous in Santiago Province. The total number was evaluated at 1.3 million in 1970, a good increase since 1948-1952 when the census revealed 739,000. This is particularly remarkable in view of the high level of mortality suffered by these animals due to a variety of parasitic and other diseases, especially hog cholera. Goats are the resource of the very poor. They feed for themselves and occasionally provide meat and milk. Sheep in small numbers yield some mutton, mostly for the urban market.

Poultry is also found everywhere. The birds fend for themselves around the huts and the product is not of high quality. The Government has supported poultry raising as a means of increasing total meat consumption. International assistance has also been available for the industry. In 1970 the number of poultry of all kinds was estimated at 7.5 million, including 7.2 million chickens.

b. Meat, Milk, and Eggs

As in most developing countries, the amount of meat commercialized and hence entered into statistics represents far less than the total amount produced in the country. The uncontrolled slaughtering taking place in rural areas is estimated to make up around one-third of all the butchering done in the island. The Dominican Statistical Office estimates that in 1964 about 158,000 cattle were slaughtered in the country, both officially and unofficially, providing 22,000 tons of meat. In the same year, 237,526 pigs were killed, yielding 8,000 tons of meat, 3,214 sheep providing 40 tons of meat and 17,341 goats resulting in 208 tons of meat. Of the total (30,248 tons) about 3,500 tons were industrially processed into hams, sausages and other meat products of all kinds. According to reports from the office of the U.S. Agricultural Attaché in Santo Domingo, by 1968 commercial production of beef alone had risen to 30,000 tons, stimulated by the prospect of a U.S. market following the certification of two local slaughterhouses by the U.S. Department of Agriculture.

The milk supply is in continuous increase, reflecting improvements in the quality of the herds as breeders are imported in greater numbers and as technology improves. In 1964 the Statistical Office of the Dominican Republic gave a figure of 186,000 tons. In the same year, FAO gave a similar estimate but by 1970 reported 265,000 tons. Powdered and condensed milk are imported at the rate of about 10,000 tons per year. Cheese is both manufactured locally and imported. Local production amounted to about 2,000 tons in 1970.

Poultry meat output has been increasing rapidly. In 1971 broiler meat production was estimated at 15,300 tons, an increase of almost 50 percent over the 1970 level and 400 percent over 1966. Lower prices for poultry meat have stimulated domestic demand. The number of eggs produced is quite uncertain and according to FAO figures seems to be increasing from an annual average of 119 million between 1948 and 1952 to 432 million in 1970. Imports of eggs occur every year and according to government statistics amounted to 20 tons or about 445,000 units in 1964. According to FAO, by 1970 egg imports had increased to 763 tons or roughly 17 million eggs, all hatching eggs from the United States. In March 1972, *Foreign Agriculture* reported that the Dominican Republic is nearly self-sufficient in both poultry meat and eggs.

4. Fisheries [6] [2]

There is little fishing done in the Dominican Republic, most of it along the southern and northern coasts. This is not a traditional occupation of the population. There are only about 5,000 registered fishermen exploiting the coastal waters. The 100-fathom line which arbitrarily separates coastal from deep-sea fishing is only about 1 mile offshore around the island. In the past this has discouraged the creation of what amounts to a new industry. In 1967 about 3,200 tons were landed which included 36 varieties of various species of fish, the dominant kinds being sardines, herring, tuna, mackerel, salmon (in the estuaries at certain seasons), cod and anchovies. Lobster fishing is a growing industry. The 1967 catch of 63 tons was five times greater than that of preceding years. Most of the catch is exported to Puerto Rico. The population is not conditioned to fish because of the refrigeration, transportation and marketing problems that would have to be solved to create a demand. The main fishing ports are Azua, San Pedro de Macorís and La Romana but many small seashore villages and towns have some part-time fishermen also. Freshwater fishing is of very small importance and a pond project started in the early 1950's does not seem to have prospered.

D. TRADE

Food is the most important item of trade. Whether domestic or foreign, from the isolated village vendor to the large import-export firm located in the capital, food in one form or another constitutes the bulk of commercial exchanges.

1. Domestic Trade [1] [2] [22]

The rural pattern of trade is not very different from that described for Haiti. Most of the items sold are agricultural products and most of the vendors are women, who carry their wares themselves, traveling by foot or by bus when an access road to the farm exists. Nonperishable goods outweigh perishable ones, such as meat and eggs, which must be consumed soon after they are available. Prices, therefore, are variable, depending upon the hour of the day. The chance to make a sale at low profit today is preferred to the risk of higher profits on another day. In the rural areas, marketing is governed by the absence or availability of roads and transportation. This causes some isolated farmers to waste considerable time and energy in going to and from the nearest market and once there, they sell their produce at low prices because they have no alternative outlet within commuting distance, a fact which is not unknown to the potential buyer. Women also sell along the roadside or at the regular marketplace. The middlemen, whether truckers or enterprising individuals, make profits over the producer and considerable differences exist between the income of the producer and that of the last person selling to the consumer—all this in spite of the well-intentioned paragraph of the 1963 Constitution guaranteeing the farmer a fair price for his products. Some of the crops are sold directly to processors.

Some villages have general stores where manufactured goods are available. All trade is on a cash basis. In the towns and cities a larger variety of sales outlets are naturally found, from the one-room *pulperia* selling objects of first necessity in the poorer quarters, to larger places vending a broader spectrum of items, from clothing to equipment. Trade is not ingrained in the way of life of the population and many of the most successful tradesmen are foreigners, such as Syrians, Lebanese, Haitians or Chinese.

Taking Santiago as an example of trade in urban areas, the food supplies are provided by a number of specialized stores selling meat *(carnicerias)*, milk *(lecherias)* or bread *(panaderias)*, or by street vendors *(ventorillos)*, or by the two major open markets of Modelo and Hospedaje. These markets are in turn supplied primarily by a number of transport entrepreneurs using anything from donkeys to buses and modern trucks. These men collect the wares of the producers (some are themselves producers) and converge on the city from every horizon. Markets are usually run by administrators who collect taxes from the sellers and assure maintenance. Each vendor occupies a site which he guards and has a right to sell if he cannot continue to occupy it. The sellers buy their goods directly from those farmers able to bring their produce to market in person or from truckers or other transport entrepreneurs. A complex credit system supports these transactions. However, the type of marketing varies with the product. Plantains are sold by the producer to the trucker while tomatoes are carried to the market by the farmer himself in crates containing about 40 kilos each, sold at about $1.00 a crate. In 1966, it was estimated that an average wholesaler in Santiago could net $12.44 a day on tomatoes and $18.63 a day on plantains. From these wholesalers, the trade passes into the hands of street vendors who load pushcarts and distribute the goods to their clientele in the cities. The movement of staples such as rice and beans continues to go from producer to wholesaler and from the latter to retailers without any evidence of government interference through stockage, imports and resale in an effort to keep prices in line.

2. Foreign Trade [10] [2] [29] [31] [32] [3] [4] [12]

The trade balance of the Dominican Republic deteriorated regularly during the 1960's. Between 1964 and 1969 some deficit occurred every year except in 1965. This situation can be explained in part by the fact that salaries, which had been kept low during the Trujillo era, began rising after the dictator's death. This availability of money led to increased purchases abroad (including food) and simultaneously lessened the competitiveness of Dominican products. In addition, low levels of domestic reinvestments of profits earned during the Trujillo period left the country ill-equipped to increase production and sales. The Dominican Republic had lived through a period of chaos and anarchy during the pre-Trujillo years which greatly facilitated his rise to power and his early popularity. This was followed by a resentment against his methods which led to his assassination. While he was in power, a period of commercial prosperity developed, during which most of the profits were dissipated unproductively. After Trujillo fell from power, there were still fewer profits to invest and more expenditures were necessary to equip the country for greater production. These expenses used up foreign exchange; hence, hoarded money was put back into circulation. At the present time, so much is being spent on capital investments (water, power, tourism) that the balance continues to lean to the deficit side, but if internal peace continues to reign, it may legitimately be hoped that the dividends from these investments will rise and tilt the scale in the positive direction.

Tables 5 and 6 list the major agricultural exports and imports. The position of agricultural exports has remained strong, representing 88 percent of all exports in 1961 and 89 percent in 1969. The export trade is based on sugar (48 percent of all exports), cocoa (11 percent), oil cakes and tobacco (both good money-makers in spite of some difficulties). The sugar trade is extremely profitable because the product is imported by the United States under a quota system which guarantees a price three times that prevailing on the world market. In an effort to broaden the base of agricultural exports, so as to lessen reliance on sugar, coffee, cocoa and tobacco, the Government is encouraging greater production of such crops as pigeon peas, peppers, cucumbers, taro, avocados and other fruits and vegetables for sale abroad. Exports of onions, garlic, meat and even rice have occurred and have encouraged the producers of food crops. Based on figures available in April 1971, a surplus in the balance of trade was expected at the end of the year.

The growth of wheat imports reflects the rise in personal incomes that has taken place and the increasing preference for breads and pastas over domestic traditional starchy foodstuffs. The list of agricultural imports shows a number of items which could be and hopefully will be produced domestically. The most important of these items is rice, imports of which have declined but remained at 13,000 tons in 1968. Returning prosperity is evidenced by the rise in purchases of wheat, a luxury item. Milk is also being imported in greater quantities. Some is donated through bilateral and international aid programs. Most of the imported milk is powdered or condensed. Although 1965 was a bad year, the restoration of order brought an upsurge in imports in the following years. Meat imports are declining as the domestic livestock industry makes progress. The numbers of live animals (breeders) imported attests to the activity of the livestock program. As potato planting increases, the amount of this tuber purchased abroad decreases. Various types of fish, especially cod and smoked herring, continue to be imported in uncertain quantities. The following table shows the financial outcome of these foreign trade operations.

Trade Balance – Dominican Republic, 1963-1968
(in millions of dollars)

	1963	1964	1965	1966	1967	1968	1969
Total export trade	174	179	125	135	156	163	184
Total import trade	160	192	86	160	174	196	210
Balance	+14	–13	+39	–25	–18	–33	–26
Agricultural export trade	158	165	109	120	136	144	–
Agricultural import trade	30	45	27	36	35	41	–
Balance	+128	+120	+82	+84	+101	+103	–

Source: Food and Agriculture Organization of the United Nations, *Trade Yearbook 1970.*

The table shows that the country exports far more food and agricultural products than it imports.

E. FOOD INDUSTRIES [2] [1] [24] [3] [6]

There are between 700 and 800 plants concerned with the processing of food in the Dominican Republic. These plants sell to 300 wholesalers who distribute the products to about 11,500 retailers. The plants are part of a broad industrial sector, some of which is in the hands of the state as a result of the confiscation of Trujillo enterprises. The Dominican Corporation for State Enterprises (*Corporación Dominicana de Empresas Estatales*–CORDE) operates some 30 enterprises representing 25 percent of all Dominican industrial activities. Some of these are concerned with food. The Dominican Mills *(Molinos Dominicanos)* could mill 400 tons of wheat a day but in 1967 utilized only 54 percent of their capacity. The wheat goes to 325 bakeries which process the flour into bread. Other outlets are the five pasta factories manufacturing noodles and spaghetti.

The Salt Refinery *(Refineria de Sal)* is capable of handling 12 tons a day but at present it operates at only 8 percent of its capacity. The Milk Industry *(Industria Lecherias)* has the capacity to handle 47,000 bottles of milk per day. There are also a small number of milk pasteurizing plants which supply the Santo Domingo market almost exclusively. There capacity is said to be over 50,000 liters a day. It is believed that about $389,000 worth of milk is sold in the Dominican Republic every year. There are also a number of plants preparing ice cream. About 200 tons of butter and over 1,000 tons of cheese are made every day.

It is estimated that a total of about 24,000 tons of vegetable oils are produced annually. The Vegetable Oil Factory *(Fábrica de Aceites Vegetales)* produces vegetable oils from soybeans and groundnuts at the rate of about 300 tons a year, although it is capable of producing 2,000 tons. Margarine is manufactured in growing quantities which may well eliminate the need for imports of the product. Industrial Chocolate *(Chocolateria Industrial)*, with a capacity of processing 100 kilograms of cocoa a day, sells $140,000 worth of chocolate a year. The Government also controls a number of other food processing firms, including liquor and rum distilleries. About 7-8 million liters of rum or almost 2 liters per person are produced every year.

The private sector has a number of enterprises, especially the 14 sugar mills operating under the auspices of the *Consejo Estatal de Azúcar*, a government agency which in this instance cooperates with the private sector, especially regarding price policies. These sugar mills include the large Río Haina plant which produced 166,000 tons of sugar in 1967 and the La Romana mill which produces 200,000 tons a year and is owned by the Gulf and Western Corporation. All these mills are concerned almost exclusively with filling the annual United States quota of 600,000-700,000 tons and meeting a domestic demand of 150,000 tons a year. Molasses is mainly exported but some is used by the local industry for a variety of purposes.

Except for clandestine slaughtering, meat is processed in over 1,000 slaughterhouses, providing the country with about two-thirds of its meat needs. Only a few of these slaughterhouses are modern and sanitary. Pork is a popular meat, and about 3,000 tons of ham, sausage, salami and other specialities are manufactured each year. A broiler industry based on imported hatching eggs is now developing. It provides some 20,000 tons of meat for local consumption every year. Tomatoes and beans are processed in rural plants which also market a variety of products like fruit juices, jams and preserved fruits and vegetables.

Rice is milled in over 50 plants which operate at a 60 percent extraction rate. The bran is exported for animal feed. There are about 24 companies producing beverages, both alcoholic and nonalcoholic. Two breweries utilize the 20,000-25,000 tons of hops that are imported yearly and have an output of about 32,000 tons of beer. Various plants produce carbonated beverages of different flavors and sugar content. There are 10 firms producing rum, while 1,000 tons of wine are derived from five small wineries.

F. FOOD SUPPLY

1. Storage [24] [1]

Little information is available on the amount of food on hand by category at a given time. These foods are in the *campesino's* hut, in the shops, in government warehouses and in importers' storage facilities. Storage space belonging to retailers of farm produce is also available around city markets, but the capacity is small and shortages are acknowledged at all levels in spite of the rapid turnover of merchandise. The staples found in these market stores consist of rice, red and black beans, and some leafy vegetables that can hold from one market day to the next. The balance on hand mentioned in government statistical tables is positive only for sugar, syrups and cocoa beans. The Government keeps prices down on certain goods estimated to be of prime necessity, but how this is done without throwing surpluses on the market is not clear and where these surpluses, if any, are housed is not stated.

The Dominican Government is promoting regional sales of agricultural products and conceivably must control some storage space, but details are lacking. A recent observer reported verbally that one of the greatest problems facing Dominican agriculture is the creation of an efficient system for gathering, storing and moving agricultural products to market. To this end, a great effort should be made to multiply the all-weather roads, expand storage space, including refrigerated facilities, and establish a market information system.

2. Transportation [1] [2]

Transportation in the Dominican Republic is primarily by road. The highway system encompasses over 9,000 kilometers of roads, half of which are paved and only one-third of which are passable all year round. The means of transportation vary from foot to pack animals to bicycle, private car and bus. The buses, which are nonscheduled, are usually loaded with farmers' wives taking their wares to market. Their large burlap bags full of goods are carried on the roof. As stated earlier, the lack of adequate farm-to-market roads is an important deterrent to the creation of a sizable food supply in the country. The lack of a centralized agency, such as a cereal board, which could regulate the marketing of basic dietary staples is perhaps a consequence of the inadequacy of the road network.

The railroad is not developed and there are no large rivers which could serve as a unifying communication network. There is only one major airport, located at Punta Caucedo, near Santo Domingo. There are 18 harbors but only eight are important to international trade: Santo Domingo, San Pedro de Macorís, La Romana, Barahona, Pedernales, Salcedo, Puerto Plata and Azua. Santo Domingo is the only one equipped with the silos and refrigeration needed to store food delivered from abroad.

III. DIETS

A. GENERAL [6] [22] [24] [1]

As in most developing countries, the Dominican diet is low in protective nutrients and proportionally high in energy staples. In 1967, the Government published a balance sheet of the foods available in the territory of the Republic in 1964 which may be optimistic in quantities but is realistic in terms of the composition of the fare. This study brings to the fore the usual discrepancy between the favorable concentration of natural resources and their uneven utilization and distribution. Incomes are generally low, both in the rural and urban areas. A study made by Norvell, Billingsley and McNeely in 1966 revealed that in the prosperous city of Santiago where 173 households were investigated, 19 percent of the families had incomes of less than $50 a month. The median income of all households was $100 a month, 60 percent of which was spent on food. Such a constraint precludes saving and the formation of capital to finance economic development. It must be remembered that a typical Dominican family includes at least five persons and not uncommonly seven, eight or nine.

A large portion or the rural two-thirds of the population lives on a marginal subsistence level. A 1969 nutrition survey (Sebrell, King et al.) disclosed that the majority of the people examined not only have poor diets but also have suffered from malnutrition all their lives. This allows the conclusion that malnutrition in the Dominican Republic is an important public health problem. As in other developing countries, this is evidenced by the high rate of infant mortality due to the synergistic relationship between malnutrition and infectious disease.

Chronic malnutrition is the result of a way of life typified by the dependency of a large family upon the output of a very small plot of land. Cash for the purchase of supplementary food is extremely limited and is obtained by selling the occasional surpluses reaped from the family plot or by hiring out as temporary fieldhands during the harvest season. Because field workers are numerous, the pay is low, seldom exceeding $1.65 per day. At best, employment is available 50 percent of the time. Malnutrition is also common in the urban areas where it is precipitated by unemployment and the lack of financial resources which cannot be compensated by subsistence farming.

The average family partaking in the diets to be described lives in a two-room house *(bohío)*. One room is for sleeping and the other for preparing meals and eating. The basic diet revolves around rice and beans, as in most Caribbean countries. Other foods frequently eaten are plantains, manioc, corn and sweet potatoes, the latter more in some regions than in others. Meat is usually represented by beef and pork although chicken consumption is increasing. Goats provide milk and meat, even in the urban areas where they are seen trotting at the periphery of the city. Table No. 7, condensed from the government study mentioned previously, gives an idea of the availability of the foods but not of their consumption. Hence, the actual intake is less than the optimistic estimate shown in the table.

In 1964, after adding imports, deducting exports, seeds, animal feed and crops allocated to industrial uses, there was an availability of cereals in the amount of 154 grams per capita per day. Rice was the main cereal, followed by wheat (in the form of bread) and corn. According to the same computation, tubers provided 198 grams of food, mostly derived from manioc and sweet potatoes. Sugar and molasses contributed 85 grams per day, mostly in the form of raw noncentrifugal sugar. Legumes are important as a source of protein, and 47 grams per capita per day are available in the Dominican markets. About 85 percent of the legumes consumed are grown locally. Nuts are valuable foods because of their protein and fat content. A variety of species exist, especially fresh and dried coconuts (in the amount of 16 grams per capita per day). Many kinds of vegetables are seasonally offered in the markets at the level of 42 grams per capita per day. The most popular are tomatoes and onions. Fruits enter into the daily diet at what may seem the enormous rate of 751 grams per capita per day. However, these are largely starchy fruits, since plantains represent about half of the consumption and bananas almost one-fourth. Avocados, oranges and mangoes are also favorites.

The meat supply totaled an average of only 50 grams per capita per day. Almost half of this is beef, with chicken and pork providing most of the balance. Eggs are scarce: an average of only 10 grams per capita per day is available, which means about one egg per week per person. Milk and milk products provide 146 grams per capita per day, mostly in the form of fresh fluid milk. Fish, which is not popular in the Dominican Republic, is available at the low rate of 17 grams per capita per day. Only 5 grams are fresh fish; the rest is imported salted cod or otherwise preserved fish.

Visible fats are present in the diet at the rate of 26 grams a day, coming mostly from groundnut or coconut oil. A variety of beverages are used, contributing an estimated 38 grams per person per day. More than half consists of beer and the rest is mainly coffee, although other beverages, especially cocoa, furnish about 3 grams of the daily diet.

B. SPECIAL DIETS [24] [21]

As expected, there is a difference between rural and urban diets. Sebrell, King et al. found that most of the fluid milk, fresh vegetables and fruits are consumed in the rural areas. This indicates a rather low overall level of economic development. As industrialization expands, these foods will be increasingly channeled to the urban trade and the farmer who wants milk or oranges will have to buy them at the nearest city supermarket. Meat is more frequently consumed in urban areas. Hence, ascorbic acid, vitamin A and calcium are available to the *campesino* but he misses energy values, proteins, iron, niacin and thiamine.

Sebrell, King et al. also found distinguishable regional differences. The eastern districts appear to have better diets than other regions and the southwest is the most unfavorably served. But the differences seem to be small and the investigators concluded that specialization of the corrective programs by area would not be justified. Pregnant women suffer most, not so much because their diets are different but because, as mentioned earlier, given a marginal consumption of nutrients their condition demands a dietary supplement which they do not receive. As everywhere else, the preschool child is also seriously victimized. Yet, considerable efforts are being made to provide better nutrition for the mass of the population. The Government of the Dominican Republic has recently opened the first of a series of economy restaurants where luncheons can be had at a cost of 25¢. It is planned to expand this experiment to other parts of the country.

C. LEVELS OF NUTRITION [24] [20] [6]

Table No. 8 shows what the intake of calories and basic nutrients should be, according to the recommended allowance of the U.S. National Academy of Sciences, and what the mean intake actually was among subjects covered by the 1969 survey made by Sebrell, King et al. These investigators found inadequate consumption of protein, calories, iron, retinol (a component of the vitamin A complex essential to visual perception), ascorbic acid, folic acid, niacin, calcium, riboflavin, zinc, magnesium, pyridoxine, alphatocopherol, vitamin B_{12} and copper. They determined that 15 percent of the population survives on the least adequate diets while another 15 percent enjoys the most abundant fare. However, even among the most favored people, instances of significant nutritional deficits of some vitamins and minerals are found.

In terms of calories, the investigators found an average intake of 1,634 for the whole country, with a maximum of 2,301 at Guaymate and a minimum of 1,062 at Mella and Angostura. The average deficit amounted to 24 percent. Moreover, 29 percent of all households examined received less than 66 percent of the recommended caloric allowance. If we consider that, on the basis of the country's overall food supply, at least 2,265 calories were available per capita in 1964 (see Table No. 7) and that, according to all testimonies, more food is available now, it becomes obvious that there must be a serious imbalance in distribution and probably an important amount of wastage. The solution to the distribution problem deserves high priority since it controls the effectiveness of food use. What is the point in increasing food supplies if the increments do not reach the consumer?

The same range of shortages was found to exist for protein. Average intakes were 18.1 percent short of recommended allowances, and in absolute numbers varied between a maximum of 68 grams per day at Guaymate and 28 grams at Mella and Angostura. This deficiency was confirmed by the biochemical study of blood samples. The 1969 investigators (Sebrell, King et al.) reported that in most areas visited, 54 percent of the children under 6 years of age had serum protein values below the acceptable level. On a national average basis, 67 percent of young children had serum albumin levels below the acceptable level. In the National District the proportion of children in this category rose to 85 percent, pointing to an increased protein nutrition problem in the urban environment. This finding is not uncommon in developing countries, following the cityward migration of recent years. The ratio is also distressingly significant among adults since 36 percent of all households investigated had less than 66 percent of the recommended protein allowance. "Less than acceptable" includes several levels of inadequacy, the lowest being "deficient." The categorization of inadequacy varies with age, sex and other circumstances. Deficient values were found in 30 percent of all children from 0 to 5 years of age, 11 percent of those aged 6-17 and 7 percent of those over 17 years of age. The northern region and National District seemed to be the most affected for all ages. The sulphur-containing amino acids (cystine, methionine and tryptophane, the last a precursor to niacin) are among the most limiting in the Dominican Republic diet, according to Sebrell, King et al. At 41 grams per day, total fat in the diet was 18 percent short of the recommended allowance, although this could be offset by the availability of natural food fats.

Calcium nutrition is not satisfactory. A daily availability of 693 milligrams was reported for 1964 while in 1969 Sebrell, King et al. found among low-middle-income groups an average per capita consumption of only 317 milligrams per day with a maximum of 541 milligrams and a minimum of 111 milligrams. Thus, even the sample with the highest calcium consumption did not reach the national average of available calcium, underlining the importance of a sound distribution system. Phosphorous was found to be consumed in significant quantities with a slight excess on a nationwide basis. Iron consumption in 1969 averaged 10.6 milligrams per capita per day against a recommended allowance of 14 milligrams and an availability of 15.4 milligrams. The investigators found that the maximum intake among their samples reached only 13.4 milligrams, while the minimum dropped to 7.4 milligrams. The shortage appears to be on the order of 24.3 percent. Thirty-four percent of the households investigated had intakes lower than 10 milligrams per capita per day and, as expected, anemia was found frequently.

The amount of vitamin A consumed averaged 943 international units per capita per day. The usual recommended allowance is 5,000 international units but lesser quantities are often considered acceptable for adults under certain conditions. However, an intake of 943 units is definitely a very low average, about 81.7 percent short of the minimum acceptable. The availability of vitamin

A is as high as 3,976 international units, on the basis of 119.4 milligrams of retinol (see Table No. 7). If all the observations on which these figures are based are correct, then a considerable amount of vitamin A is lost between the harvest of the foods available and their ingestion and assimilation by the body. Sebrell, King et al. found a generally inadequate intake of this vitamin, which is consistent with the clinical signs of avitaminosis A observed among the people examined. Yet, the plasma concentration of active principle was less than acceptable in only 10 percent of the subjects and that of formed vitamin A in only 9 percent of the subjects. Such discrepancies between deficient intakes and blood values are frequently encountered in surveys. The clinical observations often reveal symptoms that are expected, considering the inadequate consumption, but surprising when contrasted against plasma levels. Obviously, more research is needed regarding the metabolism of vitamin A.

The average consumption of thiamine on a national basis was found to be approximately 0.77 milligrams or 96 percent of the recommended allowance of 0.8 milligrams. The lowest consumption was 0.46 milligrams and the high 1.11 milligrams. In 1964, availability of this vitamin was found to be 1.17 milligrams, pointing once more to a lack of proper utilization of the resources. Biochemical studies confirmed this unsatisfactory picture by revealing that the urinary excretion of thiamine, which is a test of actual consumption, was less than acceptable among 46 percent of young children and 70 percent of those over 13 years of age. Yet, no symptoms of beriberi have been reported.

The average daily per capita consumption of riboflavin was found to be 0.66 milligrams, equivalent to a shortage of 45 percent against the recommended allowance. This is a quite common finding in underdeveloped countries. The recommended allowance is 1.2 milligrams. The 1964 availability was 1.06 milligrams. Best average intakes within the population surveyed reached 1.04 milligrams, lowest 0.26 milligrams. Again, young children below the age of 4 were the greatest sufferers with 48 percent showing a urinary excretion of riboflavin at less than acceptable levels. This situation improved among adolescents (over 13 years of age), only 16 percent of whom excreted riboflavin in unsatisfactory quantities. The clinical examinations again were consistent with the deficiencies found in the diet and in the body fluids.

The theoretical dietary supply of niacin makes 15.17 milligrams of niacin available daily to each inhabitant. Sebrell, King et al. found an actual consumption of 9.4 milligrams per capita per day. Since the recommended allowance is 14 milligrams, a shortage of 67 percent was revealed. Low values of 6.9 milligrams were found and a high of 14 milligrams, equivalent to the optimum, was recorded. Yet, the investigators discovered that urinary excretion of N-methylnicotinamide was acceptable in 93 percent of the subjects in spite of the fact that 71 percent of all people examined obtained less than 67 percent of the recommended daily consumption. The reasons for this discrepancy are not clear and could be due to many causes.

The study of ascorbic acid nutrition revealed an interesting fact, pointing to the need for biochemical assessments of nutrients in blood and urine before reaching conclusions in nutrition surveys. The national supply of ascorbic acid, also known as vitamin C, comes to 186 milligrams per capita per day, almost four times as much as the recommended allowance of 48 milligrams. Yet, actual consumption of this vitamin amounted to only 36 milligrams per capita per day. A study of its concentration in the serum showed that 64 percent of the samples-almost two-thirds of the people examined-had less than acceptable concentrations. This is explained by the fact that most of the ascorbic acid supply found in the diet is derived from plantains (132 milligrams per capita per day) and roots (45 milligrams). These foods are always eaten cooked and ascorbic acid is destroyed at temperatures éxceeding 54°C. The deficiency is further confirmed by the clinical picture (see *Nutritional Disease Patterns*).

Other important deficiencies were spotted by the investigators. Folic acid, whose role is vital in the production of red cells and in the prevention of megaloblastic anemia, was found to be consumed at the rate of only 71 percent of the daily recommended dosage with a wide range of deficiencies. Fifty-one percent of the children under 12 years of age, 47 percent of adult males and 66 percent of adult females had low hemoglobin values.

Pyridoxin, also known as vitamin B_6, was determined to be short in the amount of 50 percent. Alphatocopherol (vitamin E) was generally found wanting in the proportion of 62 percent of the recommended allowance. Finally, vitamin B_{12} presented a 70 percent deficit. Turning to the minerals, zinc and magnesium were also in significant shortage. The role of zinc in growth and development of the child appears to be more and more important as revealed by recent research. Pregnant and lactating women are always vulnerable population groups and Sebrell, King et al. reported finding the following percentages of "unacceptable" levels: thiamine 64 percent; hemoglobin 46 percent; total serum proteins 42 percent; plasma vitamin C 68 percent; and plasma vitamin A 5 percent.

IV. ADEQUACY OF FOOD RESOURCES [6] [22]

Obviously, the present food resources of the Dominican Republic do not provide good nutrition. Yet, the potential for an adequate diet is there, since 1,067,000 hectares of arable land and 828,000 hectares of pastures could easily take care of at least 4.2 million people. Moreover, the resources of the sea are still poorly exploited. With appropriate education, the right foods could be made to appear desirable. The system of distribution could be improved and the apparent large losses or wastage could be avoided or at least reduced. Unless people are made aware of the importance of nutrition, however, they will continue to suffer, regardless of their incomes. Of course, both education and food distribution are contingent upon good communication between minds as well as between places. In practice, this means education in food economics and it means better roads.

The Cibao Valley abounds in fertile soils which could make for a bountiful harvest, but some of the best land is preempted for cane. The sugar is exported and the food bought with its earnings costs far too much for the pocketbook of the ordinary man. An excellent program is now under way to teach the farmers' wives how to prepare a sound menu with local sources at acceptable prices, and the mothercraft centers and school lunch programs are rapidly improving the nutrition of children. It is true that the Republic does not import any food that it could not grow at this time and that rice imports have fallen to practically nothing from 32,000 tons a year in 1963. But imports of wheat reached 133,400 tons in 1968. Vegetable fats are still bought abroad at about the rate of 18,000 tons a year, some from the United States under concessional arrangements. Milk is still a significant item on the import list which could eventually be produced at home.

Given the potential for adequacy, it would seem that the program aimed at reaching this potential and fulfilling the promises of the land could be successfully expanded. Agriculture should be reoriented in favor of food crops at the expense of cash crops if new land cannot be found. Iodine and vitamin deficiencies could be overcome through fortification.

V. NUTRITIONAL DISEASE PATTERNS [24] [5]

A look at Tables 6 and 7 should suffice to convince anyone that serious nutritional deficiencies must exist in the Dominican Republic. We are indebted to the work of Drs. Sebrell, King et al. for much of the data on which this section is based. their 1969 survey of nutritional status in the Republic is a model of thoroughness and is rich in information and good judgement. The picture of nutritional diseases is graphically expressed in tables which give in detail findings by age group, sex and regional distribution.

In all, Sebrell and his fellow investigators examined 5,515 subjects, including 1,237 children 0-4 years of age, 1,802 children from 5 to 12 years old and 2,476 people over 12 years of age. Only 39 percent of the people examined were free of any type of lesion that could be attributed to nutritional deficiency of some sort. Among the very young children (0-4 years), 71 percent were free of symptoms. Among the 5-12-year-olds, 41 percent were without lesions and among those aged 12 or more, only 22 percent were unaffected, giving the impression that the number of malnourished people increases with age. No significant variation could be found between different districts, with the exception of the National District where the percentage of people free of lesions increased 50 percent. Very young children seemed to fare better in the urban districts of Santo Domingo and Santiago where unaffected children amounted to 72-83 percent. Elsewhere the rates among the very young ranged from 53 to 69 percent.

In a hospital survey of 400 children under the age of 4 made by DeNova between November 1966 and February 1967, 39 percent of the children were found to have severe kwashiorkor and 5.5 percent were said to have marasmus. Only 114 or 28.5 percent were diagnosed as normal, 39 (9.8 percent) were considered to have Grade I malnutrition, 87 (21.7 percent) Grade II and 160 (40 percent) Grade III.* In their 1969 survey, Sebrell, King et al. found normal children of the same age represented 25 percent of the number examined, those with first degree malnutrition 49 percent, those with second degree 22 percent and those with third degree 4 percent. Signs of protein deficiencies as expressed by depigmented and staring hair were found in 0.9 percent of the children below 4 years of age. Of course, no statistical comparision is possible between hospital data, such as DeNova's, where the sick cases are concentrated, and the results of a survey based on randomly selected samples of presumably healthy people. The two studies do confirm, however, that a significant number of children under the age of 4 have kwashiorkor, and that protein-calorie malnutrition is not an unusual occurence.

The children seen by DeNova also showed a number of skin symptoms. Thirty percent had gastroenteritis and diarrhea. Others had frequent vomiting, edema and anorexia.

Anemia is frequent in the Dominican Republic, as shown by DeNova's finding that 90 percent of the 400 children admitted to the hospital during his study had hemoglobin levels below 10 grams per 100 milliliters. DeNova also determined that 10 percent of the children at the hospital had sickle-cell anemia. Sebrell, King et al. found that 11-30 percent of all the children investigated in their survey, 12-56 percent of the males over 12 years and 10-26 percent of the females above the age of 12 had hemoglobin concentrations below 10 grams per 100 milliliters. There was a great difference in rates between districts. Children in the southwest were three times more frequently affected with anemia than children in other districts. No reason was put forward for this discrepancy. Males over 12 in the eastern districts were deficient in hemoglobin at the rate of 56 percent and females at the rate of 25 percent. An in-depth investigation of the ecological factors which are probably responsible for this phenomenon has not yet been made.

Among 0-4-year-old children, symptoms often attributed to vitamin A defi-

---

*Grade I = weight 10-24 percent below normal standard.
 Grade II = weight 25-39 percent below normal.
 Grade III = weight 40 percent or more below normal.

ciency, such as follicular hyperkeratosis, xerosis and crackled skin, and staring hair were present at the rate of 0.9 percent, 2.6 percent and 8.4 percent, respectively. Eye symptoms, including dryness of the conjunctivae, were also discovered at the rate of 0.2 percent. Various signs suggesting possible presence of scurvy in its early stages were found.

The study of growth and development and anthropometric measurements made by Sebrell, King et al. revealed that in most children the birthweight is normal but between 12 and 18 months a delay in the normal curve of growth begins to appear which persists until the age of 16. At age 14, both boys and girls appear to be underweight by 17 and 27 percent, respectively. Other anthropometric measurements confirmed this observation regarding delayed growth. Head circumference was comparable only to the lowest percentile of the norm and according to a chest/head circumference ratio developed by Jelliffe, the figure found in the Dominican Republic would indicate a widespread protein-calorie malnutrition syndrome among infants under 2 years of age. Wristbone maturation is slow compared to United States and even to Central American data. Development of stature was found to be significantly slowed down, to the point where at age 15 the children are shorter than standards by 11 or 12 centimeters.

Sebrell, King et al. found some interesting regional differences. In the National District, the Cibao Valley and the eastern provinces, cases of third degree malnutrition were more common in urban than in rural areas. This is where the large cities of Santo Domingo and Santiago are located and where the problem of nutrition among the jobless is far more serious than among the unemployed in the countryside. In the southwest, in Pedernales Province, however, they found that Grade III malnutrition was more common in rural areas. This is the least fertile province in the country and one of the poorest, in spite of the recent development of the bauxite loading facilities at Cabo Rojo.

A serious pathological picture emerges. Multiple signs usually ascribed to nutritional deficiencies are frequently found. Among the most common are symptoms of riboflavin deficiency. Conjunctival infection was present in 75 percent of the subjects seen by Sebrell, King et al., angular lesions of the lips in 2.8 percent, angular scars in 6 percent, and cheilosis in 4.9 percent. Symptoms associated with vitamin A deficiency, such as follicular hyperkeratosis and crackled skin, were found in 10.3 percent of the subjects and dryness of the skin in 3.9 percent. Redness and swelling of the gums suggestive of insufficient ascorbic availability were seen in 36.3 percent.

This picture of frequent multiple signs, not very significant in themselves but highly significant when grouped together, is further confirmed by the biochemical findings in the body fluids. As everywhere in Middle America, enlarged thyroid glands and goiter are a significant problem in certain districts. On a nationwide basis, Sebrell, King et al. found that the problem begins to exist in

3.1 percent of boys between 6 and 12 years of age and 7.26 percent of the girls in the same age group. It increases with age to what appears to be a maximum at 13-17 years among girls, of whom 20 percent are affected compared to only 10.12 percent of the boys. The occurrence among adult women is 17.81 percent. The highest endemic districts are the Cibao Valley (26.5 percent of all females) and the southwestern provinces (22.6 percent).

VI. CONCLUSIONS

The Dominican Republic has many factors in its favor, including the existence of a relatively large amount of good land, permitting both crop cultivation and pasturage, and its favorable location as an island surrounded by the resources of the sea. The problem of producing the food required for the population can easily be solved and the goal of attaining self-sufficiency in food can readily be reached. Given these facts, it should be possible to pinpoint the major areas in which profitable changes could be effected. The food deficit areas are milk, rice, fish and fats. These should be changed to food surpluses through a number of rather simple procedures, the most important of which might involve returning to food crops or to pastures some of the land that has been allotted to cash crops, especially sugar. To do this, a change of philosophy is required, and this may be the most difficult of all changes. One must accept the fact that cash crops produced with cheap labor do not convert into cheap food from foreign markets. At best, they convert into expensive food, in most cases meat, milk or processed foods which are priced above the means of the majority. They also convert into manufactured goods which usually do not fit into the way of life of the *campesino*. When the circuit is completed, sugar or coffee earn foreign exchange which, in turn, buys high quality beef, poultry, airplanes or automobiles which never trickle down to the man who produced the sugar or the coffee. The two-class system that leads to so much unrest, sometimes to revolution, is perpetuated and there is no real development in the country.

If, on the contrary, the surplus agricultural production consisted of more rice, more wheat, more vegetables and fruits, more meat and milk, the returns in foreign exchange might or might not be smaller than they are now, but the diet and income of the producer would certainly be better. Moreover, this good diet would be assured before the conversion from coffee to airplanes has taken place. The improved diet would secure for the producer the first step on the road to standard of living equalization, without which no real development can ever occur. Together with this basic change of policy, less dramatic steps could be taken. These would enhance and multiply the effect of improved diets.

The most important of these further steps is education; not the kind of education that makes a minor bureaucrat but the type that makes a clever, informed, industrious farmer and a wise and competent mother. Simultaneously with the increased acreage in food crops, communications within the rural areas and from the rural areas to the cities and maritime outlets should be improved. This would permit the export of food surpluses in increased quantities. Agricultural credit for farmers should be expanded and so should storage facilities. These would be needed to gain control of the markets, both at home and abroad. Such a program, summarized here in a few words, but full of extended possibilities, a program which would start by minimizing the price of food and giving an immediate reward to the producer of food, is well within the capabilities of a land as rich as the Dominican Republic.

BIBLIOGRAPHY

1. American University (Foreign Area Studies). *Area Handbook for the Dominican Republic.* DA Pam No. 550-54. Washington, D.C., U.S. Government Printing Office, 1966.

2. Bateman, R.H. "Basic Data on the Economy of the Dominican Republic." *Overseas Business Reports.* OBR 68-114. Washington, D.C., U.S. Government Printing Office, 1968.

3. Buck, W.F. *Agriculture and Trade of the Dominican Republic.* ERS-Foreign 330. Washington, D.C., U.S. Department of Agriculture, 1972.

4. DeMoya, C.S. "The Dominican Republic Diversifies Exports." *Foreign Agriculture,* 1970, VIII (38), 7.

5. DeNova, H.R. "Incidencia de la Desnutrición Proteino-Calórica Infantil en el Hospital de Niños Robert Reid Cabral." *Archivos Dominicanos de Pediatria,* 1969, 5 (1), 3-10.

6. Dominican Republic, Government of (Oficina Nacional de Estadistica). *Hoja de Balance de Alimentos para la República Dominicana.* No. 5. Santo Domingo, Oficina Nacional de Estadistica, 1967.

7. *Encyclopedia Britannica.* Chicago, William Benton, Publisher, 1970.

8. *FAO Monthly Bulletin of Agricultural Economics and Statistics* 1969-1971.

9. Food and Agriculture Organization of the United Nations. *Production Yearbook 1970.* Volume 24. Rome, FAO, 1971.

10. _____.*Trade Yearbook 1970.* Volume 24. Rome, FAO, 1971.

11. *Foreign Agriculture,* 1969, VII (11), 8.

12. _____, 1969, VII (36), 7-8.

13. _____, 1972, X (13), 14.

14. Inter-American Development Bank. *Eleventh Annual Report 1970.* Washington, D.C., IDB, 1971.

15. _____ . *Socio Economic Progress in Latin America.* Washington, D.C., IBD, 1971.

16. International Bank for Reconstruction and Development. *Statement of Loans–June 30, 1971.* Washington, D.C., IBRD, 1971.

17. James, P.E. *Latin America.* Fourth Edition. New York, The Odyssey Press, 1969.

18. King, K.W. "Malnutrition in the Caribbean." *The State of the Species* (A special supplement in the *Natural History* Magazine), January 1970.

19. Leung, W-T. Wu. INCAP-ICNND *Food Composition Table for Use in Latin America.* Washington, D.C., U.S. Government Printing Office, 1961.

20. National Academy of Sciences (National Research Council). *Recommended Dietary Allowances.* Seventh Revised Edition, 1968. Washington, D.C., NAS, 1968.

21. *The New York Times.* October 3, 1971.

22. Norvell, D.G., Billingsley, R.V. and McNeely, J.G., *The Internal Food Distribution System and Marketing Channels for Plantains and Tomatoes in the Cibao Valley of the Dominican Republic.* College Station (Texas), Texas A & M University, 1967.

23. Paxton, J. (ed.). *The Statesman's Yearbook 1970-1971.* New York, St. Martin's Press, 1970.

24. Sebrell, W.H., King, K.W., Webb, R.E., Daza, C.H. et al. "Nutritional Status of Middle and Low Income Groups in the Dominican Republic." *Archivos Latinoamericanos de Nutrición,* 1972, 22 (Numero Especial), 1-190.

25. United Nations (Department of Economic and Social Affairs). *Demographic Yearbook 1969.* New York, UN, 1970.

26. United Nations Children's Fund. *Digest of Projects Aided by UNICEF in the Americas.* New York, UNICEF, 1969.

27. United Nations Development Program. *Projects in the Special Fund Component as of 31 January 1971.* DP/SF/Report Series B. No. 11, New York, UNDP, 1971.

28. U.S. Agency for International Development. *A.I.D. Economic Data Book– Latin America.* Washington, D.C., A.I.D., 1970.

29. U.S. Department of Agriculture (Economic Research Service). *Agriculture and Trade of the Caribbean Region.* ERS Foreign 309. Washington, D.C., U.S. Government Printing Office, 1971.

30. _____. *Food Balances for 24 Countries of the Western Hemisphere. Projected 1970.* Washington, D.C., USDA. Undated.

31. U.S. Department of Commerce (Bureau of International Commerce). "Dominican Republic." *Foreign Economic Trends and Their Implications for the United States.* ET 71-031. Washington, D.C., U.S. Government Printing Office, 1971.

32. _____ . (International Marketing Information Service). *Best U.S. Sales Prospects in the Dominican Republic.* IMIS 69-23. Washington, D.C., U.S. Government Printing Office, 1969.

33. U.S. Department of Labor (Bureau of Labor Statistics). *Labor Law and Practice in the Dominican Republic.* BLS Report No. 343. Washington, D.C., U.S. Government Printing Office, 1968.

34. West, R.C. and Augelli, J.P. *Middle America: Its Lands and Peoples.* Englewood Cliffs, Prentice-Hall, 1966.

LIST OF TABLES

LIST OF MAPS

TABLE NO. 1

Population by Province – Dominican Republic, Mid-1967 Estimate

Province	Population	% Urban*	Density* (per sq km)
National District	725,607	79.6	491.6
Azua	95,550	20.9	42.1
Bahoruco	63,092	20.8	51.6
Barahona	97,183	43.2	43.0
Dajabón	56,624	18.7	62.8
Duarte	201,567	22.2	168.6
Elías Piña**	51,995	11.7	?
El Seibo	139,387	17.7	52.2
Espaillat	138,035	14.9	162.9
Independencia	33,479	42.1	20.4
La Altagracia	82,331	17.0	?
La Romana	47,612	61.5	13.6
La Vega	280,974	16.3	97.6
María Trinidad Sánchez	123,456	9.9	88.3
Montecristi	71,491	34.4	40.8
Pedernales	17,765	42.6	11.9
Peravia	128,609	21.6	89.3
Puerto Plata	185,895	16.5	118.3
Salcedo	90,419	12.9	189.7
Samaná	56,534	19.0	61.3
Sánchez Ramírez	130,872	7.8	108.0
San Cristóbal	333,359	15.2	90.4
San Juan	191,717	17.8	56.4
San Pedro de Macorís	71,962	33.3	80.6
Santiago	338,134	33.8	125.6
Santiago Rodriguez	46,650	12.4	53.4
Valverde	89,091	40.0	138.7
Total	3,889,390		

*Order of magnitude
**Also called San Rafael or La Estrelleta.

Sources: R.H. Bateman, "Basic Data on the Economy of the Dominican Republic."
Encyclopedia Britannica.

TABLE NO. 2

Area Devoted to Major Crops – Dominican Republic, 1948-1970
(in 1,000 hectares)

	Annual Average 1948-1952	1964	1965	1966	1967	1968	1969	1970
Corn	40	22	20	25	25	28	28	31
Rice	44	57	76	76	81	88	82	82
Potatoes	–	1	1	1	1	1	2	2
Sweet potatoes and yams	11	11	11	11	10	11	10	–
Manioc	18	15	15	15	13	14	14	–
Dry beans	27	17	21	51	41	34	43	40
Pigeon peas	27	27	27	27	27	27	27	27
Groundnuts	23	50	50	48	46	46	72	72
Cottonseed	–	5	5	3	1	1	1	1
Sesame seed	1	1	1	1	1	1	1	1
Onions	1	–	3	3	3	3	3	–
Tomatoes	–	–	1	2	2	2	2	–
Cowpeas	27	27	27	27	27	27	27	27
Bananas	18	13	20	20	20	19	13	–
Cocoa beans	–	–	134	–	–	–	–	–
Coffee	76	–	–	–	–	148	–	–
Tobacco	18	19	19	20	19	18	18	20
Cotton	–	5	5	3	1	1	1	1
Sisal	–	1	1	1	2	2	2	–
Sugarcane	100	116	120	120	142	120	135	152

Sources: Food and Agriculture Organization of the United Nations, *Production Yearbook 1970.*

FAO Monthly Bulletin of Agricultural Statistics, 1969-1971.

TABLE NO. 3

Production of Major Crops – Dominican Republic, 1948-1970
(in 1,000 tons unless otherwise stated)

	Annual Average 1948-1952	1964	1965	1966	1967	1968	1969	1970
Corn	42	43	38	43	39	40	43	50
Rice	70	143	167	178	147	181	195	200
Potatoes	4	15	16	18	20	20	21	21
Sweet potatoes and yams	95	100	99	100	97	100	86	–
Manioc	148	153	152	153	152	155	170	–
Dry beans	24	30	30	37	30	27	34	32
Pigeon peas	16	21	21	21	21	22	21	22
Grapefruit	2	2	2	2	3	3	3	3
Lemons and limes	5	7	7	7	7	6	6	6
Oranges and tangerines	34	56	56	57	58	58	58	58
Groundnuts	15	50	45	51	45	47	70	70
Cottonseed	–	3	3	2	1	1	1	1
Sesame seed	4	3	3	3	3	3	3	3
Coconuts (million nuts)	29	73	73	75	75	77	77	–
Onions	4	3	14	18	17	17	17	–
Tomatoes	4	6	22	35	57	72	76	–
Cabbages	1	–	2	2	2	2	2	–
Cowpeas	16	21	21	21	21	22	21	22
Pineapples	4	–	5	6	6	7	7	–
Plantains***	953	1,418	1,422	1,422	238	250	250	–
Bananas	208	252	270	238	238	250	250	–
Cocoa beans	30	25*	30	30	28	28	40	30
Coffee	27	40	36	44	42	44	43	45
Tobacco	19	19	19	20	18	16	21	25

TABLE NO. 3 (continued)

Production of Major Crops – Dominican Republic, 1948-1970
(in 1,000 tons unless otherwise stated)

	Annual Average 1948-1952	1964	1965	1966	1967	1968	1969	1970
Cotton	–	1	2	1	1	1	1	1
Sisal	.3	–	.4	.3	1	1	1	–
Sugarcane	4,788	5,197	6,012	6,952	7,651	5,682	6,800	8,030
Raw sugar	552	580**	691	819	668	864	1,043	1,180
Copra	1	–	–	3	5	6	3	3

*This estimate is too low. All sources consulted, including FAO, concur that 26,000 tons of cocoa were exported in 1964. The Government of the Dominican Republic gives a 1964 production figure of 41,283 tons.

**This estimate is also too low since FAO concurs with other sources that over 650,000 tons of raw sugar were exported in 1964.

Sources: Food and Agriculture Organization of the United Nations, Production Yearbook 1970.

FAO Monthly Bulletin of Agricultural Statistics, 1969-1971.

***W.H. Sebrell et al., "Nutritional Status of Middle and Low Income Groups in the Dominican Republic."

TABLE NO. 4

Number of Livestock – Dominican Republic, 1948-1970
(in 1,000 head)

	Annual Average 1948-1952	1966	1967	1968	1969	1970
Cattle	711	1,000	1,050	1,082	1,090	1,100
Pigs	739	1,200	1,250	1,275	1,300	1,330
Sheep	27	79	81	82	83	84
Goats	310	790	780	780	775	760
Chickens	1,924	6,300	6,500	6,700	7,000	7,200
Ducks	32	74	75	76	77	78
Geese	1	1	1	1	1	1
Turkeys	51	245	250	255	255	260

Source: Food and Agriculture Organization of the United Nations, *Production Yearbook 1970.*

TABLE NO. 5

Major Agricultural Exports – Dominican Republic, 1963-1969
(in tons unless otherwise stated)

	1963	1964	1965	1966	1967	1968	1969
Cattle (head)	—	—	—	—	3,000	5,100	—
Meat (fresh, chilled, frozen)	—	—	—	1,300	480	5,090	5,160
Corn (unmilled)	—	—	2,800	4,400	—	800	—
Citrus fruit	1,144	585	301	182	82	51	—
Bananas	119,750	69,080	48,020	10,620	1,450	4,080	3,220
Coconuts (in shell & dry)	4,348	5,899	4,008	4,104	6,488	5,774	4,911
Onions (fresh)	—	—	—	—	9	30	—
Legumes (dried)	650	640	230	200	250	10	—
Tomatoes (fresh)	—	220	220	100	550	680	960
Sugar (raw basis)	652,300	650,300	521,000	548,300	646,500	604,800	632,100
Coffee	27,510	34,390	24,560	25,380	22,190	23,520	27,650
Cocoa beans	23,780	26,220	22,430	25,940	23,930	25,270	23,820
Oilseed cake and meal	14,770	19,950	7,080	22,150	27,420	16,050	13,860
Tobacco	16,744	25,258	14,861	12,703	19,993	16,480	18,235
Copra	7,100	6,990	5,630	2,850	4,880	1,400	—
Cotton (raw)	670	390	650	110	—	—	—

Source: Food and Agriculture Organization of the United Nations, *Trade Yearbook 1970.*

TABLE NO. 6

Major Agricultural Imports – Dominican Republic, 1963-1969

(in tons unless otherwise stated)

	1963	1964	1965	1966	1967	1968	1969
Cattle (head)	400	200	100	200	700	500	1,000
Meat (fresh, chilled, frozen)	1,670	690	80	50	30	50	–
Dried meat	82	111	40	76	66	52	–
Meat preparations	439	826	225	380	299	291	354
Milk and cream (evaporated, and condensed)	1,440	3,330	2,900	6,310	7,020	7,810	3,910
Milk and cream (dry)	3,000	6,700	2,580	5,590	3,940	7,140	7,830
Fluid milk	–	–	–	–	–	800	–
Butter	589	612	21	51	24	203	–
Cheese	482	423	232	348	330	520	–
Eggs (in shell)	–	22	27	236	628	509	763
Cereals (total)	95,800	87,900	78,400	86,000	86,900	133,400	76,500
Wheat & wheat flour	63,400	60,200	55,400	77,300	79,200	117,400	76,500
Rice	32,300	21,900	22,100	–	–	13,000	–
Corn	–	3,900	–	400	5,500	3,000	–
Pears, grapes, apples	1,054	952	924	1,000	931	516	1,230
Raisins	266	217	107	199	164	175	–
European potatoes	2,190	2,590	1,130	2,090	580	470	930
Legumes (dried)	4,880	10,520	2,220	1,070	3,310	4,110	6,060
Onions	2,667	3,358	1,578	2,262	33	186	1,440
Hops	34	58	17	7	23	24	34
Peppers and pimentos	140	124	83	108	131	158	–
Margarine, etc.	54	254	98	210	19	14	–
Wines (hectoliters)	3,400	2,900	3,300	4,100	2,100	3,700	–
Tobacco	886	417	470	474	858	840	–
Groundnuts	–	–	–	12,800	27,560	5,370	16,000
Natural rubber	130	130	70	60	50	70	90
Fish oils	37	34	29	32	35	–	–
Animals fats	3,480	4,770	2,750	6,100	7,480	5,760	8,150
Soybean oil	–	112	3,050	4,654	7,195	18,786	11,900
Cottonseed oil	–	682	289	2,674	200	1	2,500

Source: Food and Agriculture Organization of the United Nations, Trade Yearbook 1970.

TABLE NO. 7

Availability of Foods Per Capita Per Day – Dominican Republic, 1964
Estimated Population = 3,500,00

Foods		Net Availability (tons)	Per Capita Per Day (g)	Calories	Proteins (g)	Fats (g)	Calcium (mg)	Phos. (mg)	Iron (mg)	Vit. A (mg*)	Thiamine (mg)	Ribo. (mg)	Niacin (mg)	Ascorbic Acid (mg)
Cereals	Subtotal	197,135	154	556	13.5	2.0	23	209	2.3	18	0.22	0.08	2.4	0
	Rice	108,010	84	308	6.0	0.5	7	87	1	0	0.07	0.02	1.3	0
	Corn	24,828	19	70	1.8	0.8	2	56	0.5	14	0.08	0.02	0.4	0
	Wheat flour	48,280	38	138	4.4	0.5	7	37	0.5	0	0.04	0.03	0.5	0
	Paste	9,666	8	24	0.9	0.2	3	23	0.2	1	0.03	0	0.2	0
	Others	6,351	5	16	0.4	0.0	4	6	0.1	3	0	0.01	0	0
Roots	Subtotal	252,807	198	191	1.9	0.4	43	67	1.6	19	0.14	0.06	1.15	45
	Manioc	117,961	92	100	0.5	0.2	24	32	0.7	3	0.04	0.03	0.48	27
	Others	134,846	106	91	1.4	0.2	19	35	0.9	16	0.10	0.03	0.67	18
Sugars and sweets		108,559	85	310	0	0.3	30	25	2.3	0	0.01	0.06	0.17	1
Legumes		60,160	47	142	9.0	0.7	40	118	2.9	6	0.25	0.09	1.05	5
Nuts, oilseeds	Subtotal	21,193	17	26	0.5	2.3	5	12	0.2	traces	0.01	0	1.17	0.5
	Coconuts	19,318	16	20	0.3	2.0	1	6	0.1	traces	0	0	0.07	0.5
	Others	1,875	11	6	0.2	0.3	4	6	0.1	traces	0		1.10	0
Vegetables		53,629	42	18	0.6	0.1	8	16	0.3	60	0.02	0.01	0.19	6

Fruits	Subtotal	959,412	751	478	5.0	5.0	57	144	3.3	915	0.27	0.23	3.59	132.5
	Plantains	452,654	355	274	2.3	0.4	17	80	2.0	600	0.15	0.08	1.29	52.0
	Bananas	173,297	136	90	1.1	0	9	25	0.3	28	0.04	0.05	0.6	13.0
	Mangoes	91,486	72	21	1.0	0	4	4	0.3	221	0.02	0.02	0.14	19.0
	Others	241,975	188	93	0.6	4.6	27	35	0.7	66	0.06	0.08	1.56	48.5
Meats		64,860	51	103	7.0	8.1	4	73	1.1	107	0.06	0.08	2.17	0.3
Eggs		13,419	10	14	1.0	1.0	5	19	0.2	12	0.01	0.03	0.01	0
Fish		22,319	17	39	7.2	1.0	97	64	0.4	1	0.09	0.04	1.02	0
Milk		185,925	146	115	7.0	5.1	279	167	0.6	52	0.07	0.37	0.19	1.7
Vegetable oils		34,023	27	227	0	26.0	1	0	0	4	0	0	0	0
Beverages		49,076	38	37	1.5	1.8	18	27	0.4	0	0.01	0.01	2.0	0
Miscellaneous		4,008	3	9	0.3	0.8	2	1	0	0.4	0.01		0.06	0.06
Total				2,265	54.5	54.6	604	942	15.6	1,194.4*	1.17	1.06	15.17	186.06

*1 international unit = 0.3 micrograms of retinol

Source: Government of Dominican Republic (Oficina Nacional de Estadística); *Hoja de Balance de Alimentos para la República Dominicana.*

TABLE NO. 8

*Comparison Between Availability of Nutrients, Recommended Allowance
and Findings by Sebrell et al. −
Dominican Republic, 1969*

	Amount Available[a] (1964)	Recommended Allowance[b]	Sebrell et al. Findings[c] (mean)	Shortage or Excess (%)
Calories	2,265	2,136	1,634	−24
Proteins (g)	54.5	55	45	−18.1
Fats (g)	54.6	50*	41	−18.0
Calcium (mg)	693.0	515	317	−38.4
Phosphorus (mg)	962.0	515	579	+12.0
Iron (mg)	15.4	14	10.6	−24.3
Vitamin A (IU)	3,976	5,000	943	−81.7
Thiamine (mg)	1.17	0.8	0.77	−96.0
Riboflavin (mg)	1.06	1.2	0.66	−45.0
Niacin (mg)	15.17	14.0	9.4	−67.0
Ascorbic acid (mg)	186.06	48.0	36.0	−75.0

*The minimal requirement of fat is not known. It is usually accepted that 20 to 25 percent
of the caloric intake should be supplied by fats.

Sources: [a]Government of the Dominican Republic, *Hoja de Balance de Alimentos para la
República Dominicana.*

[b]National Academy of Sciences (National Research Council), *Recommended
Dietary Allowances.*

[c]W.H. Sebrell, K.W. King et al., "Nutritional Status of Middle and Low Income
Groups in the Dominican Republic."

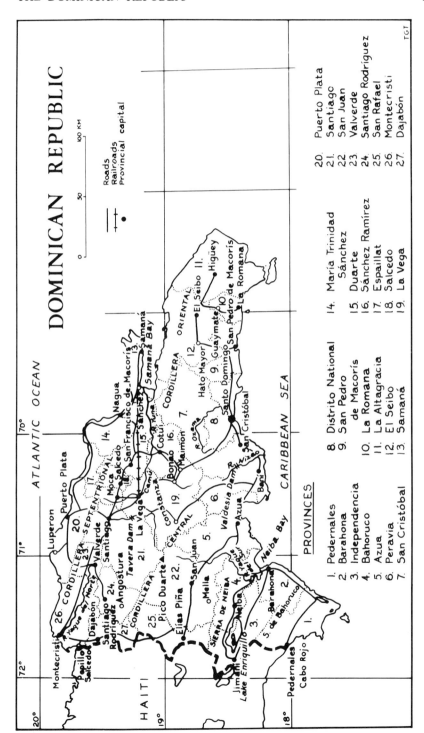

DOMINICAN REPUBLIC

ATLANTIC OCEAN

CARIBBEAN SEA

HAITI

Roads
Railroads
Provincial capital

100 KM

MAP NO. I.

PROVINCES

1. Pedernales
2. Barahona
3. Independencia
4. Bahoruco
5. Azua
6. Peravia
7. San Cristóbal

8. Distrito Nacional
9. San Pedro de Macorís
10. La Romana
11. La Altagracia
12. El Seibo
13. Samaná

14. María Trinidad Sánchez
15. Duarte
16. Sánchez Ramírez
17. Espaillat
18. Salcedo
19. La Vega

20. Puerto Plata
21. Santiago
22. San Juan
23. Valverde
24. Santiago Rodríguez
25. San Rafael
26. Montecristi
27. Dajabón

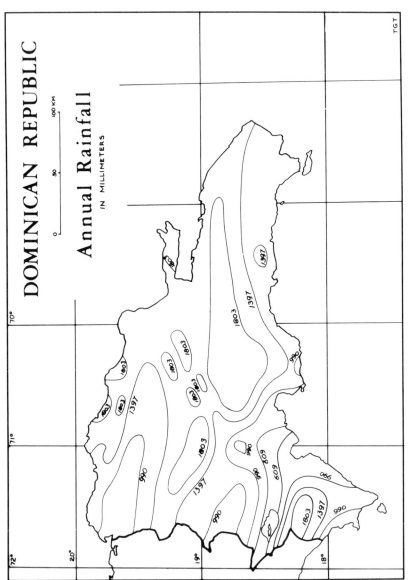

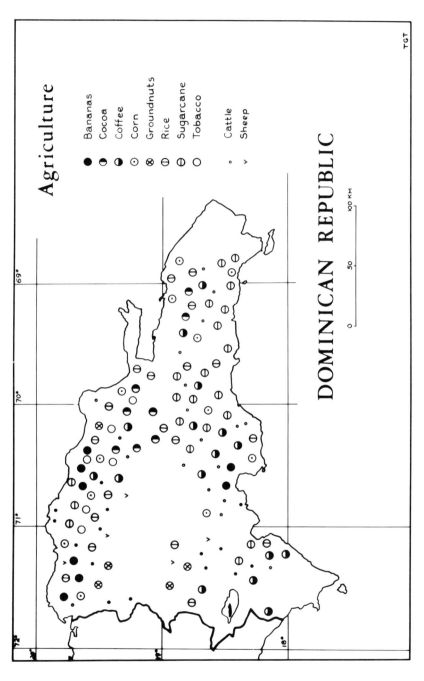

MAP NO. 3.

THE COMMONWEALTH
OF PUERTO RICO

TABLE OF CONTENTS

245

THE COMMONWEALTH OF PUERTO RICO

I. BACKGROUND INFORMATION

A. PHYSICAL SETTING [16] [42] [21] [36]

The Commonwealth of Puerto Rico lies about 70 nautical miles west of Hispaniola. Measuring about 160 kilometers in length (east-west) and averaging 56 kilometers in width, the roughly rectangular island covers about 8,891 square kilometers, of which about 886,000 hectares are land. The small adjacent islands of Mona, Culebra and Vieques (totaling 223 square kilometers) belong to the Commonwealth. Uninhabited Mona Island lies about 50 nautical miles southwest of the Puerto Rican port of Mayagüez and encompasses about 5,180 hectares of limestone plateau covered with infertile soil, poorly watered by restricted rainfall. Culebra Island lies off the eastern end of Puerto Rico, opposite the port of Fajardo, and has about 573 inhabitants. Vieques is located 10 nautical miles to the southeast of Puerto Rico and covers 16,000 hectares. This island's population of 7,210 is engaged in subsistence farming.

Like other islands in the Greater Antilles group, Puerto Rico is traversed by a central mountain spine (the Cordillera Central) fringed by coastal plains. The cordillera lies south of the island's east-west axis, rising sharply on the west coast and merging with the Sierra de Luquillo in the northeast and the Sierra de Cayey in the southeast. The southern slopes of the Cordillera reach almost to the coast and drop abruptly to a narrow but productive coastal plain. The northern slopes are gentler, leading to a broader, more fertile plain than that found in the south. The island is watered by numerous rivers, most of which rise in the mountains and drain north or south to the Atlantic Ocean or the Caribbean Sea. The major concourses are the Rio Grande de Loiza, the Rio de la Plata and the Rio Grande de Arecibo in the north.

The island can be divided into three principal geographic regions: the lowlands, the highlands and the hill country.

The Lowlands

The lowlands, which are found mainly along the coast, make up about 27 percent of the island's area. There are small inland valleys near Caguas and Cayey. When sufficient water is available, the lowlands become Puerto Rico's most fertile areas. Rainfall is abundant in the north but irrigation is required in the south, especially in the Lajas Valley where extensive irrigation works have been constructed by the Government. Most of the island's sugar crop is grown in the lowlands and pineapples are cultivated near Arecibo. Where soil fertility is lacking, the land is used for pastures. About half of the island's dairy industry is concentrated in the northern coastal lowland.

The Highlands

The rugged mountainous terrain of the central highlands covers about 36 percent of Puerto Rico's land area. In spite of gradients ranging from 30 to over 60 percent, the land in this region is extensively cultivated wherever fertility permits. Coffee is the main crop from the westernmost part of the highlands to the center, grown at the 300-900-meter level in the shade of orange, grapefruit, avocado and banana trees. Tobacco is the principal commercial crop in the humid eastern highlands, accompanied by subsistence farming and animal husbandry.

The Hill Country

About 37 percent of Puerto Rico's land area is rolling hill land. In the northeastern and north-central part of the hill country, limestone belts (similar to the Cockpit country of Jamaica) with steep cliffs, caves, caverns and sinkholes abound. Subsistence farmers cultivate vegetables and fruit, mainly pineapples and grapefruit, on small plots in the irregular valleys of the region. Some small farmers also cultivate sugarcane and tobacco.

In general, the soils of Puerto Rico suffer from erosion and exhaustion. Heavy fertilization could make the farmland productive but fertilizer is expensive since most of it is imported from the continental United States. As a result, it is used sparingly and yields are generally low. Large and small farmers alike practice crop rotation but the small farmers are seldom able to leave enough land fallow to allow real restoration of the soil's fertility. Erosion is a serious problem and is controlled primarily by making hillside plantings in crisscross furrows which slow down the runoff. Terracing is practically nonexistent and contour plowing is just beginning to gain acceptance.

B. CLIMATE [16] [42] [36]

Although Puerto Rico lies just within the tropics, the island's climate is very pleasant. The average annual temperature is 24°C. Even at higher altitudes, frosts have not been recorded, although they may occur. Warm weather is tempered by cool sea breezes. Rain-bearing trade winds bring an average of 1,890 millimeters of rain to the island each year. The rainy season extends from May to November but precipitation rarely lasts for more than a few hours at a time. There is a greater islandwide variation in rainfall than in temperature. The rain forest of Sierra de Luqillo receives an average of 4,673 millimeters each year while the Lajas Valley receives only about 762 millimeters. Tropical storms occasionally hit the island between July and October, bringing 150-200-mile-per-hour winds and torrential rains, but they rarely last more than a day.

C. POPULATION (35) (36) (17) (16) (42) (34) (2a)

The population of Puerto Rico, which was estimated to total 2.87 million in 1969, is expected to top the 3 million mark in 1972. In recent years it has grown rapidly, due primarily to improved health conditions which have drastically lowered the death rate.* Between 1901 and 1960, the island's death rate fell from 36.7 to 6.7 per 1,000 but the birth rate declined much less, giving a high rate of natural increase. The infant mortality rate is about 28.3 per 1,000 live births. Life expectancy for males in 67 years and for females 72 years.

The overall density is about 340 persons per square kilometer, one of the highest rates in the world. Emigration to the United States has provided an important outlet for Puerto Rico's population pressures with the result that the actual rate of growth is only about 1.5 percent per year. The table below shows the net flow of migration to and from the islands between 1955 and 1970.

Annual Average Migratory Movement
To and From Puerto Rico, 1955-1970

Movement	1955-1960	1960-1965	1965-1970
Emigration	−55,400	−37,000	−74,000
Immigration	+15,400	+30,000	+52,000
Net Emigration	−40,000	− 7,000	−22,000

Source: Commonwealth of Puerto Rico (Oficina del Gobernador – Junta de Planificación), *1970 Informe de Recursos Humanos al Gobernador.*

The variation reflects changing economic opportunities in both the mainland United States and Puerto Rico. It has been estimated that 64.1 percent of the emigrants are from rural areas. The pattern is to migrate from the countryside to Puerto Rican cities and from there to the mainland. Between 1960 and 1970,

---

*A significant effort has been made in Puerto Rico to control population growth voluntarily. In 1937 a law was passed which legalized the publication of contraceptive information and education in contraceptive methods. In 1969 there was an active family planning service in the Northeast Region operated by the Department of Obstetrics and Gynecology of the Medical School of the University of Puerto Rico. In other regions, a private organization, the *Asociación Puertorriqueña por Bienestar de la Familia* (Family Welfare Association of Puerto Rico), uses private physicians to provide contraceptive services.

Puerto Rico's urban population increased by 42 percent until it accounted for 57 percent of the total. The major cities are San Juan (the capital), Ponce, Mayagüez, Arecibo and Caguas. Table No. 2, showing the population distribution by regions, reveals that San Juan, the most urbanized region, is also the most populated.

The Puerto Rican population is primarily of Spanish descent with some intermixture of Negro and Indian (Arawak or Boriquén) strains. Those indigenous Indians who were not killed by disease or hard labor were soon absorbed by the Spaniards after the conquest of Puerto Rico. African slaves were introduced in the 16th century but, in contrast to the situation in most other islands of the Caribbean, the Negro population has remained the minority group. At present only about 20 percent of the population is classified as nonwhite although the "white" classification is based on sociocultural factors rather than blood lines.

Puerto Rico has two official languages, English and Spanish, but only about 400,000 people are estimated to be bilingual. The rest speak Spanish only. Spanish is used throughout the school system and English is taught as a second language. Ninety percent of all Puerto Ricans between the ages of 6 and 18 attend school. The literacy rate for the general population is at least 85 percent. About 80 percent of the population adheres to Roman Catholicism; the remainder are primarily evangelical Protestants.

The standard of living of the Puerto Rican population has improved considerably since 1947, as evidenced by the pattern of personal consumption expenditures. The table below shows the change in such expenditures, expressed in constant dollars.

Selected Personal Consumption Expenditures –
Puerto Rico, 1947 and 1970
(in millions of 1954 dollars)

Type of Product	1947	1970	Percent Increase
Total personal consumption	645.6	2,521.9	290
Food	250.9	547.8	118
Alcoholic beverages and tobacco	58.3	181.4	211
Clothing and accessories	66.2	268.0	305
Housing	54.1	268.7	454
Household operations (home maintenance)	65.1	388.8	497
Medical care and death expenses	23.4	101.8	335
Transportation	41.7	353.9	749
Recreation	37.5	212.0	465
Education	3.2	34.4	975
Other	52.5	316.0	502
	652.9	2,672.8	
Less: Expenditures of nonresidents	− 7.3	− 150.9	
	645.6	2,521.9	

Source: Commonwealth of Puerto Rico, *Statistical Yearbook.*

The table may serve to assess the level of progress. On the basis of the figures given, education heads the list in terms of increased expenditures. The Plan indicates that there is a heavy emphasis on vocational training. The smallest increase of all consumption indices concerns food, which cost the average Puerto Rican only twice as much in 1970 as it did in 1947. This is interesting, given the fact that, except for milk and milk products, more food was imported in 1970 than in 1947 and hence was more expensive. The notion comes to mind that the food budget of those who have ridden the crest of the wave of progress is higher and represents better food but that those who have not yet caught up with the momentum are, dietetically speaking, perhaps faring worse rather than better. However, in 1947 food accounted for 38.6 percent of the total personal budget while in 1970 it represented only 21.5 percent. This is a considerable improvement, as it frees 16.9 percent of the budget for the purchase of other goods and services. Indeed, for all nonfood items, 1970 consumption was four to eight times higher than the 1947 level. The importance of tourism is perhaps measured by the fact that in 1947 the consumption of nonresidents was 1 percent of total personal expenditures while in 1970 the proportion reached 5.5 percent. Mention should be made at this point of the fact that these figures represent a constant value for the dollar, hence are not distorted by the inflation that took place between 1947 and 1971.

D. HISTORY AND GOVERNMENT [42] [36] [15] [15a]

Puerto Rico, discovered by Columbus in 1493 during his second voyage to the New World, was first named San Juan Bautista. A permanent colony was not established until 1508 when Ponce de Leon brought small groups of settlers to the island. Eventually the capital city came to be called San Juan and the island Puerto Rico. Puerto Rico remained a Spanish possession from the 16th to the end of the 19th century but was the object of intermittent attacks by other European powers. French, British and Dutch raiders all tried unsuccessfully to capture the island. In July 1898, during the Spanish-American War, United States troops occupied the island and in December of the same year Puerto Rico was ceded to the United States.

A military government ruled until 1900. From that time onward, the island has had an anomalous relationship to the United States. The Foraker Act of 1900 established civilian government and made Puerto Rico neither territory nor state but a body politic called "the people of Puerto Rico" entitled to the protection officials were appointed by the President of the United States; only the members of the House of Delegates were elected by the people of Puerto Rico. The Act stipulated that Puerto Rico should be represented in the U.S. House of Representatives by an elected Resident Commissioner who, however, had no vote. In line with the American tradition of no taxation without representation, the Act exempted Puerto Ricans from U.S. federal taxes.

The Jones Act of 1917 gave U.S. citizenship to all Puerto Ricans and gave the islanders more responsibility for initiating local laws. In 1947, an amendment to the Jones Act was passed, allowing the Puerto Ricans to elect their own governor who could appoint his own cabinet, with the advice and consent of the Puerto Rican Senate. In 1950 another law was passed to allow the people of Puerto Rico to "organize a government pursuant to a constitution of their own adoption." A constitutional convention was held and in 1952 the Common-wealth of Puerto Rico was proclaimed. In 1967, a plebiscite was held to determine whether the island should continue in its association with the United States or become an independent nation. About two-thirds of all registered voters participated and 99.4 percent voted to remain associated with the United States.

Concomitant with the acquisition of a greater measure of self-government since the end of World War II, has been a tremendous drive towards economic development under a program called "Operation Bootstrap." Faced with the realization that the island's only valuable natural resource was its labor force, in 1947 the Government of Puerto Rico decided to base its future development on industry. The Government used its own meager resources to create the infra-structure—water, power and transportation—which would be needed by indus-try, and to build plants for lease to private manufacturers. Vocational education programs were established for the island's labor force. The Government then sought out mainland United States firms to establish factories in Puerto Rico. Exemption from U.S. income taxes for a specified period, plentiful labor at low rates compared to the mainland, and a pleasant climate were all major attrac-tions for U.S. manufacturers. The Puerto Rican Economic Development Admin-istration was established to seek out new industries and to assist them in starting up operations on the island. The program has had unprecedented success. In 1947, less than 10 percent of the island's labor force was employed in manufac-turing and the per capita income was estimated to be $272. By 1968 more than 143,000 or 17.6 percent of Puerto Rico's workers were employed by industrial firms and per capita income had risen to $1,123.

The structure of the Commonwealth Government closely resembles that of the mainland states. Under the present constitution, executive power is vested in the Governor, who is elected by universal popular suffrage for a 4-year term. Legislative power resides in a bicameral legislature composed of a 32-member Senate and a 64-member House of Representatives. A nonvoting Resident Commissioner is elected for a 4-year term to represent the island in the U.S. House of Representatives. The judiciary is headed by a 9-justice Supreme Court appointed by the Governor. Puerto Rico remains exempt from U.S. federal taxes.

E. AGRICULTURAL POLICIES [32] [19] [36] [41]

Although the main thrust of Puerto Rico's development plan has been to encourage the expansion of industry, attention is also being given to the improvement of agriculture. The 1969-1972 plan allocated $224 million or 6.6 percent of the total plan budget to agriculture, as shown in the following table.

Planned Government Outlays by Sector – Puerto Rico, 1969-1972
(in millions of dollars)

Sector	Dollars	Percent
Education (primary, secondary and vocational)	846	24.8
Education (university)	200	5.9
Industrial development	274	8.0
Agricultural development	224	6.6
Commercial development	32	.9
Public welfare	232	6.8
Housing	400	11.7
Transportation	396	11.6
Electricity	152	4.4
Telecommunications	6	.2
Water and sewage	155	4.5
Health	499	14.6
Total	3,416	100.0

Source: Commonwealth of Puerto Rico (Office of the Governor – Puerto Rico Planning Board), *The Four Year Economic-Social Development Plan of Puerto Rico, 1969-72.*

The primary objective in agriculture is to accelerate the rise in productivity per man per hectare. Hence, the policy is to concentrate on developing farms in limited areas of the best plains in order to increase the yield of this good land and leave less desirable soil to be improved for pastoral purposes. While the income of nonfarm families has been rising, the relative net income among farm families has declined sharply since 1950. Agricultural employment figures have also declined, with the result that farm families have a high incidence of both open and disguised unemployment. In order to bring the agricultural sector up to the level of other segments of the economy, the Government has recognized the need to accelerate crop diversification, improve the marketing system and to provide technical education in the rural areas. During the plan period, the following specific measures are being undertaken to strengthen the agricultural sector:

1. The marketing system is being closely supervised in order to ensure farmers of more adequate prices for their products.

2. A system of crop insurance is being initiated to help stabilize farm incomes and offset natural hazards.

3. Farmer participation, especially in groups, in the supply of various services needed, such as marketing and processing, is being encouraged.

4. The Government is supplying ancillary services where justified.

5. Stronger incentives and subsidies to stimulate efficiency and to increase output are being developed.

6. The managerial and technical capabilities of farmers and other agricultural personnel are being improved by providing more government assistance for agricultural education and training.

7. The Government is improving the island's infrastructure by investing in such works as irrigation and drainage to increase the productivity of the land.

8. Methods for preserving the most suitable land for agriculture are being designed and implemented.

Through the payment of incentives, farmers in some areas are being encouraged to shift away from production of coffee, sugar and tobacco to vegetables, fruits, milk products and livestock, all of which are in strong demand on the island. The capital of the Agricultural Credit Corporation is being increased by about $2 million per year in order to permit expansion of the overall agricultural credit system. Agricultural machinery services are also being expanded.

It is anticipated that direct employment in agriculture will have declined from 85,000 in 1968 to less than 50,000 in 1972 as a result of efforts to raise labor productivity and income in the agricultural sector. The Right to Work Administration assists unemployed and displaced farm workers to obtain other employment. It is hoped, however, to retain as many families in the rural areas as possible by improving nonfarm employment opportunities, community services, rural housing and other facilities. Incentives are being given for the establishment of agricultural processing enterprises in rural areas which could take up some of the unemployment slack. It is estimated that the cost of rural-urban migration, in terms of shelter, necessities, social services, etc., is about $20,000 per farm family. Therefore, the investment in making rural life more attractive is well worth making.

The Government operates an agricultural experiment station network through the University of Puerto Rico. The main station is at Río Piedras, and six substations are located in different ecological zones, specializing in research as follows:

Corozal—beef cattle, fruits, starch crops, forages;
Gurabo—dairy cattle, tobacco, sugarcane, rice;
Isabela—vegetables, fruits, sugarcane;
Fortuna—fruits, sugarcane, vegetables;
Adjuntas—coffee, fruits;
Lajas—sugarcane, livestock, rice, irrigation, drainage.
The research program of the experiment stations is oriented towards "the

development of complete packages of practices aimed at securing high and efficient production in agricultural commodities." The major focus is on products for the domestic market. A demonstration program is being carried out (Farms 75) under which it is hoped that the modern technology and efficient systems of operation developed by the experiment stations will stimulate significant increases in production by 1975.

II. FOOD RESOURCES

A. GENERAL [23] [13]

The island itself produces itself a modest percentage of Puerto Rico's food resources; the majority of the food consumed is imported from the mainland United States. The indigenous part of the diet is derived from 272,000 hectares of cultivated cropland (30.7 percent of all land) and 332,000 hectares of prairies and permanent pastures (37.5 percent of the total land area). The agricultural land thus amounts to 68.2 percent of the total available, which is a rather large portion. While it is difficult to assess exactly how much land is used for food crops and how much for cash crops, a number of sources have indicated that food crops are more widely cultivated than cash crops, a wise but uncommon practice in the tropical belt. Table No. 3 gives the most recent approximation of land use.

It is interesting to recall here that the pattern of Puerto Rican agriculture during the last century of Spanish occupation was quite unusual in the West Indies. Perhaps because of the waning of Spanish dynamism throughout the world, few aggressive sugar plantations were developed and most of the land was owned by small farmers growing primarily food crops. This situation changed, however, during the first decades of the 20th century when, under the push of American enterprise, the pattern of cash crop monoculture (sugar) was established and Puerto Rico was caught up in the economic syndrome common to other Caribbean territories. It took the pull of "Operation Bootstrap" to restore the island to a regime more conducive to good diets. This is not to say that the Puerto Rican population now has the kind of diet it should have, but the tradition of small landowners growing some food crops has, to a certain extent, come back into its own.

Considerable attention is being given to the problem of land tenure, which includes the resettlement of squatters, the awarding of life tenure to contractual tenant farmers, especially those willing to farm 2-10 hectare lots, and the granting of sugar land to cooperatives. As a result of these and other rural-oriented assistance programs (see *Farms*), the food resources of Puerto Rico are larger and better distributed than those of any other Caribbean island.

1. Agricultural Labor Force [19] [34] [35] [25] [36]

The labor force of Puerto Rico has benefited from unusually favorable circumstances as a result of the overnight creation of industry in the island. Labor laws covering standards of work, bargaining powers, health and sanitation were established in the island even before there was a substantial industrial work force. In August 1971, the total labor force was estimated at 877,000 people 14 years old or over. This represented an increase from 671,000 in 1950 and 751,000 in 1967. Employment in agriculture decreased sharply during this period from an estimated 199,000 (or 29 percent of the total work force) in 1950 to 120,000 (or 15 percent) in 1967. In 1971 the agricultural labor force did not exceed 56,000 men and women or slightly more than 6 percent of the total. The decrease between August 1970 and August 1971 was 10,000. The small size of the agricultural labor force can be explained by the existence of part-time farmers and unpaid family labor.

From 1950 to 1954 the average annual contribution of agriculture to the gross national product was 21 percent; the proportion dropped to 9 percent in 1965. In 1950 agriculture was the second largest sector after the Government and now it is the smallest. Wages are low. In the food and allied branches of industry, the minimum wage rate in September 1969 was $1.03-$1.60 per hour, compared to $2.94 on the mainland. However, this rate is still much higher than anywhere else in the Caribbean. The comparatively low level of wages has resulted in attracting a variety of industries from the mainland and has contributed to rather impressive improvements in the standards of living of the Puerto Rican population. Industry has created jobs and put money in circulation among the people who needed it most.

In August 1971 the civilian labor force numbered 3 percent more than in 1970. The civilian, noninstitutional population* 14 years old or over was estimated at 1,871,000 people in August 1971 or 49,000 more than in August 1970. The rate of participation in the labor market was 66.8 percent for males and 28.1 percent for females. In August 1971 there were 111,000 totally unemployed people (an increase of 11,000 over the figure for August 1970) and 19 percent of the employed part of the force worked less than 35 hours a week. At the same time, there were 27,000 more people than in August 1970 working in nonagricultural professions, stressing further the switch from agriculture to other kinds of activities. The unpopular sugarcane sector suffered most (4,000 defections between August 1970 and August 1971); coffee was next hardest hit (3,000 defections). In 1970 it was found that January was the best month for employment in the agricultural sector, but in 1971, strangely enough, January was the worst month.

---

*Those not belonging to the army, police or other services.

Another significant problem is the paradox of high unemployment rates combined with a high number of unfilled positions. The explanation is that the jobs available require skills which the people seeking work do not have. The highest level of unemployment is in the 16-24 age groups. The 1969-1972 plan has provisions for intensifying vocational and technical training (see *Agricultural Policies*). Increasing attention is being given to the problem of seasonal unemployment: insurance against joblessness is being promoted; work and land programs are being developed; and efforts are being made to shift workers from one zone to another according to the seasonal demand for labor.

The causes of unemployment in Puerto Rico are the same as in other developing areas, in spite of the fact that Puerto Rico is far ahead of any country in the Caribbean on the road to development. In addition to lack of skills for the kinds of jobs that are open, the lack of entrepreneurship also contributes to the labor problem. This lack of entrepreneurship has resulted in most Puerto Rican industry being imported from the United States rather than being developed locally, thus making the island dependent upon mainland companies for the creation of new jobs. The availability of welfare from public or family sources also discourages some people from seeking employment as long as a well-educated relative with a good job agrees to meet his familial obligation toward a less-favored kin. The adoption of U.S. prejudices regarding work after a certain age in skilled positions creates vacancies at the top that cannot be filled; this results in a general slowdown which hinders availability of jobs at the bottom. This kind of unemployment is a consequence of rapid industrialization, which creates more jobs for skilled workers than for the unskilled who need them most. An important factor to note is that the light industry characteristic of Puerto Rico favors the employment of women, thus changing traditional unemployment and social patterns.

2. Farms [42] [15] [15a] [39] [32] [34] [18] [23] [16]

The history of farming in Puerto Rico is of considerable interest. One of the main agricultural problems in socioeconomic development is the conflict between large and small holdings. The former are preferable for efficient productivity but perpetuate a two-class society with opposing interests. The latter are inefficient, but the owner of a small farm is his own boss and can take pride in the complete independence and freedom he enjoys within his miniscule realm. The intermediate solution to the problem, the cooperative farm, requires a great deal of technical, administrative and political sophistication if it is to succeed.

Until the time of United States involvement in Puerto Rico, there was no history of large estates owned by absentee landlords. About 80 percent of the island's arable land was owned by smallholders operating farms of about 4.5 hectares each. Forty-five years later, only 16 percent of that land was left in the hands of the smallholders, most of whom had been absorbed by a few large sugar companies established after U.S. acquisition of the island. This situation developed in spite of the famous 200 hectares law passed by the United States Congress at the time of the occupation, which made it illegal for any agricultural corporation to possess more than 200 hectares of land. In 1940, it was reported that 100,000 hectares of land were in the hands of 51 corporations, one of which held over 20,000 hectares. The large estates with illegal excesses of land used these additional acreages to graze the oxen needed for the transportation of cane, a practice which is gradually becoming unnecessary as machinery is introduced.

In 1941 the Government of Puerto Rico passed a land reform law and created a Land Authority which purchased about 50 percent of the illegal properties in excess of 200 hectares. The Land Law provided for three types of settlement programs on the expropriated land: proportional-profit sugar farms (Title IV of the Land Law); an *agregado** settlement program (Title V); and a family farm program (Title VI).

Proportional-Profit Sugar Farms

On proportional-profit sugar farms (PPF), the workers share in the profits and the Government is responsible for field management and supervision, improvement of production methods, selection of cane varieties, financing crop production, collection of the proceeds, purchase of fertilizers and equipment, irrigation and drainage, repair of farm equipment, cattle and pastures, handling of labor negotiations, representation of the estate in all legal matters, and keeping records of costs and profits. The farm manager receives a salary and a fixed percentage of the profits; each laborer receives the prevailing wage plus a share of the net profits, in proportion to the days worked. The farms range in size from 100 to 500 hectares leased from the Land Authority by the manager.

The institution of profit-sharing farms has been a qualified success. The worker's benefit under the profit-sharing procedure may amount to 15 percent of his income, but in 1962 a review of the previous 11 years found that it had not been possible to maintain efficient performances because more capital and labor was used than was economically sound. However, the institution of PPF's has been beneficial to the island because it has resulted in creating jobs and producing sugar; but it has not been demonstrated that the system as conceived is efficient.

Agregado Resettlement

Under the *agregado* resettlement program, land deemed unsuitable for sugar cultivation or acquired specifically for Title V purposes, is allocated to landless

---

*An *agregado* is a landless head of family whose sole income is derived from agricultural wage labor.

families who had been forced to sell their own farms or whose land was purchased by the sugar estates during the 40 years following U.S. occupation. The parcels distributed range from 1,000 to 12,000 square meters. The land is ceded in usufruct to the recipients, the Government retaining the title. The usufruct may be passed on to heirs.

Family Farm Program

Some of the land purchased under the Land Authority Act has been distributed to farmers in lots not exceeding 10 hectares. The method of measurement was later changed to the market value of the plot, the maximum value allowed being $5,000. The land is distributed to beneficiaries under contracts of usufruct for life against a seminannual rent to be paid to the Land Authority. The beneficiary cannot sell or mortgage the land but can bequeath it to his heirs under certain conditions. He is free to cultivate his farm as he wishes, provided he respects accepted practices of conservation and production.

In addition to the original Land Authority purchases, the Government has acquired abandoned or inadequately cultivated land which can be divided into holdings of family size farms. These have been and continue to be sold to bona fide farmers who can do them justice and who are instructed in scientific agricultural techniques. The poorest land purchased by the Land Authority is given to the Department of Forestry. In 1955 the Government owned and operated 10 percent of the island's cropland and of this share, 25 percent was planted in sugarcane.

Although production practices have changed during the last decade, the transformation from small holdings to agribusiness is slow. However, this may be advantageous since rapid changes usually involve considerable individual suffering which, so far, the population of Puerto Rico has not experienced. Gradually more intensive use is being made of the land and mechanical equipment is being introduced.

The constant diminution of the number of rural inhabitants due to migration to the cities led the Government to the conclusion that no new dwelling units were needed in the rural areas during the last 4-year plan (1969-1972). In 1964 there were 44,859 farms covering 664,389 hectares, or 14.8 hectares each. These farms included some 200,000 farmhouses, 14 percent of which were considered inadequate. About 30,000 of them will be renovated or replaced. Twelve thousand of these will be remodeled by the inhabitants themselves and the rest will be improved or replaced with government assistance in one form or another. The housing program in rural areas includes the distribution or selling of lots on which to build new houses. Some of these lots will be prepared for construction. It is estimated that 5,000 will be sold and 9,000 granted, at a total cost to the Government of about $36 million. The whole housing program is an important mechanism for economic security and capital formation. It greatly contributes to the growth of a middle class, which is the most significant benchmark of development.

As a result of many factors, including rapid population growth and increased use of land for urban, industrial and other nonfarm activities, agricultural land is becoming less and less available in Puerto Rico. The fight against erosion and the emphasis on reforestation have also contributed to restricting the amount of land available for crops. Hence, between 1940 and 1970, farmland decreased substantially. In 1971 it was estimated that agricultural land amounted to only 546,000 hectares, a 9.5 percent drop since 1969 (see Table No. 3). This, however, has not prevented the development of large-size, modern dairy farms licensed by the Department of Agriculture (see *Animal Husbandry*) as well as many smaller unlicensed dairies. The larger farms are using milking machines and possess ultramodern equipment. The most significant group of dairy farms is located around the important market of San Juan and another group is centered farther to the west in the Arecibo area on the northern coast.

3. Fertilizers and Irrigation [19] [15] [15a] [13] [18] [36] [23]

Fertilizer use has increased considerably in recent years although not quite so fast as tractor use. Between 1940 and 1964 applications of fertilizer reached over 110 kilos per hectare of farmland and 295 kilos per hectare of cash crop land. These rates are higher than those found in any other Latin American country and even higher than rates reported for the mainland United States.

As shown on Table No. 4, the amount of fertilizer applied decreased between 1960 and 1969 as a result of the policy of limiting the amount of land under crops, especially under cane, and of favoring the expansion of pastures and reforestation. The trend (see *Agricultural Policies*) is to select certain plain areas for a concentrated effort on the best soil, returning mediocre land to fallow for recuperation. Table No. 4 shows the amount of fertilizer applied on the five most important crops. Sugarcane seems to have been the most drastically restricted as shown by the size of recent applications.

The Puerto Rico Irrigation Service was established in 1908 for the purpose of increasing production in the southeast. Thirty-nine thousand hectares of land are now under irrigation. The construction of Toa Vaca Dam, a $256 million project, will provide irrigation water to arable drylands in the south and south-central part of the island through tunnels to avoid evaporation. It is thus planned to reclaim several thousand hectares of land for cultivation in accordance with intensification policies. Other water diversions from the area north of the divide are intended to intensify cultivation on good soil still further. Further improvements in the regulation of waters from the Jacaguas River, upstream from the Guayabal Dam, will be effected by the drainage of the Guayabal Reservoir.

4. Mechanical Equipment [13] [19]

As more jobs were generated in light industry through the seeding of American enterprise, it became possible to replace human and animal power on the large farms with machines on a gradual basis. Tractors and other mechanized devices were introduced into Puerto Rico only after the Second World War. In 1960, there were 3,859 tractors and by 1968 there were over 5,000 of various types in service. This gives a rate of 108 hectares of farmland per tractor. With the exception of Canada, the mainland United States and Mexico, Puerto Rico is the only territory in the hemisphere with more than 1,000 tractors, and in Central America and the Caribbean it is the only one having more than 500 in service.

C. PRODUCTION [34] [13] [41] [16]

While industrial development in Puerto Rico has made great strides in the past 10 years, agricultural production has not kept pace. The average annual increase in farm income between 1960 and 1970 was a mere 0.8 percent per year. Only in the output of milk has domestic agriculture been able to meet the increased demand for foodstuffs created by rising family incomes in the manufacturing sector. Food imports have bridged the gap between production and consumption. About 90 percent of the food consumed in Puerto Rico is imported. Output of corn, bananas, sugarcane, cowpeas and many other crops actually fell during the 1960-1970 decade (see Table No. 6) while modest increases in production were obtained for plantains, peppers and pigeon peas. The only area in which there have been substantial production increases is the livestock industry, particularly in Grade A milk output, which doubled during the decade.

There is no doubt that the picture of agricultural production in Puerto Rico is changing rapidly. Patterns of food production now include more green and other vegetables, more fruits, and more livestock products, while cash crops are receiving continuous support in the form of subsidies, incentive payments to sugarcane farmers to induce rejuvenation of plantations, and additional irrigation. Food and cash crops are intermingled on the land of Puerto Rico. Food crops are grown practically everywhere: at the periphery of sugarcane estates, in the tobacco areas, next to the pastures and amidst the coffee bushes of the central and western districts. Cash crop areas can be defined roughly as follows: sugarcane around the coastline, forming a broken ring around the island; coffee in most of the western half of the Cordillera Central; tobacco in the eastern half of the same mountain range; and animal husbandry in between, with different specialized zones. Rotation practices, according to James, are as follows: in the east-central part of the Cordillera Central tobacco is planted first, yielding two crops between January and July, then several kinds of food crops are sown, after which the land is left fallow for pasture; in the western portion of the island, which is the coffee region, citrus fruit, bananas and vanilla are grown, either with or after the coffee crop.

1. Food Crops [13] [34] [41] [19] [23] [38]

a. Cereals

The cereals consumed by Puerto Ricans are practically limited to rice, corn and wheat with rice occupying the first place in the consumption pattern. In 1970, rice was no longer being produced commercially on the island, although at one time there were some upland rice paddies. Limited experimental plantings continue to be conducted in Lajas Valley. In 1970 corn was planted on only 3,000 hectares, representing a great decrease since 1949-1950 when a yearly average of 16,000 hectares was sown. Production consequently dropped from 10,500 tons to 4,000 tons over the same period (see Table No. 6). Wheat is not produced at all in Puerto Rico, or at least not in reportable quantities. All of these cereals, even corn, are imported from the mainland at a cost of $53 million a year.

b. Legumes

Legumes consist mainly of a variety of beans and peas, such as the red kidney bean and the very popular pigeon pea *(Cajanus cajan)*, the navy bean, the chickpea, the black-eyed pea, etc. Dry beans are now planted on about 4,000 hectares, producing 2,000 tons, a notable reduction since 1950 when 8,153 hectares were sown and 2,727 tons were produced. Cowpeas, which are now sown on just over 100 hectares yielding a crop of about 56 tons, were sown on 1,498 hectares in 1950, producing 454 tons. Pigeon peas now occupy 4,000 hectares and yield 5,000 tons. This represents decline from 1950 when the crop covered 8,097 hectares and production amounted to 3,136 tons, but an increase in yield per hectare.

c. Roots and Tubers

Starchy roots and starchy vegetables in general, called *viandas*, are traditionally cultivated on small farms in mountainous regions. The yields are low because the land is not good, and hence local demand exceeds production. An important supply of these roots has to come from the Dominican Republic. Sweet potatoes were planted on over 2,000 hectares in 1964, providing a crop of 6,000 tons, a reduction from 9,643 hectares and 14,545 tons in 1950. Yams have remained relatively popular. In 1970 the area sown with both yams and sweet potatoes was given as 4,000 hectares with a joint production of around 25,000 tons. Taro *(Colocasia esculenta)*, called *yautia* in Spanish, and malanga (*Xanthosoma* spp.) are cultivated on a number of farms, yielding a crop that has remained around

15,000 tons since 1950.* Manioc is estimated to grow on 1,000 hectares and to provide a harvest of 5,000 tons of root.*

d. Fruits and Vegetables

In 1970, the production of plantains was sufficient to meet the needs of the local diet. There are about 30 varieties on the island. No external trade in this crop is reported in available statistics. Since plantains can be processed into a variety of products, some farmers grow substantial amounts for the domestic food industry. No figures are available on the size of the area planted because the trees can be found almost everywhere. This fruit is a favorite starchy food and production is on the increase from 117 million units in 1950 to an estimated 243 million in 1968.* The demand for plantains is expected to rise. Banana trees, of which there are about 15 varieties in Puerto Rico, are often planted intermingled with coffee. In 1950, the area sown in bananas was given as 17,000 hectares but it appears to have dropped to 6,000 hectares in 1968, while production, reported at 209,000 tons in 1950, dropped to 112,000 tons in 1968. The problem concerning all starchy roots, fruits and vegetables is to reduce their price and find more industrial uses for them.

Of all the fruits that Puerto Rico produces, only pineapples are being harvested in increasing amounts. Grapefruit and orange production is hardly on the increase; avocados and coconuts are losing ground. It is believed that this decline of an otherwise obvious resource is due to the lack of adequate marketing channels, the long unproductive periods between planting and economic reward, competition, both from other producing countries and from other crops, and lack of pest control technology. Other fruits include mangoes, papayas and less well-known species such as the mammee apple or *mamey (Mammea americana)*, soursop or *guanábana (Anona muricata)*, guava, custard apple *(Anona reticulata)*, papaya, pomegranate, sapodilla *(Sapota achras)*, breadfruit or *panapén (Artocarpus incisa)*, and tamarind. Acerola *(Melpighia glabra)*, the fruit of a shrub, is rich in vitamin C.

The production of vegetables, such as pumpkins *(calabaza)*, peppers, chayote *(Sechium edule)* and tomatoes, is in the hands of small farmers and appears to be rather on the increase or at least remaining constant. Large seed plantings of tomatoes and other vegetables, as well as processing facilities for tomatoes, have been established on the southern coast, but are found also in more modest amounts in other parts of the island (experimental stations). Cabbage production dropped from over 8,545 tons in 1950 to 2,000 tons in 1970. The lack of interest of the Puerto Rican farmer in vegetables is surprising but perhaps reflects the change from an agricultural to a industrial economy. Eighty-five

---

*Since figures for these crops are uncertain, they have not been entered on Tables 5 and 6.

percent of the vegetables consumed in Puerto Rico came from the mainland at a cost to the island of over $48 million a year.

2. Cash Crops [13] [19] [39] [34] [23] [26]

Cash crops are still essentially represented by sugarcane, some citrus fruits, coffee and pineapple, with tobacco on the decline. The picture regarding pineapples is especially encouraging. The fruit is of good quality and has a high level of ascorbic acid per cubic centimeter. The gross receipt from the crop in 1970 was $69.3 million, slightly below the $72.7 million earned in 1969. The acreage in pineapples has not considerably increased, but thanks to good agricultural practices, the crop has passed from 27,700 tons in 1950 to over 60,000 tons in 1968. Pineapples are now Puerto Rico's most important fruit, economically. With the exception of two small private producers, the crop is almost entirely in the hands of the Puerto Rican Land Authority. The fruit is grown on large tracts of mechancially cultivated land. Forty-five percent of the crop is sold fresh and the balance is canned in different forms. Only 5 percent of the fresh pineapple is consumed locally. Exports increased by more than 50 percent between 1961 and 1970. The other leading fruit crops are oranges and avocados. Native oranges are obtained from wild trees which are often found growing on coffee plantations.

Sugarcane was planted on 148,000 hectares between 1948 and 1952. At that time, an average of 10 million tons of cane was produced each year. The reduction in acreage began in 1960 when only 135,594 hectares were planted, although the crop remained at approximately the 1950 level. In 1964, however, the area planted dropped to 113,000 hectares and the crop fell to 7.9 million tons. In 1970 the decrease in area was more obvious: 83,000 hectares were planted, yielding 4.6 million tons of cane. The number of sugar plantations dropped from 12,317 in 1963 to 7,753 in 1968. Yet sugarcane continues to be the most important agricultural activity, apparently producing 650,000 tons of sugar a year, almost one-third of the 1948 output. However, production figures are uncertain, and FAO estimates the output at only 450,000 tons a year, down from 1,157,000 in 1948. Whatever the exact production figure, this sugar is almost entirely consumed in the United States. Mechanization, as already stated, will soon be generalized throughout the industry in contrast to the other islands of the Caribbean (see chapters on Jamaica and Barbados). Mechanization is a necessity, given the disaffection from sugar shown by labor as a result of increased industrial employment opportunities.

Coffee production is increasing, encouraged by a program of technical assistance, subsidies and credits. The area planted in 1968 covered 64,00 hectares, producing 10,227 tons. The area was exactly the same as the 1950 but is scheduled to undergo a 50 percent decrease in the current plan period. The output of these coffee plantations has remained around 10,000 tons, except for a brief rise up to 17,000 tons in 1964. The reorganization of the plantation production system is considered imperative. Plastic nets for harvesting must replace the labor force and other technological improvements are needed to keep Puerto Rican coffee competetive on the world market

Tobacco covered 15,000 hectares in 1950 and the area was gradually reduced to 2,000 hectares in 1970. The drop in production is notable, down from almost 12,000 tons in 1950 to 2,900 tons in 1970.

3. Animal Husbandry [32] [18] [34] [13] [23] [19]

a. Livestock

In the early 1950's, the livestock industry of Puerto Rico was insignificant, but since that time it has been the object of steady promotion and has grown considerably, bringing increasing benefits to the population in the form of milk and dairy products. Table No. 7 shows the growth of the herds since the end of World War II. MacPhail has stressed the ecological significance of the change which has occurred, showing the cultural fusion that has taken place in the island since the American occupation. The opportunities for change offered by new American-inspired activities have resulted in modifications of the environment, oriented in this case toward better care of the herds which, in turn, has forced new ways of life on the inhabitants, both producers and consumers. Development of livestock implies development of pastures, increased irrigation and drainage, and improvement of the marketing system which, in turn, implies new roads and transportation facilities as well as credit for the producer, all of which greatly contribute to changes in the way of life, housing and diets. The growth of the livestock industry is perhaps one of the most important factors resulting from the contributing to an increase in the standard of living. The manufacturing sector, the growth of which is said to be the most important income-generating activity since 1955, may not be the most effective in improving health and nutrition.

The current 4-year plan continues to provide for upgrading and further expanding the livestock industry. An estimated increase of 72 percent in output is expected. From June 1953, when the program of pasture melioration was authorized by the Legislative Assembly, to 1968 the amount of improved pastures rose from 2,154 to 137,000 hectares. The grazing areas are scheduled for further increase as a result of the continued transfer of land from coffee and even sugar production to pasturage. From the start of the program, subsidies were given to farmers to remove weeds, fertilize the pasture, and seed with high-quality grasses, such as Pangola, Guinea and others. Irrigation was expanded, and silos, tanks and wells were constructed to facilitate feeding and watering of the herds. The use of silage enriched with the molasses produced by nearby sugarcane estates was encouraged. Gradually, the interest of the farmers focused on cattle, especially milk cows, but some attention has also been given to beef cattle which, according to the current plan, should increase by 111 percent within the 4-year plan period. The number of bovines rose from 343,000 in 1951 to 507,000 in 1969 and the quality improved vastly as work oxen were replaced by tractors and indifferent animals by breeders from both beef and milk lines.

The swine industry also received an impetus and the herd grew from 118,000 in 1951 to 194,000 in 1969 (see Table No. 7). The number of sheep (not shown in the table) remains static at about 4,000 head. Considerable encouragement has also been given to the poultry industry since 1960, with the result that the flocks increased from 2,063,000 in 1951 to almost 4 million in 1969. This reflects the large demand for poultry meat as nutrition improves and the number of tourists increases. The number of other animals, mostly horses and goats, diminished, horses from 36,000 in 1948 to 20,000 in 1968, and goats from 32,000 to 24,000.

b. Meat, Milk and Eggs

It is estimated that the consumption of meat has increased significantly during the last two decades. The amount produced in 1969 totaled 33,000 tons against 18,500 tons in 1950. The 1969 output was two-thirds beef and one-third pork compared to 56 percent beef and 44 percent pork in 1948. Although total meat production amounts to about 12 kilos per capita per year, it is not sufficient to meet the demand, and substantial quantities are imported every year, either in the form of frozen or chilled meat or as a variety of meat products. For every 40 tons of beef produced in the island, 60 tons are imported from the mainland United States. In 1968, the cost of meat from the mainland amounted to over $77 million and meat from other countries cost $16 million.

The amount of chicken meat produced locally totals about 11,500 tons. Roughly two-thirds of this output comes from the commercial chicken and broiler industry and the other third from noncommerical farms. The trend is, of course, for the housewife to increase her purchases of the commercially produced meat to the detriment of noncommerical sources. This is understandable in view of the fact that commercial farms, which benefit from economies of scale, can sell their output for 34¢ a pound compared to 68¢ a pound charged by noncommerical producers.

The number of milch cows has risen from 139,000 20 years ago to over 200,000 in 1969, exceeding planners' expectations by 15,000 head. In 1963, the milk production of cows in licensed dairies reached over 3,000 kilograms per animal per year, which is consistent with the output of an average milch cow on the mainland. The deliveries of Puerto Rican dairies in the agricultural year 1969/1970 reached nearly 313,000,000 liters priced at 18¢ a liter. This large production is made possible by modern equipment and by the strict sanitary supervision provided by the Department of Health. The Office of Milk Industry

Regulation of the Department of Agriculture and Commerce grants a first-class certificate to those dairies following prescribed sanitary production methods. In 1960 there were 704 licensed dairy farms, 528 of which were rated first-class. However, milk was sold by 2,911 farms, indicating that there are many unlicensed operators. First-class farms sell to 13 pasteurizing plants; others sell to several hundred distributors throughout the island. The Office of Milk Industry Regulation fixes the prices at the wholesale and retail levels.

MacPhail has delineated the regional distribution of dairy farms in Puerto Rico. As expected, the dairy belt around San Juan covers the largest area and produces 40 percent of all the milk sold in the island. Next in importance is the region of the southern foothills which claims 15.6 percent of all sales, followed by the group of dairies around the town of Arecibo on the northwest coast (11.8 percent). The Caguas Valley claims 10.2 percent of milk sales and the southwestern valleys 9.8 percent. The balance of the output comes from farms spread throughout the island. The central regions of Ciales, Adjuntas and Jayuya and the adjoining area of Las Marias are the least favored in terms of milk distribution.

The following table shows the rise in production of both commercial and noncommercial milk in the past 20 years.

Production of Milk — Puerto Rico, 1950-1969
(in 1,000 liters)

Source	1950	1960	1969[a]
Commercial dairies	42,824	165,161	313,100[b]
Noncommercial dairies	103,310	124,058	72,337

[a]In 1969, a liter of commercially produced milk cost 18¢, one of noncommercial 14¢.

[b]Of the total amount of commercial milk available, 97.7 percent or 305,810,000 liters were sent to the pasteurizing plant.

Source: Commonwealth of Puerto Rico (Office of the Governor), *Puerto Rico Statistical Yearbook 1968.*

The production of eggs has also risen considerably in the last two decades, as shown on the following table.

Production of Eggs — Puerto Rico, 1950-1969
(in dozens)

Source	1950	1960	1969*
Commercial farms	144,750	4,704,143	9,499,702
Noncommercial farms	8,949,368	10,134,747	11,690,904

*In 1969, a dozen commercially produced eggs cost 51¢, and a dozen noncommercial eggs cost 64¢.

Source: Commonwealth of Puerto Rico (Office of the Governor), *Puerto Rico Statistical Yearbook 1968.*

The 1969-1972 plan provides for increasing production to 43 million dozen eggs, or more than twice the 1969 output. The plan provides for government protection of local producers against imports by purchasing their surplus eggs and strengthening regulations and inspection. It also calls for integrating the production of poultry feed with that of cattle feed by placing the aviaries next to ranches and feed mills. Poultry meat production is expected to rise under the plan by 30 percent which would bring it to about 15,000 tons a year. This could be done if the target of 22 million more chickens a year were reached. To reduce costs, the Government encourages the organization of cooperatives for purchasing equipment and marketing the output.

4. Fisheries [40] [1] [1a]

Although langoustinos, oysters, shrimp, tuna, snapper and kingfish are found in Puerto Rico's home waters, the population remains addicted to dried, salted codfish. The consumption of fresh fish is limited to the coastal population and to the large cities where tourists keep the trade alive. Inland and among most families, whatever their income, fish means and for sometime to come will continue to mean salted cod, which accounts for 35 percent of all the "meat" consumed in the island. The lack of demand for fresh fish discourages fishing and results in a scarcity. Moreover, the island is really the summit of a huge, steep-sided undersea mountain, which means that there is no shelf at the base of the island to provide an environment favorable to the survival and multiplication of most species of fish. It is believed that the waters around Puerto Rico are the habitat of only about 130 species of fish, 30 of which are considered to be first-class. Among the most common are: snapper, mackerel and groupers. However, all sources consulted agree that the fisheries, unpromising as they appear to be, have not been developed to the full extent of their limited potential.

Suarez-Caabro remarks that a sharp contrast exists between the modern, well-capitalized Japanese-supported tuna fleet operating in Puerto Rican waters and the Commonwealth's obsolete inshore fleet. However, modernization and motorization are now on their way. In 1967 a development program co-sponsored by the U.S. Department of the Interior and the Department of Agriculture of the Commonwealth was started under the Commercial Fisheries Research Development Act of 1964. A preliminary survey revealed that landings are most abundant on the west coast of the island and least abundant on the north coast. The personnel engaged in fishing include about 2,131 licensed fishermen, 38 percent of whom are full-time and 62 percent part-time or occasional. Eighty percent of the former own their boats compared to 69 percent of the latter. As expected, the west coast has the highest number of fishermen (34 percent) and the north coast the lowest (15 percent). Seventy-six percent of the fishing fleet is motorized. A variety of fishing gear is used: fishpots (62.8 percent), troll lines (9 percent), hand lines (6.2 percent), lobster pots (5.3 percent), cast net (4.7 percent), and others (12 percent).

The town of Cabo Rojo is producing 30 percent of the island's reported catch of fish and shellfish, representing 23 percent of the total value. Next come Vieques Island and Fajardo on the east coast, Guanica and Lajas on the southwest as well as Aguadilla and Mayagüez on the west, and Naguabo and Humacao on the east. These ports combined produce 66 percent of all recorded Puerto Rican seafood production. At present, fish represent 87.6 percent of the weight and 73 percent of the value of the landings. The spiny lobster is the most common of the shellfish landed (8.4 percent of the catch), followed by crab. The rest of the catch (4 percent) consists of various kinds of shellfish and turtles. A recently established commercial fisheries laboratory at Punta Guanajibo (south of Mayagüez) plans to make a variety of studies on the fishing resources around the island.* It is believed that annual production could reach 1,400 tons a year and bring an income of $800,000 to Puerto Rican fishermen.

D. FOOD INDUSTRIES [36] [1a] [27] [28]

In 1947 the basic decision was made by the leaders of the Commonwealth to bring industries from the mainland United States to the island, attracting them with cheap labor and a privileged system of taxes. The small amount of money available for this project was used to establish the resources needed by industry, such as water, power and transportation. This brilliant concept paid off handsomely, as it permitted almost instant development without the pains usually accompanying the slow and hazardous transformation from one way of life to another. The food industries are perhaps those which absorb local resources most since the majority of the other enterprises import their raw materials. Nearly 20 percent of the net manufacturing income is generated by the food processing sector of industry. As of 1971, there were 440 plants processing agricultural products and employing over 21,000 workers, not counting the 704 first- and second-class dairies (see *Meat, Milk and Eggs*) which employed 4,000 workers. Of the total 440 plants, 196 have been promoted by the Economic Development Administration (EDA) which controls 43 percent of all food processing factories. An additional 40 plants are in the process of being promoted, which will extend the EDA's control to about 50 percent of all food industries.

---

*A recent report (January 1970) indicated the presence of productive grounds from Arecibo eastward. Another (November 1970) suggested that large schools of hitherto undetected herring are swimming around the island.

Forty of the presently operating 196 plants are of U.S. mainland origin, 3 are foreign and 153 are local. Twelve more of the prospective 40 are also owned by mainland companies, while 28 are Puerto Rican. The largest number are concerned with meat products, fruit canning and preservation, vegetable canning and seafood processing. More than half of the plants are in the San Juan area. Grain mills, located in Guaynabo, Santurce, Hatoray and Catano, process imported grain—wheat, corn and rice. Food industries of all types are distributed throughout the island. Economic development advisors offer counsel on marketing and other subjects to the industrialists. The food technology laboratories of the Agricultural Experiment Station develop new processing techniques.

E. TRADE

1. Domestic Trade [19]

While in some villages trade is still carried out, as of old, at the local store or, in isolated communities, through itinerant vendors, the trend is definitely towards the development of modern commercial channels. Since most of the food is now imported, supermarkets have sprung up in many places. In 1970 they number 75 spread throughout the island. Most major cities, such as Arecibo, Mayagüez and Ponce—in addition, of course, to San Juan—have American-type supermarkets. Several food retailing chains, such as the Pueblo Company, operate in the rural towns. Food is becoming less and less indigenous and more and more American. Even local items of the diet such as *viandas* (starchy vegetables), milk and meat are bought at the supermarket. One has to go rather far into the remote parts of the island to find a *pulpería* (a small family-operated grocery store). Medium-size villages have shopping centers where more and more Puerto Ricans buy their food rather than grow it.

2. External Trade [14] [19] [31] [23] [28] [33]

Since 85-90 percent of the external trade of Puerto Rico goes to the mainland United States, it would be inaccurate to call this foreign commerce. This trade has increased rapidly since 1955. Taking fiscal years 1964 and 1968 as examples, the total value of Puerto Rican agricultural exports in 1964 was $308,641,843 and 97.8 percent went to the U.S. market (see Tables 8 and 9). The main items of export were sugar (41.1 percent of the total) and tobacco (30.9 percent). Other items included fruit, fruit products and preserves. In 1968, the total value of agricultural exports had risen to $342,530,896, of which $327,133,107 or about 95.6 percent was sold to the mainland United States market. In that year, the most remunerative export was tobacco, which represented 40 percent of all Puerto Rican agricultural exports to the U.S. Other exports included sugar, rum, various beverages, coffee, fruit and vegetable preserves as well as animal feed. The export of sugar to the United States is conditioned by the quota allotted, which in certain years cannot be filled by the local output. Moreover, sugar production is falling with the contraction of land in cane and the increased manufacture of rum, exports of which have trebled since 1950. Coffee is also an exportable item which is slowly declining in importance as coffee land is put to other uses.

In fiscal year 1964, the Puerto Rican import bill for agricultural products amounted to only $315,385,488, almost 85 percent of which benefited American farmers. Imports of agricultural products rose to $443,82,.041 in 1968 and 82.7 percent of the total was purchased from the mainland agricultural industry. The most important food item was meat, followed by milk, milk products and eggs. Tobacco is both imported and exported, but exports, which far outweigh imports are in the form of tobacco products (mainly cigars) rather than leaf tobacco and imports are in the form of leaf for processing and reexport at a profit. Tobacco imports are valued at $63 million a year.

It is clear that Puerto Rico is increasingly relying on imported food, which may be considered a sign of development since it implies the existence of incomes compatible with the high prices of imported diets. The alternative implication, of course, is malnutrition, but there seems to be less of it in Puerto Rico than in most Latin American countries. Nonagricultural trade makes up the difference between the $367 million in agricultural imports and the over $2 billion worth of merchandise purchased in the United States, and between $327 million and $1.5 billion worth of goods sold to the United States. This leaves Puerto Rico with a trade deficit of about $500 million a year.

F. FOOD SUPPLY

1. Storage [36] [23] [6]

There is no problem of food supply in Puerto Rico. Stocks of food are kept in various places of trade where they can be delivered to the consumer upon demand. No information has been found on the size of the storage containers or on the specific locations of regional distribution centers. It is, however, interesting to study the fluctuation of reserves based on 11 years (1950/51-1961/62) of storage of 33 different food items of domestic origin in all categories. Table No. 10 gives the months of highest and lowest availability of these food items during the year. The table is self-explanatory: for example, it shows goats' and pigs' meat is most available in December and least in February. Bananas of various kinds and beans are in greatest abundance in the summer but in least quantities in January and December. On the contrary, dry corn is at a peak in January and February but soft corn is harvested in June and July and is least abundant in

January. The plantains are in highest stock in the summer and in short supply in January.

A 1966 islandwide nutrition survey revealed that 66.4 percent of the families investigated had some closed kitchen storage space, but 7.4 percent had no storage space for their food, and the rest used a variety of improvised or makeshift contraptions.

2. Transportation [36] [32]

The road system has been developed considerably and the isolated communities of old are now few and far between. There are modern asphalted highways circling the island and crisscrossing each other in the interior, including major highways in the mountains. San Juan, the capital, is particularly well served, as 58 percent of the system is in this region. The Ponce area has 31 percent of the highway network and Mayagüez 11 percent of the total mileage, which now exceeds 7,680 kilometers. The road system is plied by over 36 trucking companies.

The airports are well-developed. There is a major international airport near San Juan which places the island within easy reach of any major city in the world. Another large airport is projected for construction between Ponce and Mayagüez. There are four regional as well as eight general aviation airports; the most active are at Patillo, Santa Isabel and San Sebastian. There seems to be no danger that shortages of food in one region might result in famine.

It has been claimed that no industrial site in the island is more than 2 hours away from Puerto Rico's international airport or its deep-sea harbors. The most important commercial seaports are at San Juan, Mayagüez and Ponce. Specialized ports equipped to handle petrochemicals are located at Guayama on the southeastern coast and at Guayanilla on the southwestern coast of the island.

III. DIETS

A. GENERAL [6] [37]

It is generally claimed that food consumption has substantially increased in recent years on the island of Puerto Rico as a result of rapid economic gains and that the diets compare favorably with those of Latin America. While there seems to be a broad consensus of opinion that economic gains should eventually bring about dietary improvement, several studies made before and following community development programs at Mavilla and Naranjo do not confirm this assumption. As will be shown hereunder, some changes were observed in both directions, confirming our belief that it takes more than industrial and community development to bring about dietary improvement. This will be further discussed later (see *Levels of Nutrition*).

It may be relevant to state once more that food availability is not necessarily translated into food consumption and that even one consumption survey means very little. Significant data can be obtained, however, from a number of surveys made at different times of the year in the same location so as to reflect changes brought about by the seasons. Moreover, it is the biochemical survey of the body fluids, buttressed by clinical examinations and anthropometry, which gives the most accurate evaluation of the nutritional status of a population. When all the data of availability, consumption and biological condition are combined and cover at least a year, then a benchmark is created that can be compared later with other findings. Then and only then can it be known whether the passing of time, industrialization or any other factor has brought some change and in which direction.

In 1966 Fernández and his colleagues at the University of Puerto Rico made a thorough study of Puerto Rican nutrition in a master survey* covering the whole island. Both urban and rural communities were investigated and progressively ascending income groups were studied. As expected, the categories of food consumed were very similar for all groups concerned. Variations were primarily in terms of quantity. For instance, everyone drinks coffee in Puerto Rico regardless of income; families with less than $500 a year were found to drink coffee an average of 9.6 times a week while families with $7,000 or more were found to drink it 10 times. No group drinks it less than an average of 9.6 times and none averages more than 10 times. In the whole list of 41 food items whose popularity was investigated among 848 families, no other item reached the 9-time-per-week frequency and none exceeded 10. At the other end of the popularity scale, the less-than-$500-a-year families eat seafood other than cod-fish once every 10 weeks and the $7,000 or more group once every 2 weeks, with the families of intermediate income varying between these two extremes and averaging one non-codfish seafood meal once every 3 weeks. Rich and poor alike enjoy eating salted codfish, but the poor consume it more often than the affluent (2.4 against 1.1 times a week), its popularity decreasing with wealth. The poor eat cheese once a week, the affluent almost every day (5.8 times a week). Eggs are consumed three times a week by the low income families and once a day by the well-to-do. It is interesting to note that being 14 times richer increases egg consumption only twice.

The poor eat meat in one form or another eight times a week, the affluent 14.5 times. The poor eat beans 4.9 times a week (almost 5 days a week), the well-off 4.3 times (more than 4 days a week). Plantains and bananas are very popular among both the affluent, who eat them 6 days a week, and the poor, who eat them four times a week. Rich and poor eat onions and tomato sauce almost every day. All levels eat rice, the poor a little more than the affluent who

---

*See bibliographical source No. 6.

eat twice as many potatoes and almost twice as much bread. The poor have one kind of fruit, either pineapple, mangoes or citrus fruit, once a week, while the affluent consume fruit almost every day. Desserts other than fruit appear three times more frequently on the menu of affluent families than on that of the poor. The same ratio applies to alcoholic beverages. The poor eat more lard than the well-off who, in turn, eat more butter and vegetable oils.

Milk consumption increased between 1946 and 1966 to the point where almost all age groups now drink at least two cups a day, but the preschool children from families with less than $500 a year and rural schoolchildren, grownups and old people of whatever income drink the least milk. Probably as a result of the industrialization of the dairy industry, consumption of fresh milk was found to increase with income. Evaporated milk, whole powdered milk and nonfat dry milk are used mostly by rural and poor families. This indicates that wholesome fluid milk is a luxury, a significant change from the days when fresh milk was to be had at the farm rather than in the cities.

The composition of meals was found to be better in 1966 than in 1946 in the sense that more families had foods other than coffee and bread for breakfast. The highest rate of spartan breakfasts is now among the middle-class income groups, people who have $3,000-$4,000 to spend every year rather than among the poor, and the highest rate of those skipping breakfast altogether is found among the better-off, those who enjoy incomes from $5,000 to $6,000. The proportion of people eating protein at lunch rose from less than 50 percent in 1956 to 71.2 percent in 1966. The same was observed regarding the evening meal. The addition of a protein dish to the fare was enjoyed by 75 percent of the families in 1966 rather than only 47.4 percent in 1946. The very well-off ($6,000-$7,000 a year), however, have the highest percentage of people skipping dinner altogether, not because of money, but probably because of excessive intellectual or managerial work and exhaustion in the evening.

Only minor differences in food habits were found between urban and rural families, none that could not have been expected in a community well on its way to industrialization and urbanization. Foods which originate in the rural area are channeled into the industrial circuit and processed for transformation and preservation to be sold on the urban markets at high prices. The farmer, anxious to collect as much money as possible, deprives the local market of his milk, eggs, vegetables and fruits, forcing his family and neighbors to eat more starchy vegetables and beans than their urban counterparts. The rural people also drink smaller amounts of alcoholic beverages than do the city dwellers. More and more, as in the mainland United States, the farm is becoming the basic pillar of a vast industrial complex which drains the rural areas of its products to feed the increasing urban population. Transformation of the food so that it can last through the trip from countryside to city and conditioning it for sale by retailers gradually changes its nature for better or worse. As already observable in the

United States, a good natural orange is becoming almost a rarity since the major portion of the crop is processed into frozen or canned orange juice.

B. RURAL DIETS [37]

Nutrition surveys, such as the investigation discussed above, have been made in Puerto Rico for a long time, especially during the last 10 years. Many aspects of nutrition in the island have been explored by the distinguished and experienced teams of the Department of Biochemistry and Nutrition of the School of Medicine at the University of Puerto Rico and by the Division of Nutrition of the Department of Health of the Commonwealth under the leadership of Dr. N.A. Fernández. The data gathered by these teams allows an unusual insight into the changes that occur under very favorable conditions in a community nearing the end of the transition from a subsistence to a money economy. One of the first studies of this sort was made in 1946 at the very beginning of the Puerto Rican industrial transformation by Roberts and Stefani. As a result of such investigations it was found that the improvements occurring in living conditions in the course of industrialization were more marked in certain urban sectors than in the rural areas. This led to the creation in 1960 of a Commission for the Improvement of Isolated Communities. The approach is to use graduate students from the University of Puerto Rico to stimulate community development in various areas and to survey living conditions, nutrition and health. Three isolated communities—Manzanilla, Cialitos and Santiago—were studied first under this program by Plough, Fernández et al., and revealed the following information.

1. Diets at Manzanilla, Cialitos and Santiago [22]

In June 1961 there were 70 families comprising 390 people in Manzanilla, a south shore village in the district of Juana Díaz. Their cash resources came almost solely from employment on a nearby sugar plantation. Fifty-three percent of the heads of families were laborers in the cane fields, 6 percent were self-employed farmers and 19 percent had no occupation. Thirty-five percent of the population was illiterate but 75 percent of the school-aged children attended school. Twenty-three percent of the families received welfare assistance. Only thirteen percent owned the land they occupied. Ninety-eight percent owned or occupied plots of less than 4,000 square meters (less than half a hectare). Fifty-one percent had chickens, 46 percent had pigs, 14 percent goats, 7 percent cows, 3 percent cultivated small gardens, 1 percent had fruit trees. In these mediocre but not abject circumstances, children up to 1 year of age received an average of 467 grams of milk a day, some meat or fish (4 grams), vegetables and fruits (48 grams), grain, mostly rice (30 grams), and fats (5 grams). Adults had the same diet except that they had very little meat and much more grain and vegetables. Men ate twice as much as women. All grownups used their milk in coffee. Biochemical tests proved that women as well as the children had deficiencies in calories. Iron, ascorbic acid, thiamine and, among adults, vitamin A consumption were low (see *Levels of Nutrition*). In this community each family had an average income of $682 per year which gave an annual per capita income of about $175.

Cialitos is a mountain community located "as far from the sea as it is possible to be on the island," at 500-800 meters altitude in the District of Ciales. The village is remarkable for the dispersion of its homes. While the center of the village is accessible, many houses are perched at the top of steep slopes and are of difficult access. Cialitos is a larger community than Manzanilla and at the time of the study there were 136 families totaling 824 people. Thirty-three percent were illiterate, 67 percent of school-aged children actually attended school. Forty-four percent of the families owned their farms where the main crop was coffee. Citrus fruit and animals were also raised. Although the mean annual cash income per family reached $809, 23 percent of the population is on welfare. The per capita income of the village amounted to $133. Fifty-five percent of the plots were less than 4,000 square meters but 25 percent consisted of 4 hectares or more. Livestock were also more abundant than at Manzanilla: 62 percent of the families owned flocks of chickens, 40 percent owned pigs, 1 percent had goats, and 14 percent had cows. Sixty-nine percent cultivated fruit trees and 7 percent kept small gardens. Food consumption in this financially better situated village was greater than in Manzanilla. Children up to 1 year of age were given 522 grams of milk per day, 11 grams of meat or fish, 90 grams of vegetables and fruits, 56 grams of grain (of which 34 grams were rice) and 7 grams of fats. The investigators found that more citrus fruit was eaten in season and more starchy vegetables were consumed than in Manzanilla. With the exception of vitamin A, the diets of adult men were considered to be adequate by the investigators but the diets of children and women were found to be low in calcium, vitamin A and riboflavin. In addition, children below age 1 did not appear to consume the requirement in iron, ascorbic acid and niacin.

Santiago is a community inland from the north coast of the island in the valley of the Río Camuy which gives its name to the district. This is rough land and the houses are widely separated. The village included 86 families comprising 523 people in 1961. It was in almost every way a poorer community than Manzanilla. The illiteracy level reached 44 percent and only 66 percent of the school-aged children attended school. Although the average family income amounted to $617, which mean an annual per capita income of $101, 20 percent of the population was on welfare. Thirty-three percent of the families occupied or owned plots of less than 4,000 square meters and 36 percent owned or occupied farms exceeding 4 hectares; the balance either farmed plots of intermediate size or had no land. The size of the holding, however, was not very significant because the soil in the area is poor. Nevertheless, resources for subsistence were much better than in the other two villages. Seventy-one percent of the people owned chickens, 81 percent owned pigs, 27 percent owned goats, 51 percent owned cows, 13 percent cultivated gardens and 84 percent owned fruit trees. Children in the 0-1 age group had a definitely higher intake of milk (573 grams) than in Cialitos, but less meat and fish (1 gram), fewer vegetables and fruits (48 grams), and no grain products or fats. As in Cialitos, vitamin A and riboflavin requirements were not met, even by young adults who, in all other villages, seemed to consume their quota. Women were not reaching the minimum required in any nutrient except ascorbic acid and thiamine. Children under 1 lacked iron, thiamine and niacin, but consumed enough fruit to keep them adequately fed on ascorbic acid.

It seems fair to agree with the investigators that these three surveys revealed a "less than optimal" intake of certain nutrients in all communities. The most significant shortages were in calcium, vitamin A and riboflavin. As everywhere else, young children and adult women were the heaviest sufferers.

2. Diets at Mavilla and Naranjo [4] [7] [8] [5]

In 1963, Fernández and his colleagues continued their surveys and explored the nutritional status of two more communities in rural Puerto Rico—Mavilla and Naranjo. The particular value of this research was that the same investigators were able to return to the villages after a 4-year program of community development had taken place and to compare findings with those of earlier surveys carried out in 1963. At Mavilla it was found that the amount of fresh milk consumed at any age had substantially diminished between 1963 and 1967. The intake of evaporated milk had increased in the under-2 age group but after 2 years it was nil, making a net loss in the amount of milk consumed by children over 2 years and by adults. Reconstituted dry milk was drunk in small amounts by all but the under-2 age group in 1967, less than in 1963. The amount of meat in the diet had changed very little and the quantity of codfish was the same. Fewer eggs were eaten by people of all ages except those under 2. Beans and other legumes were more abundant, the amount consumed going from an average of 20 grams per capita per day in 1963 to 41 grams in 1967. The amount of starchy vegetables per capita had increased from 14 to 35 grams a day for children under 2, but diminished considerably from 234 grams to 148 grams a day for the population as a whole. The consumption of yellow and green vegetables remained about the same. That of tomatoes in the form of preserved tomato sauce had increased from an average of 23 grams per capita per day to 34 grams. The intake of rice had increased from 116 to 176 grams per person per day but that of wheat had dropped slightly from 16 to 10 grams. The amount of sugar in the diet had not changed significantly.

In the village of Naranjo, similar data were reported except that a little more milk (average increase: 6 grams per capita per day) was consumed, a little more meat (average increase: 11 grams), but less eggs, codfish, legumes, starchy vegetables, fruit, tomatoes, rice, wheat, fats and sugar products. While Mavilla had shown a slight improvement in the overall diet with some levels of nutrients higher and some lower, Naranjo showed a definite deterioration (see *Levels of Nutrition*).

Several conclusions can be drawn from this study. The first one is obviously that no spectacular improvement can be expected in the nutrition of a population in as short a time as 4 years, except, of course, if a true starvation condition existed before, which was not the case here. When community development workers deal with a population which is well-adjusted to its ecological niche, with firmly rooted agricultural and commercial practices, it takes much more than amelioration of the environment, provision of extension services and increases in income to significantly change the nutritional pattern upon which so much of future progress depends. The Puerto Rican investigators state that intensive nutrition education based in the true needs of the people must be closely coordinated with developmental agencies serving the community if real progress is to be expected.

3. Diets at Duey Alto, Montones and Masas [10] [12] [11] [5]

Other isolated areas of Puerto Rico were investigated during the interval between 1963 and 1967. These communities also came under the plan concerning the program of the Commission for the Improvement of Isolated Communities. The sites were Duey Alto in San Germán District, Montones in Piedras, and Masas in Gurabo. The basic fare was very similar to that consumed elsewhere in the island. At Duey Alto it was found that only 20 percent of the families had incomes below $500 a year, but in spite of this, the diet lacked energy, was low in calcium, vitamin A, and riboflavin. Women and children had the hardest time, especially in meeting the requirements in protein, iron and niacin.

Barrio Montones is located about 48 kilometers from San Juan, in southeastern Puerto Rico. In 1964 the community was composed of 71 families comprising 185 persons, all in the low socioeconomic class. Access to the community was difficult over narrow dirt roads. Most of the inhabitants derived their income from farming. The main crops were (and still are) tobacco, coffee and starchy vegetables grown for cash. Thirty-three percent of the families had incomes of less than $500 per year and 16 percent received no income at all. Only 17 percent had more than $1,000 or more per year. Fifty percent of the families received at least some welfare assistance. Only 58 percent of the school-aged children actually attended school and at least 31 percent of the villagers were illiterate. About two thirds of the families owned the land they occupied but the size of plots was not reported. Beans (mostly kidney beans) and small amounts of cowpeas provided vegetable protein. Codfish represented

42 percent of all the "meat" consumed, followed, in terms of quantity, by boiled pig's feet. Rice and starchy fruits (breadfruit, green bananas or green plantains) completed the lunch menu for 94 percent of the families surveyed. Milk was available at the rate of 243 grams per capita per day, but most of it was consumed by infants, whose ration was about 64 grams per capita daily, young girls (10 to 14 years old) and men over 60 years of age. Except for this milk, the diet of infants was very much more meager than at Manzanilla, Cialitos or Santiago. Montones infants received no meat or fish, 57 grams of starchy vegetables, only 6 grams of grain products (rice and wheat) and no fats. Boys from 10 to 14 years old drank less than 1 cup of milk a day (73 grams).

In Montones, as elsewhere, caloric intake was low, not exceeding an average of 1,946 a day. The lowest intakes were found among women, infants and children. The average consumption of calcium was also low at 300 milligrams a day, as was the intake of iron (12.1 milligrams for all age groups but less than 8 milligrams among infants), vitamin A (1,599 international units) and riboflavin (1.1 milligrams). Protein (1 gram per kilogram of body weight), ascorbic acid (116 milligrams per day), thiamine (1.5 milligrams) and nicotinic acid (15.2 milligrams) intakes seemed satisfactory, although it must be remembered that in low-calorie diets, protein serves as fuel and hence may mean—insofar as tissue nutrition is concerned—less nutrient value than the food composition formula would imply. Not surprisingly, plasma protein levels were lower than norms.

At Masas, caloric intakes were low, especially in schoolchildren and adolescents. This coincided with considerable retardation of growth after the first birthday. Vitamin A intake was also low and was reflected in low plasma values. Riboflavin and calcium were consumed in smaller amounts than the required levels.

C. URBAN SLUM DIETS [9]

The diets of 544 families surveyed at Juana Matos in Catano District in 1967 revealed the low levels of consumption prevailing there. The living conditions were poor, sanitation was unsatisfactory, levels of education were mediocre. Some meat (beef, pork, poultry, fish) was available on a regular basis, but in small amounts. Starchy vegetables, a few fruits and an average of 1 egg every 3 days constituted the basis of the fare, which did not nearly provide the required minimal allowance in calories, vitamin A, riboflavin, ascorbic acid, proteins, calcium and iron. Only children between 1 and 2 years of age drank 1 liter of milk a day; from 2 to 9 years they drank about 250 grams. Pregnant and lactating women were also on short milk rations of less than a cup a day. As a result of this very spare diet, retardation of weight and height was widespread among children.

D. CHILD FEEDING PROGRAMS [34]

Considerable attention has been given to the problem of the preschool child in Puerto Rico. A system of milk stations has been in effect since the early days of U.S. involvement. Their number is fairly constant at 214 around the country. The stations give assistance to children from 2 to 8 years of age and their mothers. The case load rose from 6,503 in 1960/61 to 11,700 in 1968 but the liters of milk distributed decreased from 1,880,092 to 1,034,880. Thus the amount given to each child lessens as the number of children increases, indicating that the supply of milk in this project does not catch up with demand. The daily per capita ration dropped from 289 grams in 1960/61 to 87 grams per child in 1968. Another program which also seems to be in recession is the child breakfast program of the Department of Health. A light breakfast of milk and cereal is given to children aged 2 to 10 who do not attend school. The program served 11,409 children a day in 1961 but only 4,714 in 1968 and the number of centers dropped from 308 to 120. School lunch programs are still active. By 1968 the daily participants numbered 311,870 and 55,872,355 meals were served during the year at a cost of 43¢ per serving.

E. LEVELS OF NUTRITION [6]

The following section is based on the findings of laboratory examinations made in connection with the nutrition surveys discussed under the previous sections. Five of all the communities surveyed and four of the most important nutrients have been selected for discussion. These biological measurements quantify to a certain extent the population's state of nutrition.

Table No. 11 shows only averages for the five communities chosen and concerns itself with hemoglobin (whose presence, together with other factors, governs the prevalence of anemia), protein, carotene, vitamin A and ascorbic acid. Contributing to the averages are, of course, people in greater or smaller numbers with below normal levels of these nutrients in their blood. Their numerical importance is not reflected in averages, but their nutritional levels will be discussed in the text. These cases are either in the "acceptable," the "low" or the "deficient" categories.*

1. Manzanilla, Cialitos and Santiago [22]

Hemoglobin values were low at Manzanilla, averaging sexes. The worst cases were, as usual, among women and children. Certain age groups—20 percent of girls from 10 to 14 and 19 percent of adult women—showed values inferior to 10

---

*Acceptable — lowest rating in normal range.
Low — below normal but not deficient.
Deficient — dangerously low.

grams per 100 milliliters. Among children, 45 percent of the 2-year-olds had values below 10 grams. Total serum protein rates were generally satisfactory, with ratios between 6.6 grams per 100 milliliters and 8.3 per 100 milliliters, averaging 7.5 per 100, but very low values were found among children below 9 years of age. Thirty-six percent of the 1-year-olds had values below 6 grams per 100 milliliters, a ratio that increased steadily to 9 grams per 100 milliliters in the 6-9 age group. Serum carotene and vitamin A levels were high in adults but young children had low values. Serum ascorbic acid levels were high in all age groups. Excretion rates for thiamine and riboflavin computed in micrograms per grams of creatinine were usually low and deficient. The rates of N-nicotinamide, representing niacin nutrition, also computed in micorgrams per grams of creatinine excreted, seemed normal.

At Cialitos the mean hemoglobin levels were slightly better than those at Manzanilla. Eight percent of the children in the 6-9 age group had low levels (below 10 grams) and 10 percent of the adults (20-39 years of both sexes) suffered from less than 10 grams of hemoglobin per 100 milliliters of blood. The plasma protein levels were normal to high on the average, but 23 percent of the 2-year-olds had low values (less than 6.5 grams per 100 milliliters) and 10 percent of the women between 20 and 40 years of age also fell below the 6.5 grams per 100 millimeters mark. Serum carotene was lower and vitamin A higher in Cialitos than in Manzanilla, but the serum levels of ascorbic acid were equal in the two places. Thiamine, riboflavin and niacin were acceptable on the basis of creatinine excretion, but the percentages of low values (less than 66 micrograms per gram of creatinine) were high, both in males and females after 20 years of age. With regard to thiamine nutrition, 17 percent of males 20-39 years of age, 19 percent of females 40-59 years old, and 31 percent of females above 60 years of age were in the low or deficient category. This pattern was repeated with respect to riboflavin, where the investigators found 50 percent of the males 40-59 years of age, 54 percent of females aged 15-19, and 60 percent of the pregnant women to be below the acceptable level of 80 micrograms per 1 gram of creatinine. Niacin excretion did not show similar high percentages of low or deficient levels.

In Santiago the levels of hemoglobin were, on the whole, better than elsewhere; but among children up to 9 years of age, the percentage of cases with less than 10 grams per 100 milliliters was high, reaching 50 percent during the first year and gradually improving to 13 percent among the 6-9-year-olds (which, however, is still a high percentage). Adult females and pregnant women also had high percentages of levels below 10 grams per 100 milliliters, up to 18 percent among the 20-39-year-old pregnant women. The serum protein levels were high, but 45 percent of the 1-year-olds had less than 6.5 grams per 100 milliliters, with the ratio improving to only 10 percent in the 6-9-year-olds. Males 15-19 years old also had high percentages of low protein levels (17 percent), slightly worse than young women 10-19 years of age, of whom 16 percent showed less than 6.5 grams per 100 milliliters of protein serum. Serum carotene levels were acceptable on the average but low levels were common. Forty-five percent of the 2-year-olds and 13 percent of the 10-14-year-old males and 12 percent of the 40-50-year-olds suffered from deficiency. Serum vitamin A levels were generally good. The discrepancy between some low carotene levels and high vitamin A has been discussed elsewhere.* Few ascorbic acid levels in the serum were made, but the figures were quite low. Fifty percent of the 2-year-olds had levels below 0.2 micrograms per 100 milliliters. This improved with maturation to only 9 percent at 5 years and 0 percent by 9 years.

2. Mavilla and Naranjo [4] [7] [8] [5]

At Mavilla, average hemoglobin values were acceptable in 1963 and normal in 1967, but low values still represented 13 percent of the tests made in 1967 (compared to 14 percent in 1963). In 1963, deficient values occurred among 12 percent of the people examined, but among only 2 percent in 1967. This showed a clear improvement. At Naranjo similar results obtained. Averages were acceptable in both study years (12.5 grams and 13.5 grams, respectively) and deficient cases amounted to 10 percent of the people examined in 1963 and only 1 percent in 1967. Average protein values were 7.4 grams per 100 milliliters at Mavilla and 7.3 grams at Naranjo in 1967, entirely satisfactory levels. Values of 7.2 and 7.4 grams per 100 milliliters before community development took place were also satisfactory, but the percentage of deficient cases (protein values of less than 6 grams per 100 milliliters) were on the decrease at Mavilla from 8 percent in 1963 to 2 percent in 1967 and on the increase at Naranjo from 1 percent to 5 percent. Low values (when protein plasma is between 6.0 and 6.5 grams per 100 milliliters) increased in both places from 6 percent to 7 percent at Mavilla and from 3 to 10 percent at Naranjo without any reason for this apparent deterioration other than an increase in the number of cases, graduating from deficient to low. This was equally valid for Mavilla. Plasma ascorbic acid and values were within the normal range in both places before and after improvement. No low or deficient values were reported.

Adequacy in thiamine, riboflavin and niacin is usually measured in micrograms per grams of creatinine excreted in the urine. This technique was used in all villages surveyed. A slight improvement in thiamine nutrition was noticed at both Mavilla and Naranjo. The percentage of low values decreased from 3 percent in 1963 to 1 percent in 1967 at Mavilla and from 9 to 8 percent at Naranjo. Deficient values were not significant at Mavilla and showed a drop from 6 percent to 2 percent at Naranjo. Riboflavin nutrition measured by the same

---

*See page 178.

method indicated an increased percentage of low levels at Mavilla from 5 percent in 1963 to 8 percent in 1967 but a decrease at Naranjo from 19 percent to 14 percent. Deficient levels (the worst cases) diminished in both places from 6 percent to 2 percent at Mavilla and from 25 percent to 4 percent at Naranjo. Niacin nutrition improved markedly at Naranjo where deficient cases disappeared altogether and low values dropped from 44 percent to 8 percent. However, at Mavilla the percentage of low values rose from 7 to 17 percent while that of deficient values disappeared fully from 2 percent to 0 percent. Thus, the biological findings confirmed the food consumption data showing that the deficiencies had shifted somewhat in each village but that the general level of nutrition had not changed much.

IV. ADEQUACY OF FOOD RESOURCES [31] [32]

There seems to be no doubt that Puerto Rico has passed the point where food sufficiency is a problem. At least such a problem does not present itself in the simple terms prevailing in most developing countries. The Commonwealth is not self-sufficient in food but this is not imposed by underdevelopment—it is deliberate. The Commonwealth has chosen this way because it can afford to purchase from the mainland United States any amount of food it wishes. Puerto Rico has adopted a policy of industrialization which means that it would rather buy its food than grow it. Yet it is actively engaged in improving indigenous food production potential, aiming at quality rather than quantity. In 1963-64 the island bought $315,385,488 worth of food, mostly from the mainland, while in 1967-68 these purchases amounted to $443,827,041. In the same years Puerto Rico sold $308,841,843 and $342,530,258 worth of its own agricultural products. Hence, the supplementary food needed to survive cost $6,543,645 in 1963-64 and $101,296,145 in 1967-68. Obviously, the purchasing trend is accelerated and is in agreement with the policy originated in 1947 with Operation Bootstrap. In 1964 the cost of imported food was $2.50 per capita per year and was probably well worth it. In 1968, the cost rose to about $36.20 per capita, which indicates that either the nonagricultural sector is prosperous enough to foot the bill or that the Commonwealth is going into debt.

The preamble of the 1969-1972 Development Plan states that Puerto Rico seeks to create "a civilization of excellence." Inescapably, one thinks of Switzerland, whose prosperity is supported not by its mineral or agricultural resources, which are meager, but by the excellence of its manpower: craftsmen, businessmen, engineers and scientists. Like Switzerland, Puerto Rico is importing raw materials and exporting finished products. The policy is to continue towards more of the same by gradually reducing the land under crops and offering it for urbanization, industrialization and animal husbandry (the most sophisticated of agricultural sciences). In pursuance of this goal, Puerto Rico has encouraged the implantation of U.S. industry by offering considerable advantages in taxes and cheap labor. The results have been spectacular. The new firms were delighted to increase their profits by reducing their costs, and, by the same token, the idle manpower has been delighted to find steady jobs and increasing salaries. This bold operation was possible only because the wise Commonwealth leaders managed to extol the virtues of U.S. citizenship while preserving the islanders' cultural identity. As a consequence of this courageous and intelligent approach, the agitation of politicians who in other countries play upon a misguided nationalism to perpetuate social unrest for their own benefit has been hardly audible in Puerto Rico.

The policy, however, does have its dangers. It will work as long as the budget can afford the $36.20 per head that it costs to feed the population "at the restaurant" rather than at home, for this is, in effect, what Puerto Rico is doing: purchasing 60 percent of their beef, all of their wheat and rice, a considerable portion of their milk and eggs, most of their vegetables and fish abroad is comparable to taking the family to a restaurant to eat every day. It is possible only if the family income is sustained and this implies that international prosperity will continue, markets for U.S. industry will expand, and that tourists will maintain their high level of expenditures. As long as these conditions do continue, the food resources of the Commonwealth will remain adequate.

V. NUTRITIONAL DISEASE PATTERNS [6] [3] [2] [8] [5] [4] [24]

As expected, thanks to the relatively high level of consumption, few signs of obvious nutritional deficiencies have been discovered during the many surveys carried out in the Commonwealth. Suboptimal clinical conditions are more common than obvious diseases. Yet, certain inadequacies were found, some of which are likely to carry serious consequences. Vitamin A deficiencies were identified through a general prevalence of follicular hyperkeratosis which was present in 15 percent of the 843 people examined in 1966 and seems to have been fairly evenly distributed throughout the life span of the people, with no preference for any age group. Dryness of the skin was occasionally encountered. Four cases of xerophthalmia and three cases of Bitot spots were also seen. Ascorbic acid deficiency was a likely cause of gum inflammation in only nine subjects, while poor oral hygiene and dental caries were very common. Riboflavin deficiency was present in 15 percent of the people examined and seemed to be more frequent with advancing age. It was identified through detection of nasolabial seborrhea, angular stomatitis, corneal infection, glossitis and papillary atrophy of the tongue. Two cases of pellagrous dermatitis were observed. Ankle and knee reflexes were occasionally diminished, suggesting a possible touch of thiamine deficiency and incipient beriberi. Very few signs suggestive of protein malnutrition were noted. Hair depigmentation was seen in four persons only, dryness in six. Dental fluorosis was also seen in 1.7 percent of all persons examined.

Whatever signs of malnutrition were encountered were more frequent among the urban population than among the rural except for symptoms of vitamin C and vitamin D deficiencies. This is not surprising since urban malnutrition is the worst type. No food resources grow on the asphalt and every consumable item must be paid for. Interestingly enough, there was as high a ratio of deficiency symptoms among the higher income groups as there was among families with incomes below $5,000 a year. There was also a moderate degree of undernutrition among children and adolescents, expressed in terms of 10-20 percent underweight. A high prevalence of obesity among adult females and children was also observed. This afflicted 28 percent of the women and 12 percent of the men 19 years of age or under. Obesity also occurred among children and adolescents in families with incomes over $3,000 a year. It would be interesting to relate the epidemiology of obesity to family ties and genetics as well as to diets. Anemia was not as frequently encountered as one could have expected in a tropical area, especially where schistosomiasis and hookworm are still prevalent and compete with nutritional factors to explain the low to deficient levels of hemoglobin reported in many places. Fernández et al. report hypochromic anemia in children and infants, with rather high levels of occurrence at Montones and Masas but low rates at Naranjo and Juana Matos. De Torregrosa and De Costas found that 8.4 percent of 509 anemic children admitted to San Juan City Hospital between 1957 and 1959 had megaloblastic anemia and 16.7 percent had megaloblastic anemia associated with iron deficiency. Fifteen of the children had bone marrow pictures suggesting folic acid or vitamin B_{12} deficiency, or both, combined with iron deficiency. The same investigators found two cases of scurvy among the children, possibly due to the destruction of vitamin C through excessive cooking of food.

Anthropometry has revealed no significant differences in heights between rural and urban samples. Fernández et al. found, however, that averages were well below U.S. norms. Urban children from 2-15 years of age showed a slight retardation in growth. Rural children grow normally until the age of 10, after which they slow down and are overtaken by the urban young men whose stature is 25 millimeters higher. From the point of view of weight, the urban people seem to fare better than the rural. Infants and young adults show no significant differences between urban and rural, but both urban and rural children evidence some slowdown in weight compared to standards. This difference disappears after age 17, leading to the suspicion that the most severely underweight children in the urban areas do not make it to adolescence and adulthood.

VI. CONCLUSIONS [33] [26] [36]

The case of Puerto Rico is of particular interest because of the unusual circumstances surrounding its development. Things have happened to Puerto Rico that could not have happened elsewhere. Yet, a model has been created, the lessons of which must be considered and discussed. At a time when the problem of standard of living equalization looms on the immediate horizon of the free world and has become the fundamental task of the century, what can we derive from the Puerto Rican miracle? Is it, indeed, a miracle, can it be repeated elsewhere?

When the United States took possession of the island at the end of the 19th century, Puerto Rico was as underdeveloped as any place could be by modern standards. If the notion of gross national product had existed, which it did not, the island would have been given a very low growth rate. This was due to the fact that, except for coffee and some sugar, 80 percent of the arable land was still in the hands of the subsistence farming population; there was no industry to speak of, and in the modern sense of the word, Puerto Rico was hardly even a "developing" country. The situation improved, at least insofar as the GNP was concerned, during the first half of the 20th century, mostly because of the illegal activities of sugar companies violating federal laws. By 1970, the GNP had reached $4.6 billion, the total wages and salaries distributed amounted to $2.6 billion and personal income was computed at $3.8 billion. The standard of living has improved, the Commonwealth is almost developed.

The first lesson to be derived from this "miracle" is that its accomplishment has taken 70 years. While the famous "Operation Bootstrap" started in earnest only after the Second World War, during the 40-odd years which preceded it the groundwork for the economic boom was laid. Even the 100 years of Spanish domination contributed something to the modernization of Puerto Rico. Under a liberal Spanish policy, a good deal of education was transfused, either directly or by osmosis, and eventually the native population was in many ways and in substantial numbers quite ready to accept, even demand, something like "Operation Bootstrap." The standard of living equalization that is imperatively needed in "The Third World" if freedom, as we know it, or any reasonable facsimile thereof, is to be preserved, requires at least the length of time, under privileged circumstances, that it took to reach its present level in Puerto Rico.

The second lesson is that "Operation Bootstrap" was not the self-levitation this clever and stimulating slogan implies. "Operation Bootstrap" could exist and succeed because:

1. Puerto Rico was a part of the United States in which certain federal laws were "on vacation," especially the federal internal revenue laws and the minimum wage laws. Puerto Rico was thus the homeland of a labor force

nearly 1 million strong willing to work and capable of making a living on salaries that were much lower than those prevailing in the continental United States.

2. The Puerto Rican leadership saw the advantage to be derived from attracting industry and invested the Commonwealth's savings in the development of infrastructure, such as water, power and transportation, to further enhance the attractiveness of the island to mainland investors.

3. American industry was willing to invest heavily in factories (548 plants in 1957, 1,819 in 1970) and equipment and in the transportation of raw materials to and finished products from the island. This investment appears to have been much higher, on a per capita basis, than foreign aid grants and loans to any country in the world.

4. Even the "colonial" character of the whole operation did not attract adverse publicity, as it surely would have if any other "great power" had implanted its industry in a developing land to take advantage of cheap labor, because Puerto Rico had opted by plebiscite to remain part of the "mother country" and because the local leaders saw the long-range benefits the operation could bring to their island rather than the temporary prestige which loud opposition, based on nationalistic slogans, could have brought to themselves.

Under such nonexportable and nontransferrable circumstances, considerable changes have taken place.

While there is no doubt that the standard of living of many Puerto Ricans has improved, there is still malnutrition, misery and an urban slum problem. However, the reasons for these negative aspect of an otherwise substantial success are to be found, not in any particularly Puerto Rican complex of circumstances, but in the worldwide problem created by the overgrowth of an economy of consumption that has established cost/benefit ratios for everything except itself.

BIBLIOGRAPHY

1. *Commercial Fisheries Review,* 1970, 32 (1), 26.

2. De Torregrosa, M.V.V. and De Costas, M.C. "Megaloblastic Anemia of Infancy. Etiology and Diagnosis Based on a Study of 56 Cases in Childhood." *Clinical Pediatrics,* 1964, 3, 348-354.

2a. De Zapata, L.R. *Caracteristicas Socio-economóicas de una Muestra de Familias Seleccionadas para el Estudio Sobre el Consumo de Alimentos en Puerto Rico.* Rio Piedras, University of Puerto Rico Agricultural Experiment Station, 1970.

3. Fernández, N.A., Burgos, J.C. and Asenjo, C.F. "Obesity in Puerto Rican Children and Adults." *Boletin de la Asociación Médica de Puerto Rico,* 1969, 61 (5), 153-157.

4. _____ , Burgos, J.C., Asenjo, C.F., Rosa, I.R. "Nutrition Survey of Two Rural Puerto Rican Areas Before and After a Community Improvement Program." *The American Journal of Clinical Nutrition,* 1969, 22 (12), 1639-1651.

5. _____ , Burgos, J.C., Asenjo, C.F. and Rosa, I.R. "Nutrition Survey of Five Rural Puerto Rican Communities." *Boletin de la Asociación Médica de Puerto Rico,* 1969, 61 (2), 42-52.

6. _____ , Burgos, J.C., Asenjo, C.F. and Rosa, I.R. "Nutritional Status of the Puerto Rican Population—Master Sample Survey." *Boletin de la Asociación Médica de Puerto Rico,* 1971, 63 (4).

7. _____ , Burgos, J.C., Plough, I.C., Roberts, L.J. and Asenjo, C.F. "Nutritional Status of People in Isolated Areas of Puerto Rico. Survey of Barrio Mavilla, Vega Alta, Puerto Rico." *American Journal of Clinical Nutrition,* 1965, 17, 305-316.

8. _____ , Burgos, J.C., Plough, I.C., Roberts, L.J. and Asenjo, C.F. "Nutritional Status of People in Isolated Areas of Puerto Rico. Survey of Barrio Naranjo, Moca, Puerto Rico." *American Journal of Clinical Nutrition,* 1966, 19, 269-284.

9. _____ , Burgos, J.C., Roberts, L.J. and Asenjo, C.F. "Nutritional Status in Puerto Rican Slum Areas." *American Journal of Clinical Nutrition,* 1968, 21, 646-656.

10. _____ , Burgos, J.C., Roberts, L.J. and Asenjo, C.F. "Nutritional Status of People in Isolated Areas of Puerto Rico. Survey of Barrio Duey Alto, San German, Puerto Rico." *Archivos Latinoamericanos de Nutrición,* 1967, 17, 215-239.

11. _____ . Burgos, J.C., Roberts, L.J. and Asenjo, C.F. "Nutritional Status of People in Isolated Areas of Puerto Rico. Survey of Barrio Masas 2, Burabo, Puerto Rico." *Boletin de la Asociación Médica de Puerto Rico.* 1967, 59, 503-514.

12. _____ . Burgos, J.C., Roberts, L.J. and Asenjo, C.F. "Nutritional Status of People in Isolated Areas of Puerto Rico. Survey of Barrio Montones 4, Las Piedras." *Journal of the American Dietetic Association,* 1968, 53, 119-126.

13. Food and Agriculture Organization of the United Nations. *Production Yearbook 1970.* Volume 24. Rome, FAO, 1971.

14. _____ . *Trade Yearbook 1970.* Volume 24, Rome, FAO, 1971.

15. Hanson, E.P. *Puerto Rico: Land of Wonders.*

15a. _____ . *Transformation, The Story of Modern Puerto Rico.* New York, Simon and Schuster, 1955.

16. James, P.E. *Latin America.* New York, The Odyssey Press, 1969.

17. Kelly, W.J. *A Cost-Effectiveness Study of Clinical Methods of Birth Control.* Houston (Rice University), Unpublished Ph.D. Thesis, 1971.

18. MacPhail, D.D. "Puerto Rican Dairying: A Revolution in Tropical Agriculture." *Geographical Review,* 1963, 53 (2), 224-246.

19. McAlpine, J.D. *Agricultural Production and Trade of Puerto Rico.* ERS Foreign 227. Washington, D.C., U.S. Department of Agriculture, 1968.

20. Molina, G. and Noam, I.F. "Indicators of Health, Economy and Culture in Puerto Rico and Latin America." *American Journal of Public Health,* 1964, 54, 1191-1206.

21. Pico, R. *The Geographic Regions of Puerto Rico.* Rio Piedras, Puerto Rico, University of Puerto Rico Press, 1959.

22. Plough, I.C., Fernández, N.A., Angel, C.R. and Roberts, L.J. "A Nutrition Survey of Three Rural Puerto Rican Communities." *Boletin de la Asociación Médica de Puerto Rico,* 1963, 55 (12-A), 1-51.

23. Puerto Rico, Commonwealth of (Department of Agriculture). *Anuario de Estadisticas Agricolas de Puerto Rico 1968-69.* Santurce, Department of Agriculture, 1969.

24. _____ (Department of Health). *Vital Statistics 1970 Puerto Rico.* San Juan, Department of Health, 1971.

25. _____ (Department of Labor). *Employment and Unemployment in Puerto Rico.* Monthly Report Number 71-8. San Juan, August 1971.

26. _____ (Department of the Treasury). *Economy and Finances Puerto Rico 1970.* San Juan, Department of the Treasury, 1971.

27. _____ (Economic Development Administration). "The Food and Kindred Products Industry in Puerto Rico." San Juan, Mimeographed, 1971.

28. _____ (Economic Development Administration). *1968 Official Industrial and Trade Guide to Puerto Rico.* San Juan, Economic Development Administration, 1969.

29. _____ (Government Development Bank). *The Commonwealth of Puerto Rico—A Special Report.* San Juan, Government Development Bank for Puerto Rico, 1971.

30. _____ (Government Development Bank). *Puerto Rico Financial Facts 1971.* San Juan, Government Development Bank for Puerto Rico, 1971.

31. _____ (Office of the Governor—Puerto Rico Planning Board). *External Trade Statistics 1968.* San Juan, Planning Board, 1969.

32. _____ (Office of the Governor—Puerto Rico Planning Board). *The Four Year Economic and Social Development Plan of Puerto Rico 1969-72.* San Juan, Planning Board, 1968.

33. _____ (Office of the Governor—Puerto Rico Planning Board). *Puerto Rico Income and Product 1970.* San Juan, Planning Board, 1971.

34. _____ (Office of the Governor—Puerto Rico Planning Board). *Puerto Rico Statistical Yearbook.* San Juan, Planning Board, 1969.

35. _____ (Oficina del Gobernador—Junta de Planificación). *1970 Informe de Recursos Humanos al Gobernador.* San Juan, 1971.

36. Puerto Rico, Office of the Commonwealth of. *Puerto Rico U.S.A.* Washington, D.C., Office of the Commonwealth of Puerto Rico, 1971.

37. Roberts, L.J. and Stefani, R.L. *Patterns of Living in Puerto Rican Families.* San Juan, University of Puerto Rico Press, 1949.

38. Sanjur, D. *Puerto Rican Food Habits: A Socio-Cultural Approach.* Ithaca, New York, State Nutrition Institute (Cornell University), 1970.

39. Stahl, J.E. *The Economic Performance of Proportional-Profit Sugar Farms in Puerto Rico, 1950-62.* ERS-463. Washington, D.C., U.S. Department of Agriculture, 1971.

40. Suarez-Caabro, J.A. "Puerto Rico's Commercial Marine Fisheries: A Statistical Picture." *Commercial Fisheries Review,* 1970, 32 (3), 31-37.

41. University of Puerto Rico (College of Agricultural Sciences—Mayagüez Campus). *Basic Concepts and Program. Puerto Rico Agricultural Experimental Station.* Rio Piedras, University of Puerto Rico, 1971.

42. West, R.C. and Augelli, J.P. *Middle America: Its Land and Peoples.* Englewood Cliffs, N.J., Prentice-Hall, Inc., 1966.

LIST OF TABLES

LIST OF MAPS

TABLE NO. 1

Total Population By Age Group – Puerto Rico, 1965, 1969, 1972
(in 1,000's)

Ages	1965	1969*	1972*
0–4	369	409	423
5–9	307	360	396
10–14	316	312	338
15–19	254	290	297
20–24	214	221	241
25–29	181	200	208
30–34	162	171	182
35–39	145	159	167
40–44	138	146	155
45–49	123	134	141
50–54	108	118	126
55–59	82	99	109
60–64	68	76	85
65+	160	184	204
	2,627,000	2,879,000	3,072,000

*Estimate

Source: Commonwealth of Puerto Rico. *The Four Year Economic and Development Plan of Puerto Rico.* San Juan Planning Board, 1968.

TABLE NO. 2

Population by Region – Puerto Rico, 1965, 1969, 1972
(in 1,000's)

	1965	1969*	1972*
Puerto Rico Total	2,627	2,879	3,072
San Juan Region	1,737	1,904	2,030
Ponce Region	483	529	566
Mayagüez Region	407	446	476

*Estimate

Source: Commonwealth of Puerto Rico. *The Four Year Economic and Development Plan of Puerto Rico.* San Juan Planning Board, 1968.

TABLE NO. 3

Land Use – Puerto Rico, 1969

Use	Hectares	Total Hectares
Crops		251,000
Sugarcane	105,000	
Coffee	73,000	
Tobacco	3,000	
Others	70,000	
Pastures		332,000
Improved	194,000	
Natural	138,000	
Small plots under 1 ha*	21,000	21,000
Hills and swamps		94,000
Forests		36,000
Built-on and waste		152,000
Total		886,000

*Title V plots (see *Farms*) are not included here but are included in the total for crops.

Sources: Commonwealth of Puerto Rico (Department of Agriculture), *Anuario de Estadísticas Agrícolas de Puerto Rico, 1966-1969.*

Food and Agriculture Organization of the United Nations, *Production Yearbook 1970.*

TABLE NO. 4

Fertilizer Use by Crop and Type of Mixture — Puerto Rico, 1960-1969
(in tons of nutrient)

Use	1960	1969
Nitrogenous Mixtures		
Sugarcane	21,463	14,988
Tobacco	1,245	460
Coffee	1,839	2,115
Pineapples	555	73
Vegetables	584	719
Other crops	11	10
Unmixed	7,229	3,815
Total Nitrogenous	32,926	22,180
Phosphatic Mixtures		
Sugarcane	7,279	6,220
Tobacco	1,214	406
Coffee	1,692	1,189
Vegetables	142	17
Pineapples	692	782
Other crops	22	15
Unmixed	147	359
Total Phosphatic	11,188	8,988
Potassic Mixtures		
Sugarcane	17,329	13,273
Tobacco	1,757	619
Coffee	1,473	2,785
Pineapples	485	72
Vegetables	688	936
Other crops	11	9
Unmixed	158	351
Total Potassic	21,901	18,045

Source: Commonwealth of Puerto Rico. (Department of Agriculture). *Anuario de Estadísticas de Puerto Rico 1968-69.*

TABLE NO. 5

Area Sown in Major Crops – Puerto Rico, 1950-1970
(in hectares)

Crop	1950	1960	1964	1966	1968	1970
Rice	2,162	235	48	–	–	–
Corn	16,000	6,533	2,116	3,000	3,000	3,000
Dry beans	8,153	2,430	4,000	4,000	4,000	4,000
Cowpeas	1,498	585	104	–	–	–
Pigeon peas	8,097	4,453	4,048	5,000	4,000	4,000
Sweet potatoes	9,643	3,243	2,024	7,000	5,000	6,000
Yams	–	–	4,976			
Bananas	17,000	8,000	12,000	6,000	6,000	–
Cabbages	1,000	–	–	–	–	–
Tomatoes	1,000	–	2,000	2,000	1,000	1,000
Coffee	64,000	64,000	64,000	63,000	64,000	–
Pineapples	1,237	1,370	1,741	–	1,538	–
Tobacco	15,000	10,000	12,000	7,000	3,000	2,000
Sugarcane	148,000	135,594	113,000	107,000	90,000	83,000

Sources: Commonwealth of Puerto Rico (Planning Board), *Puerto Rico 1968 Statistical Yearbook.*

Food and Agriculture Organization of the United Nations, *Production Yearbook 1970.*

TABLE NO. 6

Production of Major Crops – Puerto Rico, 1950-1970
(in tons unless otherwise stated)

Crop	1950	1960	1964	1966	1968	1970
Rice	11,270	164	42	–	–	–
Corn	10,500	5,772	1,954	4,000	4,000	4,000
Dry beans	2,727	1,227	2,000	2,000	2,000	2,000
Cowpeas	454	304	56	–	–	–
Pigeon peas	3,136	3,407*	4,000	5,000	4,000	5,000
Sweet potatoes	14,545	7,272	6,000	6,000	–	–
Yams	11,363	13,772	21,000	21,000	24,000	25,000
Bananas	209,000	–	131,000	107,000	112,000	–
Cabbages	8,545	3,227	2,000	2,000	2,000	2,000
Tomatoes	7,864	10,045	22,000	14,000	8,000	9,000
Grapefruit	10,000	–	14,000	12,000	11,000	11,000
Oranges & tangerines	30,000	–	40,000	37,000	31,000	35,000
Coconuts (1,000 nuts)	23,000	21,500	13,000	–	13,000	–
Coffee	10,200	15,680	17,000	12,900	10,227	11,800
Pineapples	27,700	46,740	64,530	65,000	60,437	–
Tobacco	11,900	12,500	14,600	7,500	5,100	2,900
Sugarcane	10,500,000	10,750,000	7,900,000	8,586,000	5,900,000	4,630,000

*Yield doubled during decade.

Sources: Commonwealth of Puerto Rico (Planning Board), Puerto Rico 1968 Statistical Yearbook.
Food and Agriculture Organization of the United Nations, Production Yearbook 1970.

TABLE NO. 7

Livestock – Puerto Rico, 1951-1969
(in 1,000 head)

	1951	1956	1961	1966	1969
Cows	139	166	183	198	203
Young bulls	68	80	92	99	101
Bulls	63	93	109	105	112
Heifers	39	48	55	75	76
Oxen	34	28	19	18	15
Pigs	118	139	163	176	194
Goats	31	27	25	24	23
Chickens (commercial)*	223	411	1,311	2,141	2,290
Chickens (noncommercial)	1,840	1,972	1,924	1,477	1,618

*Kept in aviaries of more than 1,000 birds.

Sources: Commonwealth of Puerto Rico (Department of Agriculture). *Anuario de Estadísticas Agrícolas de Puerto Rico 1968-69.*

Food and Agriculture Organization of the United Nations. *Production Yearbook 1970.*

TABLE NO. 8

Trade in Agricultural Products By Value – Puerto Rico, 1963/64

(in dollars)

Items	Imports		Exports	
	From U.S.	From Other Countries	To U.S.	To Other Countries
TOTAL VALUE	267,607,076	47,778,412	301,535,191	7,306,652
1. Animal products	98,708,411	32,201,003	42,935,620	503,950
Breeders	2,463,706	61,551	—	73,172
Meat and meat products	48,870,433	9,863,967	—	202,665
Animal fats	8,467,986	—	—	105,230
Milk, milk products and eggs	30,816,304	1,334,829	—	36,998
Products of the fishing industry	3,627,580	20,932,350	—	54,181
Other animal products	4,462,402	8,306	—	31,704
2. Vegetable products	113,097,403	10,500,789	164,918,714	6,737,426
Cereals and cereal products	45,991,076	2,418,485	—	574,909
Fodder and animal feed	7,378,078	615,499	—	169,200
Vegetables and products	28,645,065	2,310,061	3,209,697	163,816
Fruits and fruit preparations	10,936,938	326,920	6,261,158	668,773
Nuts and nut preparations	775,703	7,041	510,434 (a)	24,800
Oils and vegetable fats	6,877,832	800,235	—	24,189
Cocoa, coffee and tea	1,860,811	185,169	3,191,160 (b)	1,306,939
Spices	358,521	242,989	—	16,932
Sugar, raw and refined	180,239	—	124,270,911	3,824
Confectioneries	5,264,703	664,334	1,577,278	244,850
Honey	26,592	—	3,599,546	1,752,625
Rum	—	—	11,238,543	—
Other beverages	4,803,845	2,930,055	11,059,987	1,786,569
3. Tobacco and by-products	55,801,262	5,076,620	93,680,857	65,276

Source: Commonwealth of Puerto Rico (Planning Board), *External Trade Statistics.*

TABLE NO. 9

Trade in Agricultural Products by Value – Puerto Rico, 1967/1968
(in dollars)

Items	Imports		Exports	
	From U.S.	From Other Countries	To U.S.	To Other Countries
TOTAL VALUE	367,289,777	76,537,264	327,133,147	15,397,749
1. Animal Products	127,568,022	53,015,646	70,383,111	1,329,939
Breeders	1,657,453	4,558	188,635	262,432
Meat and meat products	77,251,011	16,351,283	2,311	725,074
Animal fats	209,896	–	23,292	–
Milk	41,123,278	2,686,505	554,646	185,428
Fish and fish products	7,326,384	33,973,300	69,614,227	157,005
2. Vegetable products	139,721,755	23,521,618	256,750,036	14,067,810
Cereals and cereal products	53,281,951	1,639,108	1,032,874	1,418,612
Fruits and vegetables	48,286,016	7,251,084	7,721,044	1,604,483
Oils and vegetable fats	7,804,412	1,398,500	–	–
Raw and refined sugar	191,267	–	83,245,452	1,936
Honey and confectionery	4,761,979	1,972,381	2,177,967	6,804,751
Coffee, tea, cocoa	5,971,304	212,240	478,493	816,791
Fodder and animal feed	12,032,550	1,043,899	5,309,383	648,494
Other food products	33,816,582	1,026,299	385,046	2,123,985
Rum	19,060	–	22,595,265	127,823
Other beverages	9,981,301	5,407,330	2,667,196	501,471
3. Tobacco and by-products	63,575,333	3,570,777	131,137,316	19,464

Source: Commonwealth of Puerto Rico (Planning Board), *External Trade Statistics.*

TABLE NO. 10

Seasonal Indices of Stocks of Agricultural Products at Main Marketplaces – Puerto Rico, 1968

(Annual average = 100)

Product	Jan.	Feb.	Mar.	Apr.	May	June	July	Aug.	Sept.	Oct.	Nov.	Dec.
Sweet peppers	74.04	53.49	51.18	76.60	111.35	134.16	135.47	140.76	123.27	114.04	107.23	78.41
Celery	78.25	109.43	156.01	146.25	133.20	112.16	107.67	83.34	72.30	66.01	63.66	71.72
Domestic chickens	85.81	82.69	87.72	87.35	95.94	102.54	106.36	106.36	113.93	110.41	101.08	119.24
Eggplants	97.68	86.72	100.85	94.53	107.43	107.26	87.54	89.57	98.98	113.15	108.77	107.52
Goats	84.36	31.12	58.19	96.07	85.18	73.62	126.05	97.51	142.22	108.83	93.51	203.34
Pumpkins	83.04	81.53	86.79	94.09	115.21	142.12	145.75	118.54	105.49	94.37	61.62	71.45
Pigs	87.06	78.41	83.85	85.69	99.60	100.61	95.00	98.24	99.48	107.35	103.13	161.58
Coriander	108.87	105.75	102.91	85.46	86.05	99.38	95.50	88.93	87.79	93.75	107.36	138.25
Coconuts	89.75	77.19	109.57	123.08	126.80	145.45	125.83	92.99	71.35	63.24	62.77	111.98
Shallots	142.59	95.96	81.61	64.27	61.77	79.66	58.36	48.90	58.63	154.68	187.65	165.92
Bananas (large)	81.68	72.54	73.57	64.57	85.30	105.21	109.35	136.73	133.26	139.84	101.45	96.50
Bananas (Monte Cristo)	78.85	84.01	97.73	98.07	104.33	116.40	113.15	120.56	113.29	98.38	79.83	95.40
Bananas (purple)	83.03	101.95	76.46	83.08	85.64	101.67	98.33	120.08	131.90	124.16	70.48	123.22
Bananas (small)	75.42	85.29	90.37	100.82	113.46	156.82	141.00	129.91	89.54	67.62	75.58	74.17
Beans	58.47	92.19	86.87	85.70	126.31	208.84	223.89	72.56	39.55	70.99	82.23	52.40
Beans (stringless)	110.34	83.34	81.34	82.29	97.27	152.92	91.89	61.30	88.74	126.80	115.14	108.63
Eggs (domestic)	92.73	126.78	137.32	126.85	121.12	109.96	88.45	96.61	94.52	69.87	58.26	77.53
Lettuce	135.82	126.04	141.01	138.31	95.25	72.42	76.53	79.76	66.27	65.13	80.53	122.93
Corn (dry in grains)	188.99	158.18	95.13	91.24	83.46	41.03	51.31	124.17	95.65	87.66	80.42	102.76
Corn (sweet)	33.15	48.56	64.03	84.22	138.38	201.72	220.45	93.87	47.60	74.90	115.39	77.73
Malanga	97.50	138.33	179.00	153.58	116.27	98.55	93.49	55.81	56.01	52.19	67.21	92.06

Papayas (green)	85.61	73.11	79.95	76.15	100.26	137.62	119.42	107.87	98.61	94.40	107.75	119.25
Chillies	103.14	94.83	89.97	84.87	88.79	112.92	94.02	110.46	114.33	110.58	102.60	93.48
Pineapples	55.65	47.66	86.10	103.55	167.23	200.92	168.63	88.45	61.65	66.92	74.25	78.99
Plantains (first crop)	76.92	77.97	87.62	93.97	102.83	115.34	113.76	122.20	110.12	106.52	99.71	93.04
Plantains (second crop)	60.96	56.30	57.34	62.44	84.86	101.48	127.76	158.88	171.95	139.28	96.88	81.87
Tomatoes	105.80	98.76	87.83	88.58	99.80	120.07	108.83	109.88	80.10	88.13	104.35	107.87
Dasheens (yellow)	88.48	134.83	175.62	166.43	132.75	90.01	93.55	54.51	39.83	30.33	49.56	144.10
Dasheens (white)	119.23	116.13	123.31	113.08	90.22	69.92	52.15	42.27	61.27	101.22	133.44	177.76
Dasheens (Kelly)	98.24	148.21	167.99	177.41	143.80	89.41	47.99	25.69	41.53	55.12	71.46	133.15
Dasheens (purple)	82.17	92.32	114.96	110.13	121.20	119.35	122.89	105.78	87.82	82.25	77.25	83.88
Dasheens (other)	55.71	66.94	99.84	121.99	139.24	160.69	157.11	141.18	90.62	64.70	48.02	53.96
Manioc	102.65	102.25	123.90	112.50	114.29	117.19	99.09	80.77	69.70	73.88	92.63	111.15

Source: Commonwealth of Puerto Rico (Department of Agriculture), *Anuario de Estadísticas Agrícolas de Puerto Rico 1968-69.*

TABLE NO. 11

Blood Values of Certain Nutrients in Puerto Rican Villages – 1963 and 1967

Nutrient in the Blood	Mavilla 1963	Mavilla 1967	Naranjo 1963	Naranjo 1967	Manzanilla	Cialitos	Santiago	Master Survey
Hemoglobin (g/100 ml)	12.8	14.0	12.4	13.5	10.9	11.1	12.0	13.9
Plasma protein (g/100 ml)	7.2	7.4	7.8	7.3	7.5	7.4	7.4	7.5
Plasma carotene (mcg/100 ml)	–	–	–	–	112.9	99.0	84.0	111.0
Plasma vitamin A (mcg/100 ml)	–	–	–	–	52.0	60.0	85.0	62.0
Plasma ascorbic acid (mg/100 ml)	1.1	1.5	0.2	1.5	1.0	1.0	45.0	1.4

Sources: Computed from all surveys conducted by Fernández et al.

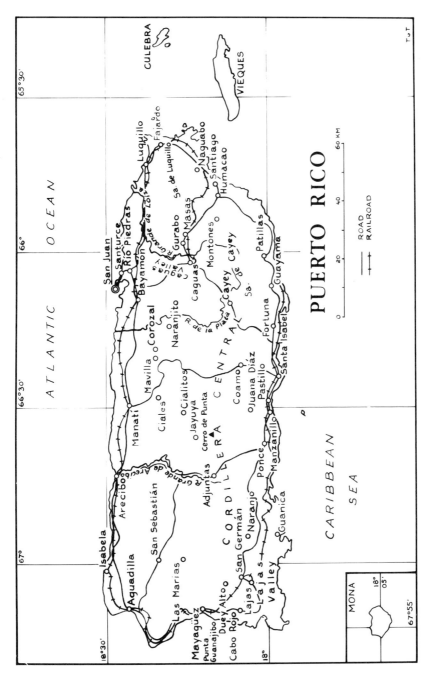

PUERTO RICO

ROAD
RAILROAD

MAP NO. 1

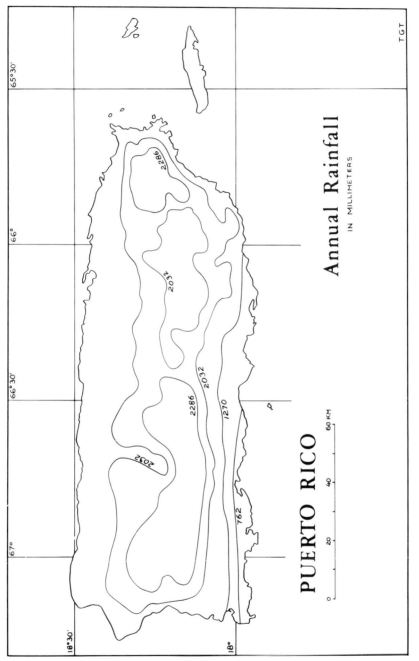

Annual Rainfall

IN MILLIMETERS

PUERTO RICO

MAP NO. 2.

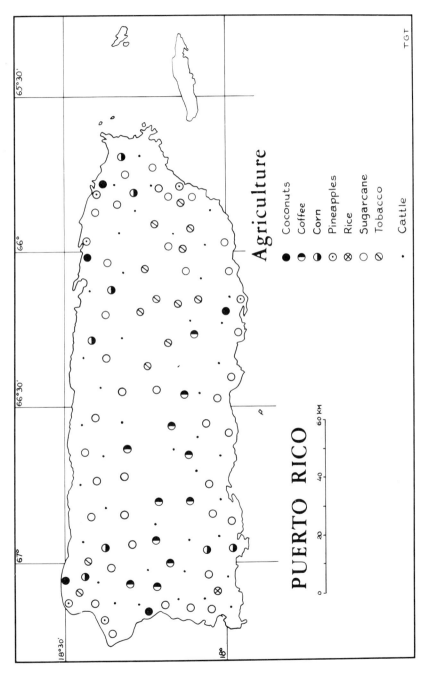

Agriculture

● Coconuts
◐ Coffee
◑ Corn
⊙ Pineapples
⊗ Rice
○ Sugarcane
⊘ Tobacco
· Cattle

PUERTO RICO

60 KM

MAP NO. 3.

THE LESSER ANTILLES

TABLE OF CONTENTS

INTRODUCTION

The Lesser Antilles are a group of West Indies Caribbean Islands extending in an arc from the Virgin Islands off Puerto Rico through the Netherlands Antilles off the coast of Venezuela. They are an artificial geographical grouping, not a political entity, as they encompass a variety of independent states and their dependencies. For ease of discussion, only Barbados, the British Leeward Islands (Antigua, St. Christopher-Nevis-Anguilla, Montserrat and the British Virgin Islands), the British Windward Islands (Grenada, St. Vincent, St. Lucia, Dominica and the Grenadines) and the French departments of Guadeloupe and Martinique will be described in this chapter. The Netherlands Antilles and the islands belonging to Venezuela will be dealt with in a later volume.

Most of the islands included here lie roughly in a square delineated by 18° and 12° north latitude and 60° and 66° west longitude. All of the Virgin Islands lie just north and Barbados just east of these limits.

BARBADOS

TABLE OF CONTENTS

BARBADOS

I. BACKGROUND INFORMATION

A. PHYSICAL SETTING [17] [2] [24] [14] [52]

Barbados is the largest (430 square kilometers) and most important of the Lesser Antilles. This ham-shaped island lies about 250 nautical miles northeast of mainland South America just over the thirteenth parallel, 59.5° east of Greenwich, making it the most easterly of the West Indies islands. It is 34 kilometers long and 22 kilometers wide. The island is of coral origin and is almost encircled by coral reefs.

The ground rises in terraced fashion from sandy beaches to a high point of 337 meters at Mt. Hillaby. Most of the island is covered by coral limestone and soils which are particularly favorable to sugarcane. The land is about 85 percent arable. Although forage crops once covered the island, only about 16 hectares remain. Various kinds of palm trees, mahogany, breadfruit, tamarind, casuarina, flamboyant and frangipani trees are scattered throughout Barbados but the island's central landscape is characterized for the most part by gently undulating land covered with sugarcane fields. Few slopes on the island are too steep for cultivation.

There are no rivers on Barbados, just gullies and a few rivulets. Most of the island's freshwater resources lie underground in limestone caverns which permit pumping of the water to the surface. There are few wild animals: some monkeys (which are an annoyance to cultivators), mongooses (which were introduced to the island in order to decimate the rat population and have now become pests themselves) and some hares occasionally killed for food.

B. CLIMATE [17] [52] [2]

The climate of Barbados is generally pleasant with temperatures averaging 24-26.5°C and rarely exceeding 30°C or dropping below 18°C. Even in the dry

season (which lasts from about December to May) the climate is tolerable due to
the ocean breezes and easterly trade winds. Rainfall varies between districts with
averages of about 1,270-1,905 millimeters (see Map No. 2). Hurricanes occasionally hit the island but none has done great damage since 1831.

C. POPULATION [36] [40] [14] [52] [2] [32]

In 1969 the population estimate for Barbados was 252,900 people. The rate
of increase is said to be about 1.1 percent a year, which is low for a developing
country, and the density at 591 persons per square kilometer is one of the
highest in the world, comparable to that of the Nile Valley. In 1968, the infant
mortality rate was 45.7 per 1,000 live births, compared to 22 in the United
States. Life expectancy at birth was 62.7 years for males and 67.4 years for
females.

Ethnically, the population is about 80 percent African, 5 percent European
and 15 percent mixed. There are a few East Indians in the country. The
inhabitants are predominantly urbanized with only about 23 percent of the
labor force engaged in agriculture. The literacy rate is high at 97 percent;
education is free and compulsory from 7-13 years of age. By religion, the
population is primarily Christian; about 20 percent of the people are Anglicans
and the remainder are mainly Methodists, Moravians or Roman Catholics.

In spite of unemployment problems, the level of living is higher than in the
Windward and Leeward islands. Per capita annual income rose from $306 in
1960 to $430* in 1967 which, of course, does not mean that every Barbadian
has that much to spend in cash every year.

D. HISTORY AND GOVERNMENT [17] [53] [14]

The early history of Barbados is obscure, but archeological findings indicate
that the island was once inhabited by a sizable population of Arawak Indians.
The Spaniards landed there in 1518 and there is evidence that they took Indians
from Barbados to Hispaniola as slave laborers. By 1536 no Indians were left.
British settlers landed on Barbados sometime between 1620 and 1625 and,
uniquely among the West Indies, the island never changed hands thereafter. The
settlers were mainly sugar planters who introduced African slaves to work their
estates. Slavery was abolished in 1834 and emancipation was completed by
1838, but without destroying the island's economy as it did in Jamaica.

---

*This figure (quoted by Buck) is different from the average family income of $300 found
by Caribbean Food and Nutrition Institute investigators. This shows once more the fallacy
of measuring development through GNP which does not show the distribution of cash
income among individuals.

Barbados was part of the short-lived West Indies Federation (1958-1965) and became an independent nation within the British Commonwealth in 1966. The Queen of England is the Head of State and the Prime Minister the Head of Government. The Governor General represents the Queen and acts on the advice of the Cabinet appointed by the Governor General with the consent and recommendation of the Prime Minister. The Cabinet is responsible to the bicameral Parliament. The House of Assembly consists of 24 members elected by universal suffrage while the Senate is composed of 21 members appointed by the Governor General: 12 on the recommendation of the Prime Minister, two on the advice of the Leader of the Opposition and seven at the Governor's discretion. The judicial branch of the Government is headed by a Supreme Court whose decisions override those of lower courts.

Bridgetown is the capital of Barbados. The island is divided into three district councils (North, South and Bridgetown City) and 11 parishes (St. Lucy, St. Peter, St. Andrew, St. James, St. Joseph, St. Thomas, St. John, St. George, St. Michael, St. Philip and Christ Church). Barbados is a member of the United Nations, the Organization of American States, the General Agreement on Trade and Tariffs, and the Caribbean Free Trade Association. It participates in the Caribbean Oils and Fats and Rice agreements.

E. AGRICULTURAL POLICIES [21] [42] [35] [2] [15]

For centuries Barbados has relied on a single crop—sugarcane—to support its economy. Of the 27,732 hectares of arable land, 24,300 are planted in sugarcane. Sugar accounts for 96 percent of the island's agricultural exports and 89 percent of its total exports, bringing an annual income of about $20 million. Barbados' food import bill, however, amounts to over $15 million per year. Therefore, without the $15 million derived annually from the tourist trade, the island would have little money to devote to infrastructure and rural development activities. The Government recognizes the precariousness of Barbados' present economic position. The island's sugar income depends to a great extent on the Commonwealth Sugar Agreement which will be up for renewal in 1975 and which may have to be abandoned altogether by the British Government when the U.K. joins the European Economic Community (Common Market). The tourist trade, on the other hand, is very sensitive to political instability and racial unrest, which so far have not plagued Barbados but could create real or imagined problems in the future. It is essential, therefore, that agricultural diversification be promoted both to decrease the island's heavy reliance on food imports and to provide new sources of foreign exchange.

Positive government actions to encourage diversification and to increase food production have included the creation of an Agricultural Development Corporation, the establishment of a Marketing Corporation and the initiation of research on food crops adaptable to Barbados. The Agricultural Development Corporation operates about 800 hectares of public or crown lands on the east coast where agricultural diversification on a commercial scale is demonstrated. Recently many Barbadian farmers have been experimenting with truck crops as a result of the Government's emphasis on varying production. Onions were grown commercially in 1970 for the first time in the island's history.

The Marketing Corporation buys and sells locally produced vegetables, fish and shrimp on the domestic market and exports yams, potatoes and fish. The Corporation promotes the formation of producers' cooperatives (it is reported that the Government admits favoring cooperatives over individuals in the awarding of grants, loans and subsidies) and provides processing facilities for food crops, fish and shrimp, as well as storage accommodations.

As a result of legislation passed in 1955, all sugar estates of 10 hectares or more are required to plant 12.5 percent of their arable acreage in food crops each year. Moreover, each estate must keep one cow or pig or five sheep for every 8 hectares of land. The sugar producers themselves have begun voluntarily experimenting with other crops, establishing a Crop Diversification Research Unit in 1965 under the aegis of the Sugar Producers Association.

The Government's concern for the nutritional status of the population has been illustrated by the establishment in 1967 of a National Nutrition Committee whose purpose is to improve nutrition in the country.

F. FOREIGN AID

1. Bilateral Aid [14]

Barbados receives no grants-in-aid from foreign governments. There is, however, a U.S. Peace Corps contingent on the island. Indirect aid is received from the United States and the United Kingdom in the form of favorable sugar quotas and Barbados is given preferential treatment by the U.K. under the Commonwealth Tariff System.

2. Multilateral Aid [41]

The United Nations Children's Fund (UNICEF), the Food and Agriculture Organization of the United Nations (FAO), The World Health Organization (WHO), the World Food Program (WFP) and the United Nations Educational, Scientific and Cultural Organization (UNESCO) give assistance to Barbados. An applied nutrition project under United Nations auspices has been underway in Barbados since 1968 at a cost of approximately $41,000. The objective of the project is the improve the nutrition of the population, particularly mothers and children, through nutrition education, training of staff and increased production of nutritionally valuable foods. By 1970, the school feeding aspect of the project had reached 10,400 children in 39 schools; 33 school gardens had been established; a pilot poultry-raising center had been initiated; and home economics had been introduced into the standard curriculum of 38 schools on the island. Education of the general public is being accomplished through the use of a mobile cinema, which shows films on nutrition, horticulture, small animal raising, etc. Courses in applied nutrition are organized for agricultural education, medical and social welfare personnel. UNICEF has provided supplies, equipment, transport and training grants under the project; FAO has supplied an expert in nutrition and home economics; WHO has provided technical advice and fellowships; and the WFP has obtained food donations for the school feeding program.

In addition to the applied nutrition program, UN agencies (UNICEF and UNESCO) have supported a $12,000 social services project aimed at improving day care facilities and increasing the understanding of the needs of the preschool child, including nutrition, and how to meet those needs.

II. FOOD RESOURCES

A. GENERAL [18] [15]

Barbados has an arable land total of 26,360 hectares, about 24,000 of which are occupied by 60-75 sugar estates, leaving only 2,360 hectares, dispersed at the periphery of the estates, for production of food crops. Domestic livestock and fish provide additional sources of food. There is a heavy reliance on food imports whose value rose constantly between 1961 and 1966 but declined slightly in the years 1967 and 1968.

A survey was conducted in 1969 by the Caribbean Food and Nutrition Institute (CFNI) to determine the state of nutrition on the island. Of the 651 families investigated, only 12 percent were found to grow part of the diet they consume. The food budget is high, amounting to a mean 51 percent of all expenditures. If the median rather than the mean is considered, the majority of the families spend 64 percent of their income on food. Further studies reveal that 10 percent of the families located in the lowest percentile spend 94 percent of their income on food while at the other end of the income scale, the most privileged sector spends only 39 percent.

The average income of the families investigated in the survey reached $300 per year. However, if the median rather than the mean is considered, the level drops considerably to $181 per annum, meaning that there are many more people below the mean than above. Mean total expenditure was $284, which is consistent with an average income of $300, but does not leave much for capital formation. The biggest source of income for 57.9 percent of the population is wages, followed by white-collar workers' salaries (9.7 percent of the population), other relatives' contributions (8.8 percent), trading profits (4.8 percent) and others. The main source of noncash income is food grown or given by relatives.

Since only about 12 percent of the families on Barbados grow some food for autoconsumption and only a small number of laborers work tiny plots for themselves on the side, it is clear that most of the food resources by far have to be purchased and only a tiny fraction of society can contribute homegrown staples to their diets.

B. MEANS OF PRODUCTION

1. Agricultural Labor Force [26] [48] [27] [6] [5] [2]

The labor problem of Barbados is governed by two major factors: the very high density of the population (591 per square kilometer) and the declining appeal of work in the cane fields. This conjuncture creates at the same time unemployment during the off-season of the sugar industry and labor shortages at harvesttime. The consequences for the production of foods and for nutrition are bound to be serious. The second most important industry is tourism, which attracts to the city as many workers as it can absorb, if not more. With the disaffection from the sugar fields, there is bound to be unemployment in the cities among the young people, who in ever-increasing numbers are deserting the hard labor of cane cutting. Only approximate employment figures are available for recent years but, out of a total labor force of about 95,000 people, it is estimated that 20,000 are in domestic and personal services, 15,000 in commerce, 12,000 in construction work and 13,000-15,000 in agriculture. A number of workers not included in the above list are self-employed.

The table below shows the changes that have occurred over the last 50 years in agricultural employment, which for 300 years provided a livelihood for the majority of the population in Barbados.

Changes in the Agricultural Labor Force – Barbados, 1921-1969

Year	Agricultural Labor Force	Total Population	Percent
1921	32,728	156,774	21
1946	24,156	192,800	12
1960	21,388	234,327	9
1968	14,848	252,931	6
1969	13,325	255,000	5

Source: *Labor Developments Abroad,* 1970, 15 (11).

The table reflects the lack of interest of the labor force in this traditional field of employment—a lack of interest which is general throughout the sugar belt (see chapter on Jamaica) but more pronounced in this small island where, paradoxically, other occupations are not readily available. At harvesttime, workers can still be imported from St. Vincent and St. Lucia, but with increasing difficulty due to the unpopularity of cane cutting. In 1969 sugar-field workers numbered

8,872 men, representing 66.6 percent of all male agricultural laborers. Fifty percent of these sugarcane workers were over 50 years of age and 20 percent were over 60. This spells the end of the industry within 10 years unless labor is replaced by cutting machines; and in that event, the unemployment rate will rise. Research is being conducted to design a harvester adapted to local circumstances.

In March 1971, the Government announced that it would soon guarantee 40 hours a week employment rather than 24 to all sugarcane workers. No information is available as to how this is to be accomplished. Reportedly, the Government wishes to train manpower to operate cooperatives.

2. Farms [53] [2] [15] [52] [18]

As elsewhere in the Caribbean, one of the most consequential problems in the history of malnutrition is land tenure. At the time the slaves were freed, almost all the arable land was owned by sugar planters. This forced the emancipated slaves to work for their former masters or leave the island. Because of this abundant cheap labor, the economy survived, almost on its old terms. It also surmounted the crises that shook the sugar industry at various times during the 19th century. In 1935, a considerable amount of the best land (over 50 percent) was still privately owned by large plantations while 70 percent of the farmers owned less than one-half hectare each. This resulted in lessening the amount of homegrown food to such an extent that its price rose to exceed that of imported food. It became cheaper to live on imported rice, cornmeal, evaporated milk and salted codfish than to buy vegetables at the nearby market. By 1935, the system had directly influenced nutrition because of the high cost of the food budget. The only way to change this situation would have been to grow more food. We shall see that diversification in Barbados is a serious problem fraught with unusual difficulties, the greatest of which is that under present conditions the Barbadian soil can produce sugarcane better and cheaper than any other crop.

There is no vacant land on Barbados. The population pressure on the one hand and the smallness of the island on the other have worked to produce a condition of full land use. There are about 250 estates of from 4 to 400 hectares each, but averaging 60-80 hectares. The smallholders also produce cane, but some of the estates produce as much as six times more per hectare than the poorly organized single farm operator. Food-producing farms are usually small plots of 1 hectare or less. These holdings represent two-thirds of all farms but occupy only 15 percent of the land. Small farms either adjoin a compound of houses which, along with a church, a school and an all-purpose shop, form a cluster-like village, or they are part of a village located on or at the periphery of a sugar estate or along a main highway, usually on rather poor land. Occasionally, dispersed houses stand on the least fertile sections of land in the country.

In 1969, it was estimated that a minimum area of 7 x 7 meters, 49 square meters could make a small but significant contribution to a family diet if adequately cultivated. It was found that while 27 percent of all families surveyed by the CFNI investigators had no food gardens, 16 percent had gardens smaller than 49 square meters. Fifty-seven of the rural families had small farms larger than 49 square meters but smaller than 1 hectare. About 46.8 percent of the holdings were located in St. Michael Parish, 23.3 percent in the northern districts, 15.8 percent in St. Philip Parish, and 14.1 percent in Christ Church Parish. Fifty percent of the farmers owned their land, 40 percent were primarily tenant farmers on leased land, and 10 percent were government employees, presumably operating on Crown land. Some 92.3 percent of the farms adjoined the house of the cultivating family. About 73.3 percent of the farmland was planted in crops, 5.4 percent was in pastures, 0.8 percent was fallow and 20.5 percent was uncultivated.

The foods produced on these farms were, in order of decreasing popularity, coconuts (on 37.2 percent of the farms), bananas (33.4 percent), limes (22.9 percent), breadfruit (22.5 percent), pigeon peas (21.7 percent), avocados (21.6 percent), and papayas (21.1 percent). Other crops included yams, sweet potatoes, pumpkins, tomatoes, etc. These crops were consumed by the farmer and his family, but surpluses of some of them, such as sugarcane, avocados, bananas, sweet potatoes, yams, okra, tomatoes and carrots, were sold in sufficient amounts to be considered commercial.

3. Fertilizers [18]

No data are available on the amount of fertilizer used on the food cropland of Barbados. It is likely that those plots of land adjoining the cash crop estates receive more fertilizer than, for instance, small detached hillside farms. Barbados as a whole absorbs 2,800 tons of nitrogenous fertilizer per year, less than in 1964 when 4,200 tons were used but not much more than in 1948-1952 when the amount was 2,100 tons per annum. The fluctuation of sugar prices on the world market may have much more to do with the curve of fertilizer application than the degree of sophistication of the farmer. Since 1966, small amounts of phosphatic fertilizer (400-600 tons) have been spread on certain lands. Potash is much needed on Barbados soils and the consumption of this chemical is similar to that of nitrogenous mixtures (2,800 tons in 1969 against 2,100 tons in 1948 and 4,800 in 1964). If this were shared between cash and food crops, about one-tenth might have been spread on legumes, vegetables and cereals.

4. Mechanical Equipment [18]

The size of food-producing holdings precludes the use of mechanical equipment. The nature of sugarcane, the primary cash crop, requires that the individual plants be placed in holes dug by hand. As yet only preliminary research has been done on the type of machines that could be used for harvesting the cane. It comes as no surprise that the number of tractors on record did not exceed 319 in 1964, the most recent year for which data are available.

C. PRODUCTION [52]

As already indicated (see page 314), food production is compulsory on certain estates but a ceiling is imposed on prices; hence, no farmer plants more than he has to and beyond what he can consume. When the land permits it, the smallholder prefers to raise sugarcane than to take a chance on selling surplus food crops. It was the fertility of the soil and the availability of cheap labor which 300 years ago launched Barbados on its monoculture career of planting sugarcane. The cane is the main money-earner for all farms, whether they be large estates or mini-plots.

1. Food Crops [52] [18] [15] [21] [6] [47]

An effort to develop the production of food crops was launched in 1963 when the Barbados Marketing Corporation was founded. This agency gives financial assistance to farmers and operates a demonstration project of 300 hectares on the east coast. Most of the food production is concentrated on roots and legumes which represent the basic staples of the diet. As shown by the following table, since 1966 there has been a slight decline in the production of most food crops.

Production of Major Crops – Barbados, 1948-1970
(in 1,000 tons)

Crop	1948-1952	1964	1966	1968	1969	1970
Corn	1	1	1	1	1	1
Sugarcane	1,464	1,760	1,860	1,284	1,400	n.a.
Centrifugal sugar (raw)	168	195	204	142	156	160
Sweet potatoes and yams	38	20	20	22	22	n.a.
Manioc	2	1	1	1	1	n.a.

n.a.=data not available

Source: Food and Agriculture Organization of the United Nations, *Production Yearbook 1970.*

The only cereal grown, and in very small amounts, is corn. It is believed that there is a considerable future for this crop; if the local demand could be satisfied from domestic production, $250,000 per year in foreign exchange could be saved. The smallness of the food plots is, of course, a hindrance to mechanical production. Pulses, mainly pigeon peas, are grown on patches in the sugar estates. About 250 tons are produced annually, but 1,200 tons are imported.

Sweet potatoes have declined, but plantings in corn and pulses are said to have increased. Unfortunately, there are no statistics on which to base a discussion of areas sown and quantities consumed. All the information available indicates that there is no shortage of vegetables or fruits in Barbados, although only 25 percent of the estates grow them. Most of those who do grow food crops focus on tomatoes, which are channeled into commercial markets. Other vegetables are raised by small producers, thus adding some cash to their income. Barbadians spend about $24 per year per capita on vegetables, and residents, rather than tourists, consume 90 percent of the homegrown supply. The following table shows the estimated output of vegetables by kind during the crop year 1967-68.

Production of Vegetables – Barbados, 1967-1968

Crops	Area (hectares)			Production (tons)		
	Estates	Smallholders	Total	Estates	Smallholders	Total
Tomatoes	49	14	63	250	73	323
Cucumbers	13	37	50	67	183	250
Cabbages	12	83	95	61	426	487
European potatoes	9	–	9	73	–	73
String beans	8	73	81	45	405	450
Carrots	8	93	101	44	478	522
Other vegetables	19	302	321	96	1,592	1,688
Total			720			3,793

Source: Caribbean Food and Nutrition Institute, *Barbados Nutrition Survey.*

2. Cash Crops [2] [18] [22] [15] [47]

Cane dominates cash crop production. From 1961 to 1965, the average annual output was 176,000 tons a year. The crop dropped to 161,000 tons in 1968, to 142,000 tons in 1969 and rose to 157,000 tons in 1970. In terms of value, the average sales after 1966 amounted to $32.6 million a year as against $8.3 million for all other agricultural products. The sale of sugar, molasses and rum has accounted for 88.2 percent of all domestic exports from Barbados. The fate of Barbados sugar after Britain enters the European Common Market is the most serious concern of the Government of Barbados. The present industry, whose agreement with Britain expires in 1975, is anxious to improve its position by updating processing techniques. This represents large capital investments which cannot be contemplated unless the future of the crop is strengthened and outlets are assured. To this end, requests are pending to the United States Government to increase its quota of purchases from the West Indies.

Sugar could be replaced at least partly by onion cultivation which could not only save the island $175,000 in imports each year but could also earn at least $1 million through exports. Local onion growers, however, are waiting for tax concessions and credit facilities from the Government to help them finance the considerable capital expenditure needed. Lack of irrigation facilities and scarcity of credit for nonsugar crops have been heavy handicaps have and come under attack by experts from the Inter-American Committee for the Alliance for Progress (CIAP). Complete reorganization of the Barbados Marketing Corporation, the sales outlet for nonsugar crops, has been recommended by CIAP.

At the end of January 1971, the Minister of Agriculture announced subsidies for feed for all animals except poultry and horses, subsidies for fertilizers, a rise in the maximum grant for irrigation facilities from $750 to $3,000, and several other improvements in existing incentive schemes. Along with diversification in agriculture, the Government is trying to get away from its excessive dependence on North America for industrial investment and for the flow of tourists. It has become keenly interested in the European market.

Other possible cash crops include fruits and vegetables, some of which are already shipped to the United Kingdom, and cereals, some of which are shipped to Antigua, St. Lucia and Trinidad.

3. Animal Husbandry [14] [18] [15]

a. Livestock and Poultry

Barbados has a livestock industry, although cattle could never compete with sugar for the use of land. The high cost of imported feed is a hindrance to the development of a locally based meat industry. Nevertheless, the Government is supporting a program to improve the quality of the local stock. An island-wide artificial insemination scheme for cattle is based at the Central Livestock Station. There are approximately 17,000 head of cattle, 42,000 head of sheep, 30,000 pigs and 20,000 goats on the island. These animals are raised on estates and small farms in groups of three or four, mostly for their contribution to the local food supply. Some ranches specialize in animal husbandry for commercial purposes. Live animals as well as some small amounts of meat, meat preparations and eggs are exported to Grenada and Trinidad.

b. Meat, Milk and Eggs

Meat production is increasing and its consumption has almost doubled since 1958, bringing the total per capita per annum availability to 24.1 kilos. The following table shows the increased preference for pork, the growing consumption of poultry, and the static availability of beef (which means, given the population increase, that either fewer people eat beef or that the same people eat less of it).

With the exception of beef, imports of meat have increased considerably during the 8 years considered. Thirty to 50 percent of the pork imported is in the form of salted meat.

Availability of Meat – Barbados, 1958 and 1966

Years	Kind of Meat	Local Product (tons)	Imports (tons)	Total Available (tons)	Per Capita Per Year (kilos)
	Beef	390	1,354	1,744	6.8
	Pork	477	560	1,037	4.1
1958	Mutton	96	81	177	.7
	Poultry	184	298	482	1.7
	Total				13.3
	Beef	390	1,350	1,740	6.8
	Pork	697	1,743	2,440	10.0
1966	Mutton	100	210	310	1.2
	Poultry	260	1,280	1,540	6.1
	Total				24.1

Source: After Caribbean Food and Nutrition Institute, *Barbados Nutrition Survey.*

Since 1966, Barbados has had a milk processing plant at Pine Hill. This is supplied by the milk of about 5,000 cows distributed throughout the estates and small farms. Production is increasing, as the Pine Hill factory received 1,800 tons of milk in 1968 against 600 tons in 1966. FAO estimates the amount of cow's milk drunk on the farm at 5,000 tons and the amount of goat's milk at 2,000 tons. To increase availability, substantial quantities of milk and milk products are imported, although in decreasing amounts every year, indicating that local production is slowly catching up with demand. The amount of evaporated or condensed milk and cream imported has dropped from 4,520 tons in 1963 to 3,480 tons in 1968, but the imports of the dry product increased from 450 tons to 650 tons during the same period.

4. Fisheries [2] [6] [15]

About 1,700 persons depend upon fishing for a living. They operate a fleet of about 500 powered boats, converted from sail with the assistance of Government loans. A shrimp fishing industry has been started by Barbados Seafoods Ltd., a company formed in 1963. The firm at present has about 28 trawlers in operation but the fleet will eventually comprise 50 vessels, fishing mainly at the mouth of the Amazon River on the South American coast.

The fishing activities of Barbados are not as intense as one would expect, given its favorable location. The fishing grounds around the island are teeming with good edible fish but the landings are not adequate to feed the population and fish is still imported in considerable amounts. A United Nations Development Program pre-investment survey revealed that in 1969 Barbados imported $1 million worth of fish and fish products. Exploratory investigations indicate that there are large unexploited resources of fish along the Guyana coastal shelf and hence that possibilities exist for Barbados and other neighboring Caribbean countries to increase their yearly production of fish and shrimp for export. There are 26 landing points on the island, about 12 of which keep records. It is believed that landings at these locations correspond to 46 percent of the total fish consumed. Moreover, a survey recently conducted in Barbados indicates that only 40 percent of all families catch fish regularly themselves. The largest proportion of these families are located in Christ Church and St. Philip parishes. The table below shows that, by and large, the availability of fish has not changed very much during the last 10 years. If estimates are correct, the total amount of fish available in 1968, both domestic and imported, amounted to 9,700 tons, which would give an annual consumption of about 100 grams per capita per day, wastage not deducted.

Annual Availability of Fish – Barbados, 1958-1968
(in tons)

Year	Availability
1958	3.6
1960	4.4
1962	6.7
1964	3.0
1966	5.8
1968	4.5

Source: Caribbean Food and Nutrition Institute, *Barbados Nutrition Survey*.

D. FOOD INDUSTRIES [21] [22] [2] [15]

Beyond the processing of cane into sugar, molasses and rum, the food industries of Barbados are not very developed. As could be expected, sugar mills form the largest part of the industrial potential. In 1966 these included 21 factories located mostly in the central highlands. This is equivalent to the number which Jamaica has for dealing with a much larger crop, indicating the relative inefficiency of the Barbadian plants. In April 1971, it was announced that a company had been formed to own and operate all of the island's sugar and molasses factories. Four have already been closed as the result of this consolidation and it is planned to shut down three more during the next few years. This concentration should help rationalize the factory capacity and substantially cut down production costs, but a sizable amount of capital is needed to expand and modernize the remaining 10 factories.

Other food industries include Barbados Seafoods Ltd., which owns a shrimp processing plant, the West India Biscuit Company, the Banks Breweries, and a canning factory at Waterford in St. Michael Parish which also exports molasses.

Other plants process vegetable fats and produce various kinds of edible oils, margarine and lard as well as soap.

The milk processing plant at Pine Hill has a capacity of 10 tons daily, but the cost of operation is high because the cattle have to be fed with imported feed. In 1968, the producer received 14-15¢ for 450 grams and the retail price of homogenized, pasteurized and packaged milk was up to 45¢ a liter, too high for the average consumer.

The Barbados Marketing Corporation operates an abbatoir capable of producing 50 tons of meat per week. The construction of a pork processing plant was considered in 1968 but no information was available on its development at the time of this writing. The economic side of the project poses a problem, since the cost of raising pigs on a commercial basis would increase the price of each animal on the hoof by 25 percent, and this would price it out of the local market.

The food industries of Barbados give jobs to 4,000 workers, of whom 1,600 are employed in distilling rum. One million liters of rum are produced every year.

E. TRADE

1. Domestic Trade [21] [2]

The Barbados Marketing Corporation was created in 1963 for the purpose of stimulating the diversification of agriculture and increasing local food production. The corporation can give financial assistance to farmers and operates a Price Support and Stabilization Program. In spite of these efforts, the amount of food grown and sold on the domestic market is only equal to the amount imported. However, because some of the imported foods, like cereals and fats, are in concentrated form, Gooding has computed that out of 231 million calories consumed per year (1968 basis), only 92 million are produced locally. This would allow 2,100 calories per capita per day, assuming a wastage rate of 20 percent. In terms of cash, the value of the food produced locally amounts to $7 million and that of the imported food $15 million.

2. Foreign Trade [2] [19] [14] [47]

Foreign trade is based on agricultural products, although their share of the export market has diminished from 97 percent in 1961 to 74.4 percent in 1968. Agricultural imports, mostly food, rose by 46 percent between 1961 and 1968 but their share of the total dropped from 32 to 26 percent. Food imports consist mainly of wheat and cereals, dairy products, milk, eggs, fruits and vegetables, meat and meat preparations, fats and oils, etc, as shown in Table No. 1. The table shows a substantial number of items that are imported and then re-exported, although the very large amount of nutritious foods imported shows that the cost of a good and well-balanced diet must be high. The beverages shown as exports consist mostly, if not exclusively, of rum while the imported beverages consist of whiskey and French wine. The intensity of the effort to become more and more self-supporting in meat is reflected in the increase in animal feed imports.

The United States is the major supplier of meat, fruit, dairy products and cereals. It buys some of the sugar crop, most of which, however, is shipped to the United Kingdom. As a result, the U.S. sugar quota for Barbados is not always filled.

One of the main sources of foreign exchange for Barbados is tourism and there are some people who wish to make it the mainstay of the economy since it brings about $15 million a year in profits. Others, perhaps wisely, realize the fickleness and vulnerability of this kind of trade, which is at the mercy of rumors, social unrest and fads.

F. FOOD SUPPLY [21]

Quite obviously, the food supply in the island itself is meager. This could create a serious situation is for any reason—war or other—the island were isolated for any length of time. This is what prompted the British Government during World War II to pass a law requiring all sugar estates to plant a minimum acreage in food. This legislation has been revised and is still on the books, although to what extent it is enforced is not clear. It is said that only 60 to 70 estates out of 250 comply with the law on this matter. Most of the food is planted between the harvesting and sowing of sugar crops, that is, from February to May and from October to November.

1. Storage [2] [52]

The Barbados Marketing Corporation has cold storage plants capable of accommodation 200 tons of meat and 12 tons of fish. There are sugar sheds on all estates and storage baskets on most farms and in most households. The size of the storage space must be more than sufficient for storing local crops because the national budget includes warehousing as a source of revenue, indicating the availability of surplus space for rent.

2. Transportation

Transportation on a small, flat island like Barbados is no problem. Facilities for moving food and other goods from one point to another are excellent and do not create any danger of distribution failure once the food is available.

III. DIETS

A. GENERAL [15] [34] [51]

The diets of Barbadians follow the general Caribbean pattern, which is based on salted codfish from New England or Canada, locally grown pulses, imported rice and fruit. If supplied in adequate quantities, such a diet could be well-balanced and satisfactory. Like most, if not all, other countries in the area, the tradition of sugar and/or banana plantations has resulted in heavily loading agriculture in favor of cash crops, with the result that food crops have been neglected and a sizable portion of the diet has to be imported. In Barbados this amounts to half the weight of all foods available, two-thirds of the cost and 60 percent of the calories. It is interesting to note that in May 1969 the cost of 450 grams of imported salted codfish was 30¢. A 450-gram portion of salted codfish would yield 500 calories and 128 grams of excellent quality protein. Rice, another imported staple of the diet, cost 10¢ per 450 grams in 1969, which would provide about 40 grams of protein and a little over 1,000 calories. Reduced to a per person cost, the amount spent on food reached 45¢ per capita per day in the district where Bridgetown, the capital, is located and dropped to 25¢ per capita per day in St. Andrew. Animal proteins uniformly represented one-half of the expenditure; cereals 15.7 percent; sugars, fruits and pulses about 3 percent each. The soft drink purchases reached 10 percent of the total spent and this could be a real problem.

The mean annual income per capita is $300 (total income divided by the number of people) while the median (the mid-point on a scale of incomes) is only $181. The figure for the lowest tenth percentile on the income scale is only $47.30. A large majority of incomes are below the mean.

Households include an average of 5.9 people per family and 48.2 percent of the members are below 15 years of age. The number of females far exceeds the number of males: 59 percent versus 41 percent. CFNI investigators found that 54.6 percent of mothers or mother surrogates are not employed and take care of their homes while the rest are part of the labor force on a fulltime or part-time basis. About 11.7 percent of the husbands or male adults are permanently unemployed and the rest do some work occasionally or on a part-time basis.

The 1969 CFNI nutrition survey showed that 77.6 percent of the houses were owned by their occupants. It also revealed that 74.8 percent of all houses surveyed had a kitchen in the house, 8.4 percent used separate structures for cooking, 9.3 percent had no kitchen, and 7.5 percent cooked in a room also used for other purposes. Seventy-five percent of the households used oil stoves; 52.4 percent had water faucets in the houses while others obtained their water from public fountains, usually less than 10 meters away.

Of the families surveyed, 27.5 percent had breakfast and an evening meal, 17.6 percent had only one meal a day around noon, 16.7 percent took their only meal in the evening, 12.9 percent had a mid-day and an evening meal, 9.7 percent had three meals a day, 9.4 percent had breakfast and lunch, 2.7 percent had only breakfast, 0.9 percent had no organized meal but took snacks whenever they could and 2.5 percent could not be recorded. Sixty-two percent of the families did not bother to prepare meals for men at work or for children. About 70.5 percent of the children under 5 years of age ate more often than the adults, 25.5 percent ate as often and 4 percent less often.

Considering the picture as it emerges from the statistics, Barbados appears to be a country where a higher level of adjustment of the people to the land has been achieved than in much of the developing world. Food is available; its cost, although high, is not exorbitant and there are no distribution problems. Hence, there is a good potential for acceptable diets. Yet, as we shall see, families do not meet their nutritional requirements.

The 1969 CFNI investigators computed that 2,334 calories, not counting alcoholic beverages, and 64.6 grams of protein were available to each Barbadian per day. Cereals provided 39.8 percent of these calories, sugar 17 percent, oils and fats 10.9 percent, meat and fish 10.7 percent, milk and milk products 6.5 percent. Similarly, the largest source of protein was again cereals (19.8 grams), meat (16.5 grams), milk and cheese (8.6 grams), fish (8.1 grams) and pulses and nuts (4.6 grams). Rice with 84.1 grams per day was the largest single source of protein available.

A detailed study of the daily per capita consumption of 12 food groups was made during the CFNI survey, which revealed the preferences shown in Table No. 2. The table shows that imported European potatoes are almost as popular as domestic sweet potatoes. The amount of fruit eaten is minute and the detailed list of fruit shows that imported items (canned and dried fruit, apples and pears) represent one-third of the total consumption of fruit, an interesting fact given the excellence and abundance of tropical fruits in Barbados. Imported evaporated milk is the most popular of milk products, which may be explained by the difficulty of keeping fresh milk refrigerated. Yet, there is evidence that costly prestige imported foods are preferred over local products, an aspect of nutrition not uncommon in the developing world. Nutrition requirements and consumption values of the population were determined by the researchers involved in the 1969 survey on the basis of FAO and WHO standards. These are shown together with intake as percentage of requirement in Table No. 3.

It may be of interest to mention a few special dishes which, however, one should not construe as being eaten every day by every family. Sweet potatoes grow all year round. Some ripen in 6 weeks, some in 14 weeks, while other varieties require up to 8 months for maturity. Eaten broiled, baked or boiled, they are essential ingredients of a dish known as "pudding and souse," made from the meat and intestines of pigs. In the days before American and Canadian flour were as fully available as now, sweet potatoes and manioc plants were the standby "bread" of the islanders. At Christmas time, sweet potatoes are in great demand for *pone,* a dish made of grated, pressed sweet potatoes mixed with sugar and spices and baked in the oven to form a sort of plum cake. To wash it down, the Barbadians consume a potato beverage called *moby* made from the expressed liquor of either the red or the white potato. It is a cooling, pleasant drink, especially when mixed with water.

The basis for a planter's breakfast is called a "pepper pot" and includes leftover chicken, turkey and beef. This dish originated in the days when plantations were great distances away from towns and from each other. The stew was prepared in large batches and protected against deterioration by adding cassareep, an herb from Guyana. The pot was brought to the boil every 24 hours and thus would keep for weeks. Now the pepperpot is a Sunday brunch dish. Since the mixture is very peppery, sliced sweet potatoes, breadfruit and manioc cake are served with it. A large planter's breakfast might also include a whole suckling pig, supplemented with fried fish, black pudding and souse. Souse is marinated pork doused with vinegar, cucumbers and onions. All this food is washed down with planter's punch (rum and fruit juices).

B. SPECIAL DIETS [15]

The CFNI investigators studied the diets of four groups considered to be "at risk" from a nutritional point of view: 1) pregnant women; 2) lactating women; 3) infants from weaning to 2 years of age; and 4) children from 2 to 5 years of age. Unfortunately, the number of individuals available in each category was small but the indications collected from these numbers are valuable. The data show that except for protein and vitamin A, the average intake of all nutrients was much below requirements. However, the value of the protein ingested varied unevenly for each of these special cases. Intakes of calories and vitamins by these four groups were particularly low. As with other population groups, the maximum found for each nutrient was high above requirements, but the minimum was never above 32 percent of the requirement and in the case of ascorbic acid ran as low as 1 percent (see Table No. 4).

1. Diets of Pregnant Women

On the basis of the small numbers studied, the diets of pregnant women seem to be quite deficient in everything except vitamin A. The investigators found that, by and large, people considered certain foods to be good for pregnant women: meat, milk, fruit and fruit juices, and green vegetables, which is a fairly good list. Rice, rice flour, sweet potatoes, yams and cornmeal were considered undesirable. Almost half the pregnant women interviewed took iron pills regularly; others did not bother or forgot to take them. Forty percent of the pregnant women practiced pica, eating chalk because they liked it and because, they claimed, it eased "stomach burn."

2. Diets of Lactating Women

During lactation the same foods which were popular during pregnancy were continued but cornmeal and wheat flour or other cereals were restored to the diet. Pepper, rum and other alcoholic drinks were avoided because they could harm the baby.

3. Diets of Infants

The CFNI investigators found that the nutritional requirements of infants were generally not met, either through ignorance or through the lack of appropriate foods. Caloric needs were met for only 46 percent of the infants studied (see Table No. 4). This, of course, is serious because in a situation of caloric deficit, the protein intake, whatever it may be, is burned for energy and does not help tissue development. Maximum protein consumed (the highest individual in the sample) was 277 percent of needs for infants. Potatoes, carrots, fish, eggs, meat, milk and pumpkins are considered good for infants and children. The amount, however, must be small, otherwise there could be no real malnutrition in children in Barbados.

Child care is of special interest as it governs diet, health and further development. As many as 53.4 percent of the mothers were found to take care of their children by day; hence, that proportion of mothers did not work. This almost exactly matched the number of fathers residing with the family and contributing to its budget. Slightly over half of the families had both father and mother living in the home, the father earning money and the mother taking care of the children. When the mother is not at home, a grandmother or older sister takes care of the infant and in this situation malnutrition is more likely to develop.

Ten percent of the mothers began breast feeding their infants immediately after birth, 40 percent the day after birth, 23.8 percent the second day and 5.1 percent after the second day.* Fifty percent of the mothers gave glucose and water pending the rise of milk in the breast; 25 percent gave only water; a few gave bush tea. Some of these bush teas can be dangerous (see chapter on Jamaica). The investigators found that 48.6 percent of women breast fed at night and gave three or four bottles a day. Weaning takes place early in Barbados. At 3 months 25.3 percent of the mothers have stopped breast feeding; at 6 months the figure has risen to 48.3 percent and at 9 months to 82.8 percent. Only a very small number continue to breast feed for 2 or 3 years. Many women (34.6 percent) assert that the child weans himself when he wants to.

A number of proprietary mixtures are given as breast milk substitutes. The most popular brand in 1969 was Lactogen, given by 31.9 percent of the

---

*The remaining 21.1 percent were unaccounted for.

mothers, and the second most popular was Klim, purchased by 15.3 percent. Diluted cow's milk comes only third on the list of breast milk substitutes, with 9.1 percent of the mothers surveyed using it. Other women favored diluted goat's milk, diluted donkey's milk and even undiluted cow's, goat's or other animal's milk. In addition to these milk formulas, bush tea, fruit juices, eggs, chicken, mashed fish, bread, peas and spinach are among the items that may be given to the child. Sweet mint, orange peel and flowers are common herbs used for making bush tea. Ninety-three percent of all families interviewed by the CFNI team used cod liver oil and 63 percent used vitamin preparations. Many children (35.6 percent) had snacks at least three times a day and 76.4 percent had at least two snacks.

Of all people interviewed, 74.4 percent felt that eggs were good for children. Fish was considered to be beneficial by 84.9 percent of the people, although a few felt it caused worms. Fifty-four percent felt that meat was good for children 6-12 months of age, but some felt that only gravy should be given. Some doubt as to the virtues of dried skim milk existed in the minds of quite a number of mothers (24.7 percent) and only 54.1 percent were in favor of it. Many mothers (36 percent) were against feeding peas to children less than 1 year of age and they gave some sound reasons: the peas are indigestible; the children cannot chew them and could choke on them, etc. While some of these real inconveniences could be corrected by the way the peas are prepared, it is certainly true that if given to infants in the same form they are given to adults, peas can lead to difficulties. Yet, about one-third of the mothers saw merit in their consumption and presumably would use them extensively if the Government would show them how to prepare them. Spinach was considered to be good for children by 72.8 percent of the mothers. Fruits like papaya, avocados and coconuts, and their jellies were deemed good; sardines were not.

4. Diets of Preschool Children

The CFNI found that 50 percent of the preschool children did not meet their caloric requirements and the danger of this situation regarding the waste of the protein ingested is the same as for infants. Among the more adequately fed 50 percent, on the other hand, the highest protein consumer in the sample reached over twice his normal requirements (201 percent).

5. School Feeding Programs

School feeding programs were initiated in Barbados in 1937, with each child receiving a morning snack consisting of three-eighths pint of reconstituted skim milk and two yeast biscuits. In 1962, a hot lunch program was initiated. Since 1967 the World Food Program has provided wheat flour, skim milk, cheese, meat, butter and dried fruit for the program. By 1970 over 10,000 children in 39 schools were participating in the school lunch program.

C. LEVELS OF NUTRITION [15]

Table No. 3 shows that the average levels of nutrition for all the groups sampled in the island were nearly adequate or better in five of the most important nutrients: proteins, calcium, iron, vitamin A and thiamine. The adequacy in protein is gratifying and that in vitamin A is unusual in tropical countries (except for those using red palm oil for cooking). This is the result of the high consumption of sweet potatoes. The caloric level was slightly below normal and, as usual, the riboflavin intake was low. The low levels of vitamin C found are not surprising given the small amounts of fresh citrus fruit consumed (see Table No. 2).

Table No. 3 also shows the differences existing between the various districts. Christ Church, which is a rich tourist area, had the best diet of all. Its inhabitants appeared to have more than satisfactory levels of nutrition except in riboflavin and, to a small degree, in ascorbic acid. The parishes of St. Andrew and St. Philip, which are rural or mostly rural, were the worst off in terms of calories, calcium, thiamine, riboflavin and niacin intakes. Vitamin C was very low in St. Andrew at 58 percent of requirements. The reasons for these differences have not been investigated. It is enough for the moment to state that considerable variations exist between households.

The table below shows the percentage of families whose members met their respective nutrient and caloric requirements on a per capita basis.

Families Meeting Their Caloric and Nutrient Requirements – 1969
(in Percent by Parish)

Nutrient	Christ Church	St. Philip	St. Michael	St. Andrew	St. Joseph	Average
Calories	49.3	38.9	33.3	23.8	40.0	35.2
Protein	78.9	61.1	62.1	47.6	53.3	61.1
Calcium	73.7	27.8	42.2	19.0	46.6	41.7
Iron	47.3	33.3	40.9	42.5	26.6	39.5
Vitamin A	68.4	72.2	71.2	33.3	60.0	64.0
Thiamine	52.6	33.3	39.3	28.6	53.3	40.3
Riboflavin	42.1	16.7	22.7	4.7	20.0	21.6
Niacin	21.0	16.7	13.6	9.5	6.7	13.7
Vitamin C	47.3	38.9	37.8	4.7	33.3	33.8

Source: Caribbean Food and Nutrition Institute, *Barbados Nutrition Survey.*

This table is interesting because it shows the relatively small number of families meeting their nutrient requirements in certain cases. For instance, in Christ Church Parish, 49.3 percent of the families obtained sufficient calories, but in St. Andrew only 23.8 percent were equally fortunate. Widespread differences also existed in calcium and vitamin A intake between Christ Church and St. Andrew and in niacin between Christ Church and St. Joseph.

The following table shows that the best-fed household enjoyed 429 percent of the caloric requirements while the worst-fed had only 33 percent of the recommended allowance. The same widespread differences are shown for vitamin A: 537 percent versus 8 percent. Thus, ample evidence is afforded that presumably large pockets of malnutrition exist, even when the mean seems satisfactory. Overconsumption exists in a small category and underconsumption in an important segment. The primary reason for these widespread differences is not necessarily money, although income plays a role. More probably tradition, education and availability of certain kinds of foods are the bases of the discrepancies.

Maximum and Minimum Percent Satisfaction of Caloric and Nutrient Requirements Among Households on a Per Day Per Capita Basis – Barbados, 1969

Nutrients	Maximum	Minimum
Calories	429	33
Protein	423	33
Calcium	477	16
Iron	525	21
Vitamin A	537	8
Thiamine	451	27
Riboflavin	259	16
Niacin	334	23
Ascorbic Acid	429	3

Source: Caribbean Food and Nutrition Institute, *Barbados Nutrition Survey.*

Another misleading aspect of nutrition is protein consumption. This seems high if measured by the average available or even the range between parish averages, but proteins are important chiefly because of the quality of the constituent amino acids. Some of these amino acids cannot be synthesized in the body with other molecules, hence have to be provided by the diet. The presence of these ready-formed compounds in the protein molecules ingested imparts quality to the protein. Further studies by the 1969 investigators found that at least 12 percent of the households in St. Michael, where the capital city of Bridgetown is located, and up to 28 percent of those in St. Philip, received less than 10 percent of the needed amount of quality protein.

In summary, although the average intakes of calories and nutrients reached 100 percent or more of requirements, only 64 percent of the families investigated consumed all of the vitamin A requirements, 40 percent consumed all the calcium, iron and thiamine they needed, 33 percent received their requirement of vitamin C, 22 percent their requirement of riboflavin, and only 14 percent their requirement of niacin. This permitted the investigators to say that in at least one third of the homes diets need improvement in quantity and quality, while in another third the quality of the menu needs to be ameliorated. It seems to be mainly a problem of education since quality foods exist on the island and could be secured in greater quantities. This applies especially to pulses, fish and fresh fruit.

IV. ADEQUACY OF FOOD RESOURCES [47][21]

The problem of growing enough food to feed the people of Barbados received a partial solution when, during the Second World War, it was made compulsory to grow food and raise some livestock on 12 percent of the agricultural land of all estates. The levels of production are such that enough food to provide a good diet for all would be available if the food were adequately distributed and if the least prosperous segment of the population were better educated in nutrition. The Diversification Research Unit of the Barbados Sugar Producers Association made some valuable suggestions at a conference on protein foods for the Caribbean held at Georgetown, Guyana, in 1968.

It has been said that the production of milk, meat, eggs and poultry from domestic sources could be increased, that yields from the acreage planted in vegetables could be improved, and that more corn could be produced even if none of the new so-called "miracle" hybrids were used. Farmers are now guaranteed a market for all the corn they can offer. Production of pulses, however, is handicapped by the cost of labor and the small size of the fields which can be sown in legumes. The Government is well aware that an increase in the production of homegrown foods is the most obvious solution to the problem of malnutrition but it will require some public education to lead the farmers to a change of habits.

V. NUTRITIONAL DISEASE PATTERNS [15][53][39]

It is of interest to note that the health services of Barbados are exceptionally good for a developing country. There are three main health centers and a number of subcenters where mothers can receive advice and where children can get early treatment. Environmental sanitation is good; 95 percent of the houses have facilities for sewage disposal and piped water is available in 50 percent of the homes.

Malnutrition was the cause of over 12 percent of all infant deaths in the 1930's and the rate of infant mortality in those days was 217 per 1,000 live births. However, in recent days few clinical signs suggestive of malnutrition can be detected. The only significant symptom of nutritional deficiency observed by CFNI investigators in 1969 was follicular hyperkeratosis, found in 12.9 percent of the 2,121 people examined. Other symptoms included pale conjunctivae (3.7 percent), lack of fat (3.6 percent), muscle wasting (2.3 percent), skin dryness (2 percent), enlarged livers, which could be due to other causes (1.1 percent), thyroid enlargement (1 percent), bleeding gums (5 percent), angular stomatitis (6 percent) and nasolabial seborrhea (0.6 percent of adults). The three last signs point to riboflavin deficiency and prescurvy conditions (among those with bleeding gums). The deficiency in ascorbic acid among a population which could have as much of that vitamin as it wants is interesting. The explanation probably lies in the fact that very small amounts of fresh citrus fruit are consumed and that canned fruit and juices are preferred. Unless fortified, the last two must contain very little vitamin C because ascorbic acid is a thermolabile vitamin which can be lost in the process of sterilizing and conditioning the product.

Among children, very few cases of protein-calorie malnutrition and rickets were soon during the CFNI survey. Thus, an overall picture arises of a population where undernutrition rather than malnutrition is found and where only light degrees of clinical visible pathology have been reached. On the basis of the age/weight relationship, the prevalence of protein-calorie malnutrition and its degree has been assessed: 15.3 percent of the children 5 years old or under weighed only 60-80 percent of the standard. Of the infants in the first 6 months range, 14-16 percent were 20-40 percent underweight. After the age of 6 months those underweight increased to 38 percent. The proportion of underweight children fell during the second, third and fourth years and by the fifth year had dropped to 7 percent. Very severe cases, corresponding to a weight of less than 60 percent of the standard, occurred during the second half of the first year when 10 percent of the children examined showed the condition. True, full-fledged kwashiorkor, however, was not observed. One-third of all schoolchildren seen were moderately underweight. A few cases of severely underweight children were noted in all age groups up to 15 years. Among adult females there was a high incidence of overweight and obesity: 40 percent of those examined had a ratio of weight for height of 120 percent or more.

In 1959 Standard, Lovell and Harney made height and weight comparisons between groups of present-day Barbadian children and groups of London children in 1905 and 1912. The Barbadian children were found to fall between the two lots of London children, slightly better placed for height and for weight than the British children at the beginning of the century but not as good as those of the late 1950's.

Another sign of malnutrition is the chest-head measurement ratio. This quotient is considered normal when above 1 after 12 months of age. The 1969 CFNI survey showed rates below 1 in 37 percent of the cases during the second year, 39 percent during the third year and 27 percent during the fourth year. These findings support the diagnosis of moderately severe protein-calorie malnutrition in these children.

Levels of serum albumin in the blood of children of both sexes and adults were found to be normal by the CFNI investigators. Anemia was commonly found among 33 percent of preschool children, 9 percent of school-aged children, 19 percent of adult women and only 1 percent of adult men. Among the children's group 11 percent and among the adult women 6 percent had severe anemia with hemoglobin levels below 9 grams per 100 milliliters. These anemias are probably due to iron and folate deficiencies, because hookworm infestation does not occur with any frequency on the island. Most anemia cases among preschool children were found in Christ Church and St. Philip parishes where 42 percent of the children examined were anemic. In St. Michael and the northern parishes, 28.8 percent and 25.8 percent, respectively, revealed anemia. The investigators found a significant relationship between income levels and percentage of people meeting their iron requirements through their diets.

The younger groups of the population exhibited considerable dental decay. Only three out of 411 children between the ages of 10 and 15 showed complete dentition. Periodontal disease is common; thus, the loss of teeth begins in school-aged children and continues until middle age. Qualified dentists are seldom consulted and one-third of the population has recourse to nonqualified practitioners.

VI. CONCLUSIONS

The situation in Barbados is typical of most of the small Caribbean islands and can be summarized as follows. The food resources are inadequate because most of the arable land is used for sugar. This single cash crop is at present the only one that can remain competitive on the world market while at the same time permitting moderately high salaries at home. A high salary level is essential to permit the purchase of imported foods which cannot be dispensed with because there is not enough land to grow both remunerative cash crops and adequate amounts of food crops. Thus, a vicious circle is established which has created a way of life that cannot be changed before a failure-proof new system has been found. If one were allowed to speculate, one could say that the new system should be based on the mechanization of the sugar industry. This would create a labor surplus, some of which could be used for production of food crops and some for developing the fishing industry, but the everlasting problem of breaking established food habits would still have to be overcome.

LIST OF TABLES

LIST OF MAPS

TABLE NO. 1

Agricultural Trade – Barbados, 1961 and 1968
(in $1,000)

	Exports		Imports	
Items	1961	1968	1961	1968
Live animals	70	50	47	48
Meat and meat products	23	6	2,671	5,416
Dairy and eggs	28	2	2,344	2,630
Cereals and preparations	142	196	3,101	3,405
Fruits and vegetables	130	141	1,744	2,509
Sugar	2,197	1,908	211	334
Raw sugar	16,355	16,304	–	–
Animal feeds	55	10	1,309	2,665
Beverages	1,448	1,483	785	1,243
Oils and fats	214	31	1,079	1,317
Other	51	19	–	–
Tobacco, fibers, etc.	–	–	285	478
Miscellaneous	542	577	737	690
Coffee, tea, spices	–	–	616	1,020
Total agricultural trade	21,255	20,727	14,929	21,755
Total trade	21,821	27,821	46,817	84,012
Agriculture as percent of total trade	97	74.4	32	26

Source: Food and Agriculture Organization of the United Nations, *Trade Yearbook 1969.*

TABLE NO. 2

Per Capita Daily Consumption of Foodstuff Items – Barbados, 1969
(weighted average)

Item	Grams per Day
Cereals	
Rice	84.1
Bread	47.2
Other	74.4
Roots and tubers	
Sweet potatoes	47.7
Potatoes	39.5
Other	57.4
Sugars	56.0
Pulses, nuts and seeds	
Split peas	10.1
Pigeon peas	5.0
Other	0.88
Fresh vegetables	
Onions	14.7
Tomatoes	6.8
Other	30.3
Fresh fruits	
Citrus	6.6
Mangoes and papaya	6.5
Other	7.9
Canned and dried fruit	4.0
Meats	
Poultry	28.3
Pork	16.1
Other	37.6
Fish	
Fresh	38.5
Salted cod	9.6
Other	4.9
Eggs	13.6
Milk and cheese	
Evaporated	90.4
Fresh	30.8
Other	44.8
Fats and oils	
Butter	8.0
Cooking oils	7.7
Other	11.0
Miscellaneous	
Orange and grapefruit juice	9.7
Cakes	4.0
Other	12.3

Source: Caribbean Food and Nutrition Institute, *Barbados Nutrition Survey.*

TABLE NO. 3

Average Per Capita Daily Requirement and Intake of Calories and Nutrients – Barbados, 1969
(Comparison of Nutrient Intake as Percentage of Requirements)

	Christ Church (19)*			St. Philip (18)*			St. Michael (66)*		
	R.**	I.	I. as % of R.	R.	I.	I. as % of R.	R.	I.	I. as % of R.
Calories	2,344	2,550	108	2,296	2,076	90	2,279	2,110	92
Protein (g)									
Total	59.2	78.4	132	56.4	59.5	105	58.2	65.6	113
Animal	–	43.1	–	–	32.7	–	–	37.1	–
Fats (g)	–	78.7	–	–	69.2	–	–	64.3	–
Carbohydrate (g)	–	383.0	–	–	305.0	–	–	324.0	–
Calcium (mg)	554	683	123	582	445	76	539	561	104
Iron (mg)	11.8	15.7	132	10.8	11.2	102	11.0	13.8	125
Vitamin A (mcg) (Retinol)	645	924	143	634	845	133	640	941	147
Thiamine (mg)	0.93	0.86	92.4	0.91	0.85	93	0.91	0.88	97
Riboflavin (mg)	1.16	1.03	89	1.26	0.82	65	1.25	0.95	76
Niacin (mg)	14.4	14.4	100	14.3	10.6	73	14.3	12.4	87
Vitamin C (mg)	45.8	42.5	93	44.4	39.4	89	44.4	41.7	94

TABLE NO. 3 (Cont.)

Average Per Capita Daily Requirement and Intake of Calories and Nutrients – Barbados, 1969

(Comparison of Nutrient Intake as Percentage of Requirements)

	St. Andrew (21)*			St. Joseph (15)*			Total Survey (139)* (weighted average)		
	R.	I.	I. as % of R.	R.	I.	I. as % of R.	R.	I.	I. as % of R.
Calories	2,305	1,960	85	2,344	2,181	93	2,296	2,151	93.7
Protein (g)									
Total	55.2	57.9	105	59.8	59.8	100	57.8	64.8	112
Animal	–	31.3	–	–	30.3	–	–	35.9	–
Fats (g)	–	54.7	–	–	67.6	–	–	65.8	–
Carbohydrate (g)	–	305.0	–	–	336.5	–	–	328.2	–
Calcium (mg)	565	490	87	536	436	81	550	539	98
Iron (mg)	10.9	12.7	117	11.1	12.5	112	11.1	13.4	121
Vitamin A (mcg) (Retinol)	602	556	92	669	829	124	637	856	134
Thiamine (mg)	0.92	0.88	95	0.94	0.94	100	0.91	0.89	98
Riboflavin (mg)	1.26	0.77	61	1.28	0.80	63	1.26	0.92	73
Niacin (mg)	14.6	11.2	77	14.9	11.6	77	14.4	12.2	85
Vitamin C (mg)	39.7	22.9	58	46.7	40.0	85	44.7	38.5	87

R=requirement
I=intake

*Number of families surveyed.

**Requirements in the five parishes differ because of differences in sex and age groups.

Source: Caribbean Food and Nutrition Institute, Barbados Nutrition Survey.

TABLE NO. 4

Average Per Capita Daily Nutrient Requirement and Intake of Infants and Preschool Children – Barbados, 1969

Nutrient	6-23 mo*					24-60 mo**				
	Requirement	Intake	Intake as % of Req.	Max. % Satisfaction	Min. % Satisfaction	Requirement	Intake	Intake as % of Req.	Max. % Satisfaction	Min. % Satisfaction
Calories	1,266	577	46	121	18	1,597	792	50	105	23
Protein, total (g)	19.2	18.8	98	277	26	24.7	23.3	95	201	32
Calcium (mg)	566	427	76	306	19	550	339	62	280	12
Iron (mg)	6.4	4.6	76	211	10	7.7	5.0	64	175	18
Vitamin A (mcg) (retinol)	266	365	143	717	11	286	396	138	1,072	3
Thiamine (mg)	0.51	0.28	56	169	15	0.64	0.32	50	170	15
Riboflavin (mg)	0.70	0.60	86	310	14	0.88	0.45	52	241	12
Niacin (mg)	8.35	3.43	41	118	6	10.53	3.95	38	109	7
Vitamin C (mg)	18.4	17.4	95	270	2	23.6	15.2	65	497	1

*25 children in sample.
**46 children in sample.

Source: Caribbean Food and Nutrition Institute, *Barbados Nutrition Survey.*

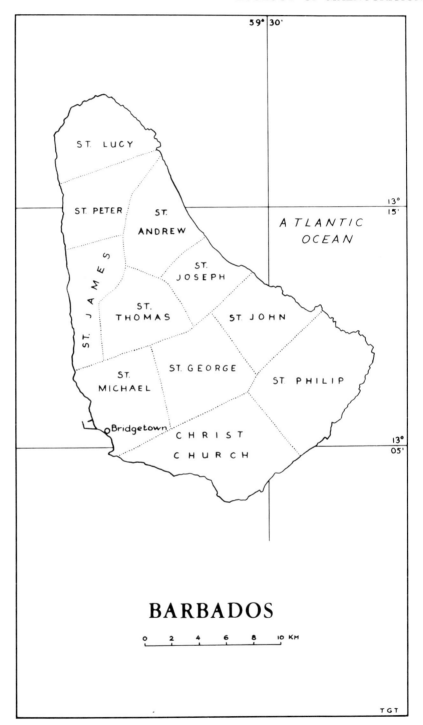

BARBADOS

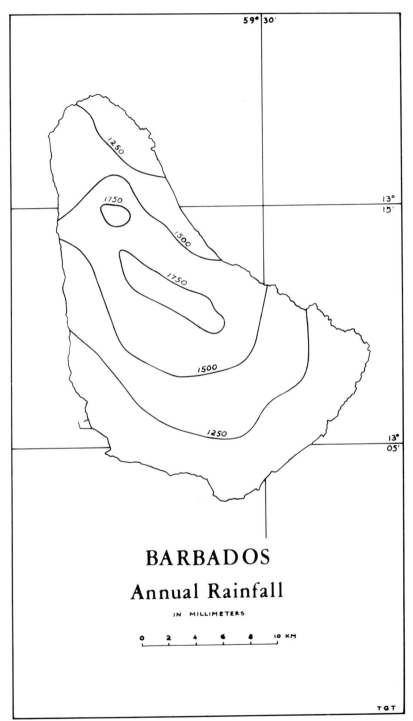

BARBADOS

Annual Rainfall

IN MILLIMETERS

0   2   4   6   8   10 KM

MAP NO. 2.

THE LEEWARD ISLANDS

TABLE OF CONTENTS

THE LEEWARD ISLANDS: ST. CHRISTOPHER-NEVIS-ANGUILLA

I. BACKGROUND INFORMATION

A. PHYSICAL SETTING [10] [52]

St. Christopher (popularly known as St. Kitts), Nevis and Anguilla are located in the northern part of the Leeward Islands (see map on page 373). Oval-shaped St. Kitts is 176 square kilometers in size, Nevis measures 129 square kilometers and Anguilla only 90 square kilometers. The terrain of St. Kitts rises toward a central mountain range which peaks at 1,200 meters (Mount Misery). At the southeastern end of the island is an arid region with a huge salt pond. The lower mountain slopes are planted with sugarcane while the upper areas are wooded. Nevis is also mountainous, rising to a central peak of 1,100 meters (Nevis Peak). Although the soil on Nevis is less fertile than on St. Kitts, Sea Island cotton and subsistence food crops are planted in the lower regions. As on St. Kitts, the upper slopes are forested. Both St. Kitts and Nevis are of volcanic origin and are separated from one another by a channel about 3.2 kilometers wide. Anguilla is a dry coralline and limestone island less than 26 kilometers long and only about 5-6 kilometers wide at its broadest point. In contrast to the other two islands, Anguilla is relatively flat and covered with low shrub. Although some subsistence farming is practiced, the island is generally not suitable for agriculture due to the shallowness of the soil and the lack of rain. Fishing and boat-building are the main activities on the island.

B. CLIMATE [14] [10]

On St. Kitts and Nevis the average annual temperature is about 26°C. Annual rainfall on St. Kitts ranges from about 1,000 millimeters along the coast to over

2,000 millimeters in the high areas of the interior. On Nevis the mean annual rainfall approximates 1,000 millimeters (see map on page 373). Anguilla's climate is similar; cloudy skies and rain are infrequent with precipitation averaging 1,000 millimeters per year. Prolonged drought has been a threat to agricultural production on Anguilla in recent years.

C. POPULATION [10] [36] [40]

The 1966 population of the islands was 57,617, divided as follows: St. Kitts, 37,150; Nevis, 15,072; Anguilla, 5,395. The principal towns are Basseterre on St. Kitts (15,897) and Charlestown on Nevis (1,530). Most of the inhabitants are of African or mixed descent. English is the official language and Christianity is the predominant religion. The rate of population increase on the islands is 2.4 percent, the infant mortality rate was 59.3 per 1,000 live births in 1968 (compared to 22 per 1,000 in the United States) and life expectancy at birth is about 58 years for males and 62 years for females.

D. HISTORY AND GOVERNMENT [10] [14] [36]

Columbus discovered St. Kitts and Nevis in 1493. The first British colony in the West Indies was founded at St. Kitts in 1623 and a French settlement was established on the island in 1624. The British settled Nevis in 1629 and Anguilla around 1650. Possession of Nevis and St. Kitts was a matter of dispute between Britain and France throughout the 17th and 18th centuries; only Anguilla remained continuously in British hands. Nevis and St. Kitts were finally recognized as British holdings under the Treaty of Versailles in 1783.

As of 1967 the three islands were to be administered together as one of the six West Indies Associated States* and known officially as St. Christopher-Nevis-Anguilla. Basseterre on St. Kitts was named the capital of the three-island state. Soon after statehood, the inhabitants of Anguilla became dissatisfied with the Basseterre administration and in 1969 voted to secede from the union. The political status of this island has not yet been settled, awaiting the findings of a West Indian Commission of Inquiry.

The West Indies Associated States do not form a federation; each state is separately associated with the United Kingdom in a relationship similar to the one which exists between Puerto Rico and the United States. Each state enjoys internal self-government, but defense and foreign affairs are administered by Great Britain. Each is governed by an Administrator, appointed by the Queen, who is assisted by an Executive Council consisting of a Chief Minister, three other ministers, one other member appointed by the Administrator on the recommendation of the Chief Minister, and the Principal Law Officer. The Chief

---

*The other members are Antigua, Dominica, St. Lucia, St. Vincent and Grenada.

Minister is appointed by the Administrator from among the elected members of the Legislative Council. The states share a common Judicial and Legal Service Commission and Police Service Commission.

E. AGRICULTURAL POLICIES [14] [10]

Like most of the West Indies islands, St. Kitts, Nevis and Anguilla are heavily reliant on food imports to satisfy the needs of the local population. In spite of an increasing demand for food crops within the islands, production of vegetables and roots has not risen accordingly. On Nevis, the Government has initiated a program to stimulate increased output of beef and vegetables. On both Nevis and St. Kitts, small family farms are encouraged through subsidies for land clearing and provision at cost of fencing supplies, fertilizers and citrus seedlings. Except for meat animals, however, the Government provides no price supports or guarantees for farm produce. A 5-year development plan has been proposed by the Ministry of Agriculture to stimulate livestock production and crop diversification.

F. FOREIGN AID

1. Bilateral Aid [10]

The United Kingdom provided budgetary aid to the three-island state of St. Kitts-Nevis-Anguilla in the amount of $823,000 in 1966 and $625,000 in 1967, and allocated about $500,000 in development aid for the 1968-1970 period. In addition, the Colonial Development and Welfare funds allocated $1,860,000 from 1965 to 1968 and allotted $1,250,000 from 1968 to 1970.

2. Multilateral Aid [41]

Since 1962 the United Nations has supported an applied nutrition program in St. Kitts-Nevis-Anguilla at a cost of $15,600. The Government has established a Nutrition Coordinating Committee and appointed a fulltime nutrition officer to work on the project. Under the program, nurses, schoolteachers and agricultural extension officers have received training in nutrition education. Nutrition education campaigns have been carried out in several communities and classes in nutrition have been held for 4-H Club members. Nutrition activities and school gardens have been initiated at a number of pilot schools. UNICEF has provided supplies and equipment as well as training grants while FAO has supplied a home economist and WHO a nutrition advisor.

A small-scale child feeding program was initiated with UNICEF help in 1954 and has continued. Skim milk powder and corn-soy-milk blend (CSM) have been distributed by UNICEF through primary schools, dispensaries and health centers. The Government supplies supplementary foods. About 10,500 schoolchildren and 7,000 mothers and preschoolers are reached each year.

II. FOOD RESOURCES

A. GENERAL [18]

The food resources of St. Kitts-Nevis-Anguilla come from a total of 35,000 hectares of which about 16,000 are arable. Fifty large estates covering 6,000 hectares, all in sugarcane, occupy the best land. Some marginal land at the edge of the forests is rented out to smallholders. Cotton, which used to be an important resource at the turn of the century, now is limited to less than a few hundred hectares.

B. MEANS OF PRODUCTION

1. Agricultural Labor Force [14]

The labor force, comprising 6,500 people, is engaged mostly in sugar and cotton work. The growing tourist trade is absorbing some of these workers. When the labor force cannot find employment, it emigrates in large numbers to Trinidad, the Dutch Antilles, Great Britain and the Dominican Republic.

2. Farms [52] [23]

On St. Kitts most of the land is in large estates, virtually all concerned with sugarcane and occasionally cotton cultivation. The Government leases small plots of 1 hectare each of farmers promising to grow a small amount of food. The success of this measure is not known. On Nevis most of the agriculture is in small holdings, although there are five large coconut estates which operate their own small ranches. Much of the land is now fallow or taken over by new growth on which cattle graze. On Anguilla, where the soil is poor and water availability limited to rainfall, only a few tracts of land are cultivated by individual families. Crops consist of pigeon peas, some cabbages and other vegetables.

C. PRODUCTION

1. Crops [23]

On St. Kitts and Nevis food crops—cabbages, tomatoes, cucumbers, roots and legumes—are grown on farmers' plots and between sugar crops on cane land. Except on Nevis, the amount produced is inadequate to meet the needs. Cotton and coconuts supplement sugarcane as cash crops.

2. Animal Husbandry [23]

Although the Government encourages the cattle industry by providing stud service and giving technical advice, livestock-raising is of minor importance on St. Kitts where most of the land is devoted to sugarcane and cotton. However, just outside Basseterre the Government operates a livestock farm and dairy. The cows on this farm produce about 300 tons of milk each year, almost all of which is supplied to the island's hospitals. On Nevis, livestock-raising is more important. Landless farmers often raise cattle, grazing them on any available unoccupied land. A large portion of the land devoted to cultivation of Sea Island cotton is unused 6 months of the year and transient cattle herds feed on the weeds. Much of the owners' time is spent moving the animals from one watering point to another in a nomadic fashion unusual on a small island. Cattle are also kept on coconut estates. Animal husbandry is a major agricultural pursuit on Anguilla where there were 1,200 cattle, 3,000 sheep, 5,500 goats and 1,680 pigs in 1961.

3. Fisheries [23]

Fishing is an important activity on all three islands. About 800 tons of fish are landed each year on St. Kitts, including most of the catch brought in by Nevis fishermen, and approximately 80 tons are landed on Anguilla. The fishing vessels used are primarily sailboats and rowboats. The Government operates two experimental motorized vessels. The catch on all three islands could be increased considerably if power boats were introduced and cold storage facilities were expanded. The major species caught include bonito, barracuda, kingfish, mackerel, snapper and skipjack. Spiny lobster is an important resource for Anguilla fishermen and the catch is mainly exported to Puerto Rico, St. Thomas and St. Martin.

A toxic substance has been reported in fish caught in certain places off St. Kitts where a blue-green algae abounds, and some fatalities from eating these contaminated fish have occurred. Recent studies have identified the Eastern Caribbean as one of the foci of ciguatoxin, a type of poison which builds up over a period of years in the muscles and organs of a number of fish with differing ecological habits. Whether or not this is the substance found in the toxic fish off St. Kitts and whether or not there is a relationship between the toxin and the algae found in the area has not yet been substantiated. But the phenomenon does pose a problem for the fishing industry.

D. FOOD INDUSTRIES [23]

Food industries in the three-island state are very limited. On St. Kitts there is a cottonseed and coconut oil extraction plant, a brewery and an abbatoir. The primary industrial activity on the island is a sugarcane processing plant which, in addition to its main function, provides routine mechanical service for the town of Basseterre. Labor shortages pose a problem for all these enterprises. At Charlestown on Nevis there is a vegetable oil processing plant. The main industrial activity on Anguilla is the manufacture of salt through solar evaporation of seawater. There is a carbonated water bottling plant on the island with a capacity of 1,200 bottles a day.

E. TRADE [19] [10]

The farmers on Nevis grow enough food for themselves, an unusual feature in the area, and they are even able to export fruits and vegetables to St. Kitts. The value of all imports for the island triplex reached $9.6 million in 1967 with agricultural products accounting for only 16 percent. Agricultural imports consist essentially of food, such as milk, flour, rice, meat and alcoholic beverages. Exports, 93 percent of which are agricultural, brought an income of $5.3 million in 1967, leaving a deficit of $4.3 million. Anguilla exports a negligible amount of cotton, grown on a few isolated plots. The island survives economically by exporting salt and laborers who hire out in the Dutch oil islands and send remittances home.

III. DIETS

A. GENERAL [23] [5]

In 1961 the U.S. Interdepartmental Committee on Nutrition for National Defense (ICNND) conducted a nutrition survey of some of the West Indies islands, including St. Kitts, Nevis and Anguilla. The ICNND investigators found that the diets of the inhabitants of St. Kitts, Nevis and Anguilla were characterized by a greater consumption of roots, tubers and sugar and a much smaller consumption of breadfruit and bananas than were the diets of St. Lucians in the Windward Islands. The following table gives the average daily per capita consumption of foodstuffs in the major towns of the three islands, as calculated by the ICNND group.

The consumption of cereals was greatest at Basseterre on St. Kitts and at Valley Road on Anguilla. Total vegetable consumption was highest at Basseterre, Charlestown (Nevis) and Old Road (St. Kitts), while roots and tubers were eaten in greatest amounts at Charlestown. Fruit was most heavily consumed at Charlestown and the lowest intake was at Valley Road. Fish consumption was highest at Old Road and Valley Road and lowest at Basseterre. Although fish intake was not as high on Nevis as on the other two islands, it was more important than meat as a source of animal protein for the Nevis islanders. As a matter of fact, meat consumption was low everywhere except at Basseterre, the capital and industrial center of the state. Milk and milk products were substantial elements of the diet at Charlestown, Valley Road and Basseterre. The highest intake of

Average Daily Per Capita Consumption by Food Groups in Principal Towns –
St. Kitts-Nevis-Anguilla, 1961
(in grams)

| | St. Kitts | | | Nevis | | Anguilla |
Item	Basse-terre	Molyneux-Tabernacle	Old Road	Charles-town	Cotton-ground	Valley Road
Cereals	315	247	307	229	266	350
Dried legumes	10	8	9	7	17	10
Green vegetables	27	4	21	27	1	–
Other vegetables	15	8	7	5	4	14
Roots and tubers	68	32	37	29	49	39
Mangoes	18	–	45	123	32	–
Breadfruit	–	130	11	40	51	31
Other fruit	73	54	104	53	68	25
Fish	35	95	123	68	71	121
Meat	134	17	18	16	16	10
Milk and products	206	127	124	265	131	225
Eggs	15	5	10	3	2	–
Fats	23	28	13	23	25	63
Sugar	29	76	84	53	55	78
Miscellaneous	2	5	12	9	4	3

Source: Interdepartmental Committee on Nutrition for National Defense, *West Indies Nutrition Survey.*

eggs was at Basseterre, but that amounted to only about two per capita per week. Fat intake was much higher at Valley Road than anywhere else and lowest at Old Road. This greater consumption of fats together with the high consumption of cereals on Anguilla accounts in large part for the higher caloric intake recorded at Valley Road.

The next table indicates the nutrient composition of these diets.

Average Calculated Daily Per Capita Nutrient Intake by Principal Towns –
St. Kitts-Nevis-Anguilla, 1961

| | St. Kitts | | | Nevis | | Anguilla |
Nutrient	Basse-terre	Molyneux-Tabernacle	Old Road	Charles-town	Cotton-ground	Valley Road
Calories	2,087	1,792	1,742	1,645	1,876	2,036
Protein (g)	84	69	88	62.5	89	69
Carbohydrates (g)	273	282	248	259	267	302
Fats (g)	71	46	49	44	55	73
Calcium (mg)	376	310.5	467	411	453	355
Iron (mg)	9.6	7.8	8.6	6	7	7.6
Vitamin A (IU)	3,884	1,106	4,834	6,470	2,560	1,148
Thiamine (mg)	.7	.5	.85	.55	.8	.7
Riboflavin (mg)	.93	.92	.72	.82	.9	.6
Niacin (mg)	14	7.5	10.4	6.85	8.45	11.2
Vitamin C (mg)	22.8	27	20	34	26	14

Source: Interdepartmental Committee on Nutrition for National Defense, *West Indies Nutrition Survey.*

The table shows that the diets at all locations, except perhaps Basseterre, were marginal and the suspicion is strong that many individuals, especially children, found themselves deprived of at least some of their requirements in basic nutrients. Caloric intake was adequate only at Valley Road, although at Cotton-ground and Basseterre 99 percent of the requirement was reached. At Charles-town, however, only 85 percent of the recommended allowance was met, meaning (since this was the average) that quite a large number of people must have had intakes far below their needs. Protein intake was nearly adequate quantitatively in three of the six locations investigated (Cottonground, Old Road and Basseterre), but low in the others. Given the general shortage of calories compared to requirements, however, some of the protein must have been used for fuel and thus was unavailable for tissue repair. Thiamine, riboflavin and vitamin C intakes were below recommended levels at all six stations. Vitamin A consumption was deficient at Molyneux-Tabernacle on St. Kitts and at Valley Road on Anguilla. Iron intake was very low in all places.

B. LEVELS OF NUTRITION [23]

In spite of the low intakes described above, biochemical analyses of blood samples revealed that plasma levels of many nutrients seemed to be sufficient to maintain tissue saturation and thus to support apparent health. Many explanations can be offered for these discrepancies. First of all, the metabolic pathways of many nutrients are not yet completely understood. Moreover, the tests were made only once. Seasonal resurveys might have revealed higher intakes at other times of the year, thus enabling the body to store nutrients over the period of scarcity.

It was found that quite a number of children below 15 years of age had poor values of plasma vitamin A: 25 micrograms per 100 milliliters on the average on St. Kitts, 5 micrograms per 100 milliliters on Nevis and 44.4 micrograms on Anguilla. Yet the plasma levels of carotene, the most important precursor of vitamin A, were not correlated with vitamin A levels; they were often higher and sometimes lower. Carotene occurs in many foods and when transformed into vitamin A, is stored in the liver. The body draws upon these stores when needed, provided they are stocked. Carotene levels reflect only the intake from the diet and vitamin A levels the availability of stores. When the latter are low, the levels in the blood are low. Hence the findings at St. Kitts, Nevis and Anguilla indicated a lack of reserves which has a greater significance than would a temporarily deficient intake of carotene.

By contrast, vitamin C, although inadequately supplied by the diet at the time of the survey, was found to be adequate in the plasma on St. Kitts and Nevis but not on Anguilla where the consumption of citrus fruits and fresh vegetables is lower. Riboflavin and thiamine, however, were both excreted in amounts suggesting inadequacy. The clinical expressions of these deficiencies in terms of symptoms are shown on the table opposite.

IV. NUTRITIONAL DISEASE PATTERNS [23] [1]

Anemia is quite common in the territory. The ICNND survey showed that 90.5 percent of all male children between the ages of 5 and 9 had hemoglobin values below 12 grams per 100 milliliters, which is considered low. Somewhat better values obtained before that age and after. Among females between 10 and 15 years of age, 87.5 percent had low values (below 12 grams). Among those over 15 years old, the situation improved and only 52.3 percent remained in the "low" category. Comparing males and females between the ages of 15 and 44, it was found, not surprisingly, that only 16.7 percent of the males showed levels lower than 12 grams per 100 milliliters. Pregnancies and menstruation among the females may account for the difference.

The following table shows the prevalence of the various clinical signs of nutritional deficiencies as identified by the ICNND investigators. This table is only indicative of the health problems resulting from faulty nutrition. It does not measure the size of the problem.

Percent Prevalence of Clinical Signs of Nutritional Deficiencies
St. Kitts-Nevis-Anguilla, 1961
(males and nonpregnant, nonlactating females)

Clinical Sign	Deficiency Presumed to Cause Symptom	Percent Prevalence		
		St. Kitts	Nevis	Anguilla
Nasolabial seborrhea	Riboflavin	13.9	17.9	22.5
Angular lesions of the lips	Riboflavin	5.0	15.3	2.2
Angular scars of the lips	Riboflavin	16.6	25.1	13.2
Swelling of the gums	Vitamin C	0.5	0.3	0.9
Papillary atrophy of the tongue	Riboflavin and/or niacin	3.4	2.0	5.6
Enlarged thyroid	Iodine	27.1	16.6	22.1
Follicular hyperkeratosis	Vitamin A and/or vitamin C	0.6	2.1	4.3
Bilateral edema	Thiamine	0.8	0.3	–
Bilateral loss of ankle jerk	Thiamine	1.8	2.6	1.7
Depigmentation of hair	Protein	6.6	2.0	10.4
Other		13.9	17.6	13.9

Source: Interdepartmental Committee on Nutrition for National Defense, *West Indies Nutrition Survey.*

The various findings of the ICNND survey indicate that Anguilla is the least well-fed of the three islands. It has the highest level of symptoms suggesting protein-calorie malnutrition among children. All three islands have a serious goiter problem.

Ashcroft, Buchanan, Lovell and Welsh have studied the growth of infants and preschool children in the three islands and have compared their findings with those for African, English and American infants and children. They found that the mean birth weights in St. Kitts and the mean rates of growth during the first 3 months were similar to those in the other countries considered, but between 4 and 12 months the rate of weight increase was lower in St. Kitts infants than in their English and American counterparts. The investigators believe that the recent tendency of mothers in the territory to reduce the length of time of breast feeding, under the pressure of social and economic conditions, explains the difference. They also suspect supplementary feeding to be inadequate, but the distribution of free skim milk should help to improve the situation.

V. CONCLUSIONS

The conclusion of this review of available data is that St. Kitts, Nevis and Anguilla, like most other Caribbean islands, are faced with the present sugar crisis and have little choice but to develop tourism to sustain their economy and improve their diets. When the sugar industry was most prosperous, the cane estates increased their acreage at the expense of the plots of land previously farmed for food crops. As the acreage in food crops dwindled, the quality of diets deteriorated. At the present time, it looks as if the resources brought by sugar are diminishing but the amount of food produced is not increasing. Contrary to what has happened in places like Jamaica and Trinidad where alternate resources were available (e.g., bauxite and oil), these small islands have little if anything to turn to when the sugar industry reaches a ceiling. Meanwhile, the population is increasing, hence, the temptation to expect salvation from tourism. Yet, this demands an investment which is not always easy to come by and there is much competition as most Caribbean islands are attractive to visitors. For these reasons, the future of these small islands is bleak.

THE LEEWARD ISLANDS: ANTIGUA

I. BACKGROUND INFORMATION

A. PHYSICAL SETTING [17] [14] [52] [36]

The island of Antigua, with its dependencies of Barbuda and Redonda, is located in the northeastern Caribbean, east of Nevis (see map on page 373). Antigua covers 280, Barbuda 160 and Redonda 2.6 square kilometers. The terrain of Antigua is generally flat, although low hills rise in the southwest. The island is noted for its fine sandy beaches which attract many tourists. The coastline includes a number of natural harbors, but none deep enough for steamships. There is a manmade deep-water harbor which opened in late 1968. Freshwater resources are scarce, necessitating desalination plants to provide drinking water for the hotels.

West and Augelli recognize three geographical regions: the eroded volcanic southwest where hills rise to a maximum of 400 meters (at Boggy Peak); a central plain about 5 kilometers wide which extends in a north-southeast direction for about 16 kilometers; and a low-lying limestone belt which covers the rest of the island to the sea.

B. CLIMATE [24] [52]

Average temperatures in Antigua range from a low of around 19°C in April to a high of about 22°C in August and September. Summer heat is tempered by trade winds. Rainfall is extremely irregular and a drought in 1969 prevented maturation of the sugar crop. Rainfall areas correspond to the three geographical regions: in the southwest volcanic region precipitation generally exceeds 1,250 millimeters per year; in the central plain area, it averages 1,250 millimeters; and in the limestone belt about 1,000 millimeters (see map on page 00). This geographical irregularity in rainfall restricts agricultural activities to two-thirds of the island's small area.

C. POPULATION [14] [40] [36]

The population of Antigua numbers about 61,000 and that of Barbuda 1,000; Redonda is uninhabited. Most of the Antiguans and Barbudans are of African descent. The population is growing at the rate of 2.1 percent per year. Life expectancy at birth is 60 years for males and 64 years for females; the infant mortality rate in 1968 was 45.4 per 1,000 live births (compared to 22 per 1,000 in the United States). The largest city is the capital, St. John's, with 13,000 inhabitants.

D. HISTORY AND GOVERNMENT [36] [52]

Antigua was discovered by Columbus in 1493. In 1632 the British began colonizing the island but a brief period of French occupation followed. In 1667, by terms of the Treaty of Breda, the island became a formal possession of Great Britain and has remained so ever since.

Since 1967 Antigua has been one of six West Indies Associated States and its governmental structure is similar to that described for St. Kitts-Nevis-Anguilla. Antigua is a signatory to the Caribbean Rice Agreement and is a member of the Caribbean Free Trade Association (CARIFTA).

E. AGRICULTURAL POLICIES [42] [14]

The Antiguan economy is supported by sugar, molasses, cotton and tourism, but agriculture has been severely curtailed in recent years because of persistent droughts. The Government is encouraging diversification of agriculture with special emphasis on such food crops as vegetables and fruits, mainly for the hotel trade. The policy is also to promote the milk and poultry industry for the same market.

F. FOREIGN AID

1. Bilateral Aid [14] [21a]

Antigua receives foreign aid from both the United Kingdom and the United States. Between 1965 and 1968 the U.K. provided $2.3 million in development aid, and in 1967 the U.S. granted a $6 million loan for construction of a deepwater port.

2. Multilateral Aid [41]

The United Nations Children's Fund (UNICEF) has supported the Government's child feeding program since 1954. UNICEF has provided transport costs for dry skim milk and corn-soy-milk blend (CSM) donations used in the program. About 6,500 primary and secondary schoolchildren receive yeast-fortified milk and cookies each year while approximately 2,000 preschool children and mothers are given dry milk rations or CSM every two weeks during the year.

II. FOOD RESOURCES

A. GENERAL

The food resources of the island are mostly imported, since local production is limited and increasingly tourist- rather than subsistence-oriented.

B. MEANS OF PRODUCTION

1. Agricultural Labor Force [52] [14]

The labor force numbered about 20,000 people in 1966. In normal (not too dry) times, 4,500 inhabitants are cane cutters or sugar plant workers. Between sugar seasons, these laborers are engaged in maintenance of existing water supplies (catchments, pipes, wells) or in creating new sources (artificial ponds). The growth of the tourist industry is absorbing more and more of the labor force, reducing the number of hands available for sugarcane work.

2. Farms [18] [52]

Out of the total land area of Antigua and its dependencies, which amounts to 44,000 hectares, 26,000 hectares (almost 60 percent) are considered to be arable farmland: 8,000 hectares are devoted to production of sugar,* cotton and food crops; 3,000 hectares are pastures and the rest lies fallow or is used for minor crops. The arable land is subdivided into 6,000 farms of sizes averaging 2-3 hectares each. The houses are clustered into more than 60 rural settlements and villages.

3. Mechanical Equipment and Fertilizers [18]

In 1968 there were 153 tractors and two mechanical harvesters in use on Antigua, mainly for sugar and cotton production. There is no information on the utilization of fertilizers.

---

*Cane is raised on small estates and also as a cash crop on the small plots of individual farmers.

C. PRODUCTION

1. Crops [18] [14]

Sugar and cotton have traditionally been the two main crops grown on Antigua but persistent droughts in recent years have severely affected production. Sugar was sown on about 5,000 hectares between 1953 and 1957 when an average of 215,000 tons were harvested each year, but between 1965 and 1968 both acreage and output were steadily reduced until only 1,000 hectares were planted and 12,000 tons harvested. The 1969 harvest amounted to nothing, but 5,200 hectares were planted in cane in 1970 in anticipation of a resurgence in 1971 due to improved moisture conditions.

Sea Island cotton has also been a victim of drought as well as of declining demand. Due to diversification efforts, some corn, sesame, soybeans, pigeon peas, onions and tomatoes are grown. Small banana groves are in production here and there.

2. Animal Husbandry [18]

Antigua has a 7,000-head herd of cattle, including 4,000 in-calf heifers kept primarily for milk. Four thousand tons of milk are reportedly produced from local cows each year. Three thousand pigs, 6,000 sheep and 6,000 goats are also kept. Some of the meat and milk consumed by the population is derived from these livestock.

3. Fisheries [52] [19]

Fishing is an important activity on Barbuda where the land is suitable only for pasture and small-scale subsistence farming. However, the catch does not meet the demand, resulting in the importation of fish and fish preparations valued at $400,000 each year. Like most other Caribbean waters, the sea around Antigua has been explored by the Caribbean Fishery Development Project. The Barbuda bank has revealed the existence of exploitable fish resources in the area. The existence of ciguatera fish poisoning has been reported only occasionally.

D. FOOD INDUSTRIES [3]

Food industries are limited to a sugarcane factory and to a recently built arrowroot plant. The U.S. firm of Nebraska Consolidated Mills is negotiating to construct a flour and feed mill on Antigua and a brewery is being built by other investors.

E. TRADE [14] [47]

The food resources of Antigua are not adequate to feed the population. Neither can they satisfy the tourist trade, which is becoming the most important, if not the only, source of income. Hence food imports are growing at a rapid pace and the U.S. share of this market is expanding. Poultry, eggs, meat and meat products, corn, fruits and vegetables are purchased increasingly from the United States. Rice is imported from Guyana, wheat and flour from Canada, coffee and tea from the U.S., animal and vegetable oils and fats from Denmark.

Exports are limited to sugar which was valued at $3.4 million in 1963, but only $1.3 million in 1965. During the following 4 years there was no crop.

F. FOOD SUPPLY [19]

It is difficult to assess the food supply of a territory which relies on imports for most of its dietary needs. These imports include live animals brought in as breeding stock or as animals for slaughter. Between 1963 and 1967 the annual value of all food imports settled around $3.8 million. Meat and meat preparations accounted for $600,000-$800,000. Dairy products reached $500,000 in 1967 and cereals $800,000. This last item had reached $1.1 million in 1965. Surprisingly, fish imports amount to $400,000 and fruits to $600,000. Most of the above imports are intended to stock the hotels and restaurants catering to tourists.

III. DIETS [5]

No quantified information is available on the diets of Antiguans since there has never been a nutrition survey of the island. One can only speculate that with more and more people coming into contact with tourists, either directly or through employment in hotels and restaurants, the food habits must be changing rapidly. Basically, the diet consists of imported fish, sweet potatoes, yams and pulses, but in what quantities is not known. The June 1971 *Barclay's Caribbean Bulletin* reported that while roots and tubers were available in abundance, vegetables were scarce.

IV. NUTRITIONAL DISEASE PATTERNS [50]

Little is known about the prevalence and incidence of nutritional diseases on Antigua. Uttley has stated that between 1949 and 1962 skin disorders and vitamin deficiencies were seen in more than 1 percent of all patients examined in hospitals and dispensaries on Antigua.

V. CONCLUSIONS

One conclusion is inescapable: Antigua will lose all significance as an agricultural producer as the tourist resource grows in importance. It is probable that there will come a point when all that is left of local output, especially fruit and milk, will be sold to the tourists while the rest of the population will learn to feed itself on imported foods.

THE LEEWARD ISLANDS: MONTSERRAT

I. BACKGROUND INFORMATION

A. PHYSICAL SETTING [14] [36] [52]

Twenty-seven nautical miles southwest of Antigua lies Montserrat or "Saw Toothed Mountain" as it was named by Christopher Columbus (see map on page 373). This rugged little island covers 101 square kilometers and encompasses three volcano groups, one of which reaches 1,000 meters in altitude. The sulfurous Soufrière volcano is smouldering but otherwise inactive. Although the island's rugged terrain makes farming difficult and the soil is badly eroded, agriculture is by necessity the mainstay of the economy due to the lack of natural resources.

B. CLIMATE [52]

The climate of Montserrat is similar to that found on other islands of the Leeward group. Rainfall varies from over 1,770 millimeters in the upland areas to less than 1,270 millimeters along the coast (see map on page 373).

C. POPULATION [3] [40]

In 1969 Montserrat's population totaled 15,000, about 3,000 of whom lived in Plymouth, the capital city. The annual rate of growth is about 1.6 percent. The 1969 infant mortality rate was 37.9 per 1,000 live births (compared to 21 in the U.S.). Life expectancy at birth is 50 years for males and 55 years for women. The literacy rate is said to be fairly high. Most of the inhabitants are of African or mixed descent. Unemployment is a problem, as elsewhere in the Caribbean, and there is a considerable amount of emigration.

D. HISTORY AND GOVERNMENT [3] [52]

Montserrat was colonized in 1632 by Irish settlers from nearby St. Kitts, but like St. Kitts and Nevis, the island was fought over by the British and French during the 17th and 18th centuries, finally becoming a recognized British colony. Since 1967, the island has been a member of the West Indies Associated States (see page 348).

E. AGRICULTURAL POLICIES [14]

The Government has initiated a 5-year (1966-1971) agricultural development program aimed at clearing land, preventing erosion, increasing the use of fertilizers and insecticides, conducting research, providing agricultural credit, facilitating ownership and rental of agricultural land and establishing a government farm machinery pool. In addition, price controls have been put into effect for a number of domestic food commodities.

F. FOREIGN AID

1. Bilateral Aid [41] [14]

Montserrat is heavily dependent upon grants-in-aid from the United Kingdom. The Canadian Government assists the island's teacher training program.

2. Multilateral Aid [41]

United Nations assistance to Montserrat has included a health services project initiated in 1962, a child feeding project started in 1954 and an education program begun in 1966. Under the health project, an integrated health service has been established, including maternal and child health, environmental sanitation, communicable disease control, health education and medical care. As a result of the project, by 1970 the number of cases of malnutrition had been reduced and the infant mortality rate had fallen from 114 per 1,000 live births in 1960 at 37.9 in 1969. UNICEF has provided equipment, health education materials, teaching aids and transportation while WHO has given advice and guidance as necessary.

UNICEF has covered ocean freight costs on donated skim milk powder and corn-soy-milk blend (CSM) for the Government's child feeding program. Approximately 1,250 mothers and preschool children and 2,000 schoolchildren benefit from the program annually. UNICEF and UNESCO have helped augment the island's staff of trained teachers by providing basic equipment for a training center, teaching aids, home economics equipment, training grants, and advice from visiting experts.

II. FOOD RESOURCES

A. GENERAL [18]

The food of Montserrat is derived from about 4,000 hectares of cultivable land, from the sea around the island and from imports, which are on the increase now that the tourist trade has become the island's most important economic resource.

B. MEANS OF PRODUCTION

1. Agricultural Labor Force [3]

The labor force comprises about 5,000 people, some working on estates, most for themselves. Due to lack of jobs, many emigrate to find employment on other islands. At the same time, Montserrat suffers from a skilled labor shortage due to the exodus of an estimated 4,000 people to the United Kingdom in past years.

2. Farms [3] [14]

There are three large estates, each covering more than 25 hectares. The rest of the arable land is split among 3,000 small farms averaging 1-2 hectares each. The Government believes that 4,500 more hectares could be put into production either as cropland or as pastures but the rugged terrain has been severely eroded and one can see that a substantial investment would be needed which might not bring the expected returns.

3. Fertilizers and Mechanical Equipment [18]

There is no information on the use of fertilizers on Montserrat. In 1965 it was reported that 24 tractors were utilized on the island.

C. PRODUCTION

1. Crops [18] [3] [14]

The major food crops on Montserrat consist of bananas, mangoes, avocados, breadfruit, limes, pumpkins, cabbages, groundnuts, sweet potatoes, yams, vegetables, especially carrots and tomatoes (10 percent of which are exported), and sugarcane processed into rum for domestic use. The major cash crop is cotton, which is raised both by smallholders on their tiny plots and by estates. At times a small surplus of cottonseed is available for export. Cotton holdings were severely damaged by winds between 1966 and 1969 causing 500 hectares out of

613 to be abandoned to other uses, partly the growing of vegetables (carrots and tomatoes) which are now exported in increasing quantities.

2. Animal Husbandry [52] [18]

There is a herd of 4,000 head of cattle which provides meat and milk for the local population and occasionally some surplus for export. There are about 26,000 poultry on the island and an unknown number of goats.

D. AGRICULTURAL INDUSTRIES

There is a cotton ginnery on the island operated by the Government, a rum distillery, a lime juice factory, a tomato paste factory, and an oil press to treat cottonseed when it is available.

E. TRADE [3] [14]

In recent years Montserrat's exports have dwindled to about $200,000 a year by value while imports have risen to $4 million. These imports are either construction materials which could be considered an investment to attract the tourist trade, or food needed to satisfy both the domestic population and the tourists. The most common food items imported are flour, beef, poultry and pork.

F. FOOD SUPPLY

At present, Montserrat is far from being self-sufficient in food. The Government is well-aware of the importance of this aspect of development and has an agricultural program for expanding food crops for domestic use. However, in recent years it has been impeded by an unusual succession of bad weather factors. If climatic conditions were to improve, the picture could change.

III. DIETS

There are no quantified data on diets in Montserrat. Montserrat natives are fond of turtle steaks, frogs' legs (which they call "mountain chicken") and "goat water," which is a kind of goat's meat stew.

IV. NUTRITIONAL DISEASE PATTERNS

There are no published data on nutritional deficiency diseases on Montserrat. The availability of meat and milk, as well as other locally grown sources of animal protein, may help support a good level of nutritional health.

V. CONCLUSIONS

It appears that a sale of accumulated stocks of Sea Island cotton which took place recently may reopen the market for that commodity. Hope for the future of the island's economy, however, seems at present to rest mainly with tourism. This important but fickle market could result in stimulating local farmers to increase food production.

THE LEEWARD ISLANDS:
THE BRITISH VIRGIN ISLANDS

I. BACKGROUND INFORMATION

A. PHYSICAL SETTING [7] [17] [52]

\

The British Virgin Islands lie at the northwestern extremity of the Leeward chain, about 60 nautical miles east of Puerto Rico and 140 nautical miles northwest of St. Kitts, astraddle latitude 18°25' N at longitude 64°30' W (see map on page 373). The group encompasses over 40 islands totaling 130 square kilometers of land area. The islands can be divided into four groups: a southerly series terminating in the island of Virgin Gorda; a parallel group including Great Thatch, Tortola and Beef Island; a northwesterly cluster which includes the Tobago Cays and Great and Little Jost van Dyke; and the island of Anegada which lies about 30 miles north of Virgin Gorda. Only 15 of the islands are inhabited. Except for Anegada, which is a relatively flat coral limestone formation, the islands are hilly. The highest point is almost 600 meters on Tortola. There are no rivers on the islands and most are too arid for agriculture with soils too light for sustained cultivation. Most of the available cropland is located on Tortola, Jost van Dyke and Virgin Gorda. On Tortola there are remnants of rain forest but no stands of trees. Molybdenum and copper deposits have been found on Virgin Gorda.

B. CLIMATE [7] [3] [52]

The climate in this island group is subtropical. Winter temperatures vary from 21°C to 27°C and summer temperatures from 25°C to 31°C, but the heat is moderated by trade winds. Average rainfall at Road Town, the capital city located on Tortola, is 1,325 millimeters but precipitation varies throughout the islands and in many places is too slight to sustain agriculture.

C. POPULATION [7] [14] [36] [40]

In 1969 the total resident population of the British Virgin Islands was estimated at 13,500, increasing at an annual rate of 2.7 percent. Life expectancy is about 50 years for males and 55 for females. Europeans comprise only about 3 percent of the population, the rest being of African or mixed descent. About 85 percent of the inhabitants live on the island of Tortola, 8 percent on Virgin Gorda, 4 percent on Anegada and Jost van Dyke and the rest are scattered throughout the other populated islands. Education is free and the literacy rate is high.

D. HISTORY AND GOVERNMENT [7] [36]

The Virgin Islands were discovered in 1493 by Columbus, who named them after St. Ursula and her 11,000 virgins. For a time, the islands were occupied by Dutch and then British buccaneers. In the mid-18th century the European powers began competing for control over the islands. A British charter was granted in 1773 and the islands have been British ever since.

The British Virgin Islands are a British colony with an administrative framework similar to that of the West Indies Associated States (see page 348). An Administrator is the Queen's representative, responsible for defense and internal security, external affairs, public service, the courts and finance. He presides over an Executive Council consisting of himself, two ex-officio members and three ministers appointed from among members of the legislature. The Legislative Council is composed of two official members, one nominated member and seven elected members.

E. AGRICULTURAL POLICIES [7] [14]

The economy of the British Virgin Islands has traditionally been based on agriculture (primarily livestock-raising) and fishing, although tourism is becoming increasingly important. Efforts are being made to expand livestock production by using drought-resistant Pangola grass. The Government runs a stock farm at Road Town and operates a pasturage area of over 100 hectares where livestock are matured and then resold to local stockmen or exported. An agricultural loan scheme has been instituted to assist farmers.

F. FOREIGN AID

1. Bilateral Aid [7] [14]

Great Britain is the source of bilateral aid for the British Virgin Islands (B.V.I.). Between 1965 and 1968 the British Colonial Development and Welfare funds granted $160,000 and loaned $74,000 to the B.V.I. Government. The islands benefit from British Commonwealth trade preferences. Canada has provided personnel, equipment and drugs for the health services program of the B.V.I.

2. Multilateral Aid [41]

Since 1968 UNICEF and WHO have assisted the Government of the B.V.I. in reorganizing and improving its health services, with emphasis on the development of maternal and child health services and environmental sanitation. UNICEF provides supplies, equipment and transport while WHO has given advice and fellowships.

II. FOOD RESOURCES

A. GENERAL [7]

In 1961 it was decided to base the future economy of the British Virgin Islands on tourism rather than agriculture since the dividends derived from the former are larger than those coming from the latter. Moreover, various factors militate against agricultural development: rugged topography; smallness of holdings (less than 2 hectares each); and uncertain rainfall (some droughts, as in 1965, are very serious).

B. PRODUCTION

1. Crops and Animal Husbandry [7] [14] [18]

Cash crops consist of limes, coconuts, bananas, and sugar for the manufacture of rum. The basic food crops are rice, corn and wheat. Livestock-raising appears to be more suitable than crops as an export and domestic investment. Special efforts are being made to develop this resource through the importation of drought-resistant Pangola grass. In 1968 the livestock population consisted of 6,000 cattle, 2,500 sheep, 12,000 goats and 5,000 swine. There is a feedlot where animals are matured and resold and a stock farm at Road Town.

2. Fisheries [13] [52]

Coastal fishing is practiced, primarily on the expansive reefs around Anegada, but no deep-sea fishing is carried out. The vessels used are 16-22 foot open boats with outboard motors, and the techniques employed are handlining and pot fishing. Various types of reef fish and lobster are caught. A Fisherman's Council assists in regulating the price of fish. Loans to fishermen are made under a fisheries credit scheme. Most fishermen work part-time at some other job.

Brownell states that the industry will have to be diversified to include deepwater fishing if it is to succeed economically. The slope at the edge of the Anegada shelf is reported to be productive in nine species of snappers, nine species of groupers and five other types of fish. In the shallower areas along the northern margins of the shelf, many pelagic fishes, such as dolphin, little tuna and blackfin tuna, are found. At present, however, these fishing grounds are out of range for most native boats. Improved vessels and techniques adapted to the environment would have to be developed to enable fishermen to take advantage of these potential fisheries.

C. TRADE [7]

The British Virgin Islands export food at about the level of 2,000 head of cattle a year worth over $80,000, 23 tons of fresh fish worth about $12,000, some fresh fruit worth $3,900, vegetables worth $1,900 and 1,500 liters of rum valued at $1,800. Wheat flour and pulses are imported from Puerto Rico because local production is inadequate.

III. DIETS AND NUTRITIONAL DISEASE PATTERNS [40]

There is very little information about diets or the actual state of nutritional health in the British Virgin Islands. Infant mortality at 70.1 deaths per 1,00 live births is still high, giving reason to suspect some level of malnutrition among those who cannot afford proper foods or who do not know the importance of the diet to child development.

IV. CONCLUSIONS

If the plan for development of tourism succeeds, the British Virgin Islands will become another international playground and lose their personality as a distinct national entity.

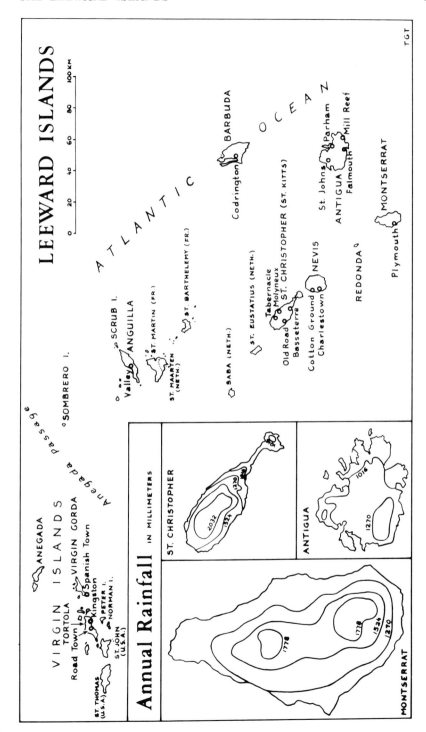

THE WINDWARD ISLANDS

TABLE OF CONTENTS

THE WINDWARD ISLANDS: GUADELOUPE AND MARTINIQUE

I. BACKGROUND INFORMATION

A. PHYSICAL SETTING [17] [36] [52] [21b]

The French Department of Guadeloupe consists of two large islands (Basse-Terre and Grande-Terre) separated by swamps and a narrow channel (called Rivière Salée) plus five smaller island dependencies (Marie Galante, Les Saintes, Desirade, St. Barthélemy and part of St. Martin*). The total area covered by all these islands is 1,702 square kilometers. Grande-Terre and Basse-Terre combined cover 1,510 square kilometers, while the remaining islands account for 192 square kilometers. The twin islands of Guadeloupe proper lie at the intersection of 16°15' north and 61°35' west (see map on page 422). Grande-Terre, the northeastern twin, is flat and low-lying with its highest elevation reaching only 150 meters. Grande-Terre, like the adjacent islands of Marie Galante and La Desirade, is mainly limestone. The island has been cleared of its original forest and now only intermittent patches of scrub remain. Extensive mangrove swamps line the Rivière Salée. Basse-Terre, by contrast, is high and rugged, centered on a chain of volcanic peaks and ridges which increase in height to the south. La Soufrière, a dormant sulfurous volcano, is the highest peak on the island (1,623 meters). Towards the west coast, the ground slopes steeply but on the eastern side of the mountain ridge the land descends gently to the Rivière Salée. Basse-Terre is drained by over 70 streams. A dense tropical rain forest characterizes the mountain region. The eight islands of Les Saintes lie off the southern coast of Basse-Terre and are also of volcanic origin. The islands of St. Martin and Barthélemy lie at the northwestern end of the outer Lesser Antilles, about 100

---

*France administers only about two-thirds of St. Martin; the remaining one-third belongs to the Netherlands.

377

miles north of Guadeloupe. Both have rugged terrain. Hills on St. Martin rise to 440 meters and on St. Barthélemy to 330 meters.

Martinique lies on the eastern Caribbean between the British islands of Dominica and St. Lucia and covers an area of 1,100 square kilometers (see map on page 422). Its topography is mountainous, reflecting the island's volcanic origin. The highest point is Mt. Pelée in the north (an active volcano) which rises gently to 1,518 meters. An older volcanic massif, Pitons du Carbet, dominates the center of the island and reaches 1,300 meters. Mt. Pelée and the western slopes of the Pitons du Carbet are raked with ravines. The island is drained by numerous streams and several large rivers flowing toward the western coast. No virgin forest exists on Martinique but in the south, scattered scrub woodlands are found and some luxuriant secondary forest exists on the slopes of the mountains.

B. CLIMATE [17] [52] [21b]

The climate on Guadeloupe varies considerably in spite of its small area, due to differences in altitude. Seasonally, the temperature varies only from a maximum monthly average of 28°C in June to a minimum of 24°C in January; however, the mountains are always considerably cooler than the low-lying areas. Average annual rainfall on Grande-Terre is limited to 1,000 millimeters in places and serious droughts are a problem during the dry season, which lasts from January until May. In the mountainous parts of Basse-Terre, however, well over 2,500 millimeters of precipitation fall each year due to the pattern of northeast trade winds (see map on page 00). The mountain summits are cloud-enveloped most of the time. Hurricanes are a likelihood during the rainy season (July-November).

On Martinique there is little variation in temperature throughout the year. In the lowlands the maximum monthly mean is 28°C (in June) and the minimum is 25°C (in January). The mountain regions are characterized by somewhat lower temperatures. Annual rainfall in the lowlands averages between 1,016 and 2,032 millimeters. On the mountain slopes, precipitation increases, reaching 4,572 millimeters on the western side of Mt. Pelée (see map on page 422). The rainy season occurs from July to November with occasional hurricanes. The period January-April is usually dry.

C. POPULATION [40] [52] [17] [21b]

The 1969 population of Guadeloupe and its dependencies was 324,000 with a yearly growth rate of 2.8 percent. The density is about 181 persons per square kilometer. In 1967, the infant mortality rate was 49.6 per 1,000 live births. Life expectancy for Guadeloupe and Martinique combined is 62.5 years for men and 66.5 years for women. Most of the inhabitants of Guadeloupe live in rural areas.

The largest town is Pointe-à-Pitre on Grande-Terre (29,538 inhabitants in 1967) and the second largest is the capital, Basse-Terre (15,690), located at the southwestern end of the island of the same name. The inhabitants are mainly of African extraction. The mulatto population is extensive due to centuries of intermarriage between the descendants of African slaves and French settlers. Only the islands of Les Saintes and Barthélemy have predominantly European populations. The ethnic composition of Guadeloupe's inhabitants has been further diversified over the years by the immigration of East Indians and Syrians who came to work as laborers, artisans and traders.

In 1969 the population estimate for Martinique was 332,000 with an annual increase of 1.6 percent and a density of 302 per square kilometer. Infant mortality in 1967 was 37.1 per 1,000 live births. As on Guadeloupe, the population is mainly of African or mixed descent.

D. HISTORY AND GOVERNMENT [17] [52] [36] [21b]

The twin islands of Guadeloupe were discovered by Columbus in 1493 but the Spanish made no attempt at settlement since the islands were populated by fierce Carib Indians who themselves had driven out the previous Arawak inhabitants. In 1635 settlers representing a chartered French company occupied Guadeloupe in spite of strong Carib resistance. The Caribs were gradually annihilated with the result that when the plantation system was established on the islands, African slaves were imported to work the fields. In 1674 possession of Guadeloupe passes to the French crown. There followed brief periods of British occupation, but the islands were restored to France by the Congress of Vienna and have remained French possessions ever since. St. Martin was divided between the Dutch and French in 1648. The French portion was ceded to Sweden in 1784 and returned to France by plebiscite in 1877.

In 1946 Guadeloupe with its dependencies became a Department of Metropolitan France. Its inhabitants enjoy all the rights and privileges of full French citizenship. Guadeloupe is represented in the French National Assembly by three deputies and in the Senate by two senators. Local government is headed by a Prefect; a General Council of 36 members is vested with local legislative authority. The Department is divided into two arrondissements comprising 34 communes. Each Commune is administered by an elected Municipal Council.

Martinique was discovered in 1502 by Columbus. Like Guadeloupe, it was occupied by Caribs who had displaced the original Arawak inhabitants. It was not until 1635 that European settlement was attempted, when a colony was established for a French chartered company. The island became a crown possession in 1674. Martinique was attacked time and again by English and Dutch forces and was held intermittently by the British between 1762 and 1814 when it reverted to France as a result of the Congress of Vienna. Like Guadeloupe,

Martinique became a Department of France in 1946. The island sends three deputies and two senators to the French Parliament. Local government is headed by a Prefect and local law-making authority is vested in a 36-member elected General Council. Martinique is divided into two arrondissements and 34 communes, with each commune administered by a Municipal Council elected by popular vote.

E. AGRICULTURAL POLICIES [14] [21b]

The economies of Guadeloupe and Martinique are essentially agricultural. The French Government's policies are aimed at expanding production of all crops grown on the islands. Price supports and guarantees are provided only for sugar and sugarcane, although subsidies are paid to farmers for the creation of new pastures, the purchase of breeding stock, and production of vegetables. Subsidies are also provided for agricultural exports to non-EEC* countries.

F. FOREIGN AID

Being departments of France, Guadeloupe and Martinique receive no foreign aid.

II. FOOD RESOURCES

A. GENERAL [18] [43]

The food resources of the two islands are inadequate to feed all the inhabitants and the growing number of tourist visitors. In Martinique the total land area amounts to 110,000 hectares, of which 32,000 are cropland and 20,000 pastures and savannas. In Guadeloupe the total area is 178,000 hectares, of which 60,076 are cropland and 14,500 are pastures and savannas (see table opposite). The interior of Grande-Terre in Guadeloupe is largely unexplored and consists of dense jungle. It is estimated that over 20,000 hectares at the periphery of the core could be used for agriculture.

While in Martinique almost all the agricultural cropland is used, some leeway still exists in Guadeloupe which is being constantly developed through successive plans. In Martinique expansion of one crop means the contraction of another, but this is not necessarily so in Guadeloupe. Some fishing is done around the islands but not enough to supply them with industrial quantities.

---

*European Economic Community (Common Market).

Land Use in Guadeloupe and Martinique, 1966

| | Martinique | | Guadeloupe | |
| | Area | | Area | |
Category	(1,000 ha)	Percent	(1,000 ha)	Percent
Cropland	32	29.2	49	27.5
Pastures and savannas	20	18.2	18	10.2
Forests and jungle	26	24.6	56	31.4
Usable agricultural land	2	1.8	20	11.2
Built-up or waste	30	26.2	35	19.7
Total	110	100.0	178	100.0

Source: Food and Agriculture Organization, *Production Yearbook 1969.*

B. MEANS OF PRODUCTION

1. Agricultural Labor Force [52] [43] [47a] [21b]

Because the population increase is high, the labor force grows rapidly and jobs have to be found for more and more young people reaching adult age. By now, the labor force must number about 100,000 on each island, with about 48 percent working mostly in agriculture. Since 1960 a special law has permitted funding of a variety of agricultural projects as well as construction to increase the tourist potential. Yet there is underemployment in the off-seasons for cane cutting and processing, and pineapple canning. During these months, many otherwise employed laborers fish or grow vegetables on their own plots—a privilege that is protected by law, so that estates and industrial plantations cannot compete.

To ward off the social consequences of unemployment, the Government subsidizes the labor force in many ways. In Martinique, salaries paid by the Government amount to 42-45 percent of all salaries paid on the island. In some years, the social security deficit incurred by the islands has to be made good by the central office in Paris. As a result of this policy, the standard of living of the population rose rapidly until the mid-1960's. The levelling off of government spending in recent years has slowed down the process.

Until 1968, when civil unrest in Paris led to a 38 percent increase in wages in continental France, the French Government attempted to raise the minimum wage level in Guadeloupe and Martinique to the level of metropolitan France. Although the Government now finds such a goal unrealistic, given the large proportion of island workers who are at the minimum wage level or below, the prevailing wage rates in Guadeloupe and Martinique are still considerably higher than in nearby English-speaking islands and social security benefits are more extensive. Nevertheless, chronic unemployment is a problem.

The higher wages paid in Guadeloupe and Martinique result in higher production costs for the islands' tropical products. This is compensated for the some degree by the fact that the islands benefit from a protected European market for their sugar and a protected French market for their bananas.

2. Farms [80] [18] [52]

There are three types of farms on the islands, although the pattern is somewhat different for each: large estates, tenant farms and small owner-operated farms. Usually the large estates are run by the owners who are, for the most part, descendants of old families who established themselves in the area during the 18th century. Some are run by resident managers, but in those cases the owners visit their plantations often, especially now that air transport has brought the Department within a few hours of the metropolis. Tenants, also called *colons,* operate smaller estates and pay rent with a fraction of the cash crop. They often grow vegetables commercially and own a few cattle. In the same manner, many small owner-farmers also grow a combination of cash and food crops and raise a few livestock. Farms over 100 hectares cover 60 percent of the total area in Martinique; the concentration is less in Guadeloupe. *Colons* and small farmers often hire out on the large plantations during the busy season. Between seasons, certain plantation owners allow some of their workers to use estate land for food crops.

3. Fertilizers and Mechanical Equipment [18] [47a]

About 6,000 tons of nitrogenous and an equal amount of phosphatic fertilizers are spread on Guadeloupe estates, as well as 19,000 tons of potash. On Martinique 9,000 tons of nitrogenous and 10,000 tons of potassic fertilizers are used each year.

The problem of keeping the work labor-oriented rather than machine-oriented is acute. The French Govern.:ent controls the import of machinery to avoid overly rapid mechanization of the large plantations. On most of the land area (Basse-Terre in Guadeloupe and all of Martinique except the Lamentin Plain), the terrain is too rugged to permit tractors to operate, in any event. On Guadeloupe 576 tractors were in use in 1968 and on Martinique 466 tractors were available in 1966.

C. PRODUCTION

1. Food Crops [18] [43] [52] [14] [21b]

Both islands cultivate a large variety of crops, both for domestic consumption and for export. Food crops include roots, pulses and vegetables. The only cereal grown is corn. Little if any is cultivated in Martinique, but about 1,000 hectares are planted in corn in Guadeloupe, producing 1,000 tons yearly. Sweet potatoes and yams cover about 3,000 hectares in Guadeloupe and in Martinique, bringing a crop of 3,000 tons a year in each Department. More is probably grown but not recorded. Manioc is also a food resource, estimated at 5,000 tons per year in Guadeloupe and 3,000 tons in Martinique. Tomatoes (3,000 tons a year in Guadeloupe), onions, cabbages and beans are grown on special plots or interspersed with bananas or cane. About 3,500 hectares are devoted to these food crops in Martinique and 6,500 hectares in Guadeloupe.

2. Cash Crops [43] [18] [14] [47a] [52] [21b]

The major cash crops on both islands are sugarcane and bananas. Since the soils suitable for each are well-identified, there is no competition between the two. In Martinique the area covered has diminished during the last decade but production has more than quadrupled. Thanks to better practices in Guadeloupe, the crop has increased tenfold while the area covered has remained the same. As a result of soil improvement and better planting conditions, however, there is a great difference in yield between the large estates and the smallholdings. Cane is harvested from January to June. Five to 10 percent of the crop is available for domestic consumption on each island. One thousand hectares are used to grow cane for the manufacture of rum, of which there are two kinds: cane juice rum, which is consumed locally, and molasses rum (industrial rum), which is exported.

Principal Cash Crops – Guadeloupe and Martinique, 1961-1969
(area in 1,000 hectares – production in 1,000 tons)

| | Martinique | | | | Guadeloupe | | | |
| | Area | | Production | | Area | | Production | |
Crop	1961	1969	1961	1969	1961	1969	1961	1969
Sugarcane	14.0	6	89	400	25.0	25.0	167	1,700
Bananas	7.5	12	146	230	8.5	8.0	165	180
Coffee	.2	–	.02	–	2.5	.5	–	.2
Cocoa	.3	–	.15	–	.5	–	.11	.1
Pineapples	.6	–	11.5	19	–	–	1	–

Sources: U.S. Department of Agriculture, *French West Indies: Agricultural Production and Trade.*
Food and Agriculture Organization of the United Nations, *Production Yearbook 1969.*

Bananas, which occupy 12,000 hectares in Martinique and 8,000 hectares in Guadeloupe, represent the second most profitable cash crop, yielding 230,000 tons in Martinique and 180,000 tons in Guadeloupe. The fruit is grown mainly on large estates. In Martinique its expansion was made to the detriment of cocoa, coffee and some sugarcane. In Guadeloupe it is grown mostly on the slopes of the Soufrière on Basse-Terre.

To make good some of the losses caused by winds or drought, coffee shrubs and cocoa trees are planted between banana trees. Twenty tons of coffee and 150 tons of raw cocoa are harvested in Martinique and 200 tons of coffee and 100 tons of cocoa in Guadeloupe. Other cash crops include pineapples, which are grown mostly on Martinique (19,000 tons), although a few are cultivated on Guadeloupe (1,000 tons). Vanilla, surplus vegetables, and fruits contribute some financial returns to farmers either on the domestic or world market.

3. Animal Husbandry [43] [14] [18]

There are quite a few livestock and poultry of all kinds in the islands. Unfortunately, the animals are not in very good condition, but they do provide some fresh milk, meat, and eggs. Basically, the cattle are Zebu, Brahman and Sahival but other breeds have been imported, mostly French Charolais and Swiss Browns. The industry is being promoted by the Government which has imported good Pangola grass *(Digitaria decumbens)* to improve pastures and has established artificial insemination centers in both departments. Most of the herds are divided between tenants and smallholders but some herds are also in the hands of Asian Indians who form a separate community, living apart from others in a section of Grande-Terre in Guadeloupe. In Martinique the efforts to develop animal husbandry have been quite successful and almost all the meat consumed is of domestic origin.

On Guadeloupe there were 76,000 cattle in 1968, yielding 2,000 tons of meat and 10,000 tons of milk. In addition, there were 21,000 pigs, 4,000 sheep, 16,000 goats, 450,000 chickens, 7,000 ducks and 3,000 turkeys. Four million hen's eggs are produced annually. On Martinique the cattle herd numbers 40,000, including 18,000 milch cows. About 3,000 tons of beef are produced and 4,000 tons of milk. Other livestock include 30,000 pigs (yielding 2,000 tons of pork), 25,000 sheep, 10,000 goats, 410,000 chickens and 26,000 ducks.

D. TRADE [19] [21b] [47a] [14]

The trade of Guadeloupe and Martinique takes two forms: 1) a purely domestic exchange of local goods between smallholder producers and urban consumers; and 2) the sale abroad, primarily to metropolitan France, of local agricultural products (mainly sugar, bananas and pineapples) and the importation of equipment and foodstuffs, mostly from France. Local producers channel their vegetables, non-exportable bananas, rum, fruits and, as the case may be, surplus milk to nearby markets or to intermediaries. Products for sale abroad are collected by exporters. Bananas are shipped to France in fast, refrigerated vessels. The fruit is harvested green when it has reached acceptable weight and size. One of the problems limiting the islands' foreign trade is the absorptive capacity of the French market, which is the destination for the entire export banana crop.

In Guadeloupe, the value of agricultural products exported between 1964 and 1969 varied from $31 million to $36.8 million, averaging $34 million annually. This trade represented 95 percent of all exports from Guadeloupe. In 1969, the breakdown among agricultural exports was as follows: bananas and pineapples, $11.4 million; sugar and molasses, $18.8 million; rum, $2.8 million. In Martinique, fluctuation in yearly income from exports ranged from $28.5 million to $43 million over the same period, giving an annual average of $35.8 million. For both islands, 1965 was the most remunerative year. As in Guadeloupe, Martinique's agricultural products represent 95 percent of all export trade. In 1969, bananas and pineapples earned $24 million, sugar and molasses $4 million and rum $4.8 million. As stated previously, France is the major recipient of the islands' exports. However, the United States participates to a small extent in this overseas trade. In 1968, Guadeloupe sold 56,559 tons of sugar to the United States.

Imports consist mainly of live animals, foodstuffs, construction materials and machinery. Agricultural products account for 24 percent of all imports by value in Guadeloupe and 21 percent in Martinique. It is interesting to note that fresh milk, cream, butter, cheese and eggs are imported in substantial quantities: $3.3 million worth was imported by Guadeloupe in 1969 and $4.3 million worth by Martinique. Fresh, chilled or frozen meat accounted for over $1.7 million of Guadeloupe's import bill in 1969 and $2.1 million of Martinique's invoice. Wheat and wheat flour imports are significant at $2.9 million worth in Guadeloupe and $3.5 million worth in Martinique in 1969. In addition, Guadeloupe imported $2.1 million worth of rice. This cereal is less popular in Martinique which purchased only $700,000 worth abroad in 1969. Both islands have trade deficits of over 300 percent.

E. FOOD INDUSTRIES [43] [47a] [21b]

Industries are almost exclusively concerned with the processing of agricultural output. Sugar manufacture is obviously the most important industry. There are more than 15 sugar mills and 30 distilleries in Martinique and over 12 mills and 26 distilleries in Guadeloupe. In addition, a flour mill, a margarine plant and an animal feed mill have been completed. Other food industries include dairies preparing pasteurized milk, slaughterhouses, and beer and carbonated drink plants.

III. DIETS

Little or no information is available on diets in Guadeloupe and Martinique. As far as is known from personal experience, the diets are generally adequate enough to prevent visible deficiencies but, as elsewhere in the Caribbean, pockets of malnutrition exist occasionally, as revealed by the local survey discussed below.

IV. NUTRITIONAL DISEASE PATTERNS [37]

In 1968 Perronnette made a study of the weight profiles of children in rural Martinique. This was done in the village of Le Robert on the Atlantic coast of the island, an area that was particularly well-chosen because it has an urban center, rural surroundings where people work on small farms, a few large estates producing sugarcane and bananas, and a small but active fishing population. The total population approximated 15,000 people, including 2,000 children from 0 to 6 years and 5,000 school-age children. The weight of the children was analyzed by groups of 100 and by 1-year intervals. All the usual statistical safeguards were respected. The analysis showed that of 1,500 children examined, 27 percent were below the expected range of weight, 5.4 percent were beyond the standard and 67.6 percent were within the normal range. This can be interpreted to mean that about 27 percent of the child population in that area suffers from some degree of malnutrition, a finding which is consistent with other surveys made in the West Indies. The investigator also found that boys were more frequently underweight than girls. Protein-calorie malnutrition in preschool children was observed frequently and constituted the most common deficiency disease diagnosed. The synergism between malnutrition and infection was also noted by this investigator.

V. CONCLUSIONS

The situation of these two departments of France is unusual. As part of Metropolitan France, their economies are strongly integrated into that of the home country. No major food deficiency should occur without being compensated by imports from the metropolis. No foreign aid is necessary, for its equivalent is built into the overall system. Three hundred years of close association has resulted in making the majority of the population as completely assimilated into the French culture as is possible, thus eliminating most of the problems which otherwise can crop up when two separate cultures join in an unequal relationship.

THE WINDWARD ISLANDS: DOMINICA

I. BACKGROUND INFORMATION

A. PHYSICAL SETTING [17] [8] [52]

The island of Dominica is located between the French islands of Guadeloupe and Martinique near the intersection of parallels 15°N and 61°W (see map on page 422). Dominica is about 36 kilometers long and 25.6 kilometers wide, with an area of 751 square kilometers. It is the most rugged of the West Indies islands with high (for that region) mountains and thick forests, making much of the island inaccessible. A central mountain ridge runs from north to south with the high land concentrated in the south where it terminated in cliffs. The highest point on the island, however, is in the north at Morne Diablotin (1,205 meters). Numerous rivers provide drainage and power. The island's soil is of volcanic origin, weathered in spots to red tropical clay. Although rich, the land is porous and easily eroded.

B. CLIMATE [8] [52]

Mean monthly temperatures range from 25°C to 32°C. The cool season lasts from December to March and the hottest month is July. The dry season occurs from February to May; the remainder of the year is rainy with average annual precipitation ranging from 1,750 millimeters along the coast to over 6,000 millimeters in the highlands where luxuriant tropical vegetation prevails (see map on page 422).

C. POPULATION [8] [40] [52]

In 1969 the population of Dominica was estimated to be 74,000 with an annual rate of increase of 2.7 percent and a density of 99 inhabitants per square kilometer. The infant mortality rate is about 44.7 per 1,000 live births and life expectancy is approximately 57 years for males and 59 years for females. The population is mainly rural; the largest town is the capital, Roseau.

Most of Dominica's people are of African or mixed African and European descent. There is a small Black Carib community of about 400. The European ancestry of the inhabitants is both French and British. Although English is the official tongue and is generally understood, a French patois is the leading spoken language. Most of the populace adheres to Roman Catholicism, but there are also Anglican and Methodist communities of long standing.

D. HISTORY AND GOVERNMENT [8] [52] [17]

Dominica was sighted by Columbus on Sunday *(dominica)*, November 3, 1493. Due to the hostility of its Carib Indian inhabitants, the island was not colonized by Europeans until the mid-18th century when the French began establishing coastal settlements. The island was seized by the British in 1759, recaptured by the French in 1778 and ceded to Britain once and for all by the Treaty of Paris in 1783. Since 1967 Dominica has been one of the six West Indies Associated States (see page 348).

E. AGRICULTURAL POLICIES [8] [14]

The Government of Dominica has initiated a program of subsidies to encourage farmers to increase agricultural production. The Government will provide up to 50 percent of the capital investment needed for new agricultural endeavors, especially small swine and poultry projects. Animal breeding centers have been established where stud fees are subsidized. In addition, swine and beef cattle breeding stock are available to farmers at reduced cost. Citrus growers can obtain spraying services at subsidized rates. There is an agricultural Marketing Board empowered to purchase, grade, pack, transport, store and export all agricultural commodities, but so far its activities have been limited to citrus fruit and bananas. The formation of cooperatives and credit unions for agriculture and fishing is being promoted.

F. FOREIGN AID

1. Bilateral Aid [8]

From 1945 to 1968 allocations to Dominica from the British Colonial Development Welfare funds totaled $9,857,083.

2. Multilateral Aid [41]

UNICEF and WHO have assisted the Government in establishing integrated health services throughout the island, including a system of maternal and child health centers. UNICEF has given supplies, equipment and transport; WHO has provided advisors and fellowships. In addition, UNICEF has covered ocean freight costs of skim milk powder and corn-soy-milk blend (CSM) donated for the Government's child feeding program. An average of 6,500 mothers and children are reached through maternal and child health centers and schools each year.

II. FOOD RESOURCES

A. GENERAL [18] [8]

The island's food resources come from a total land area of 75,000 hectares, 60 percent of which is owned by the British Crown. Only 23,000 hectares are under agricultural production.

B. MEANS OF PRODUCTION

1. Agricultural Labor Force [8]

The labor force was estimated at 24,249 in 1965 (13,743 males and 10,506 females). With a population increase of 2 percent a year, it may have reached 27,000 by 1971. It is believed that agriculture is the main employer with 7,000-8,000 wage earners and 5,000-6,000 self-employed farmers. Five thousand workers are employed in road-building and manufacturing and another 1,500 in transport and commerce.

2. Farms [14] [8] [52]

There are about 9,000 farms, most of them freehold, covering 17,000 hectares of cropland and 2,000 hectares of pasture. In addition, some 200 estates make up another 4,000 hectares. There is some subsistence agriculture in Dominica. The island is larger than the others in the Lesser Antilles chain, hence land is relatively abundant and this allows some farmers to practice shifting cultivation, as in Africa. The difficulties of communication have caused the population to congregate in 10 or 12 villages on the west coast. The two main cities of Roseau and Portsmouth are not linked together by any direct road, and although separated by about only 35 kilometers, it takes six or seven times longer than it should to drive from one to the other.

3. Fertilizers and Mechanical Equipment [18]

No information is available on the utilization of fertilizers in Dominica. In 1968 it was reported that 84 tractors were in use on the island.

C. PRODUCTION

1. Crops [18] [14] [52] [8]

Such food crops as do exist consist mainly of sweet potatoes, yams, some corn, vegetables and fruit. Most of the fruit is exported but some is consumed locally. Unlike most other islands of the West Indies, Dominica does not have soil suited to sugar cultivation. Bananas are the primary cash crop and are cultivated on 6,000 hectares. Cocoa is cultivated on a small scale (2,400 hectares) by individual smallholders. Limes and other citrus fruits are grown on 720 hectares and coconuts on 4,000 hectares (often mixed with bananas on plantations).

2. Animal Husbandry [18] [8]

There is a herd of 3,000 head of cattle and the Government is encouraging its maintenance and development through provision of studs and subsidies. There are 7,000 pigs, 5,000 goats and 3,000 sheep. One thousand tons of milk are produced annually, most of it consumed locally.

D. FOOD INDUSTRIES [8] [4]

The food industries of Dominica consist mainly of fruit and vegetable canning factories, poultry meat processing plants, lime juice extraction plants and vanilla processing firms. Since 1966 a local company, assisted by FAO, has been processing fats and oils from copra.

E. TRADE [14]

The island relies to a considerable extent on food imports, which consist primarily of meat and meat products, flour, cereals, animal feed, frozen poultry, pulses, dairy products, eggs, fruits, vegetables, sugar, tea, coffee, oilseeds, nuts and vegetable fats. Exports are limited to the products shown in the following table. The table shows that meats, cereals and dairy products represent more than 52 percent of all agricultural imports.

Exports and Imports of Agricultural Products
Dominica, 1969
(in $1,000)

Exports	Value	Imports	Value
Oranges	22	Live animals	6
Other citrus	208	Meat and meat products	696
Bananas	5,112	Dairy and eggs	548
Mangoes	15	Cereals and prepared foods	662
Lime juice	382	Fruit and vegetables	283
Cocoa beans	116	Sugar and preparations	462
Vanilla beans	*	Coffee, tea, cocoa, spices	78
Coconut oil	209	Animal feeds	136
Copra	30	Miscellaneous foods	215
Other	59	Beverages	459
		Oilseeds	6
		Cotton	2
		Oils and fats	57
		Miscellaneous	50
Total Agricultural Exports	6,153	Total Agricultural Imports	3,660
Total Exports	6,995	Total Imports	12,356
Agricultural as % of Total	88	Agriculture as % of Total	30

*Less than $500.

Source: W.F. Buck, *Agriculture and Trade of the Caribbean Region.*

III. DIETS

Quantitative information is not available on diets in Dominica which makes it impossible to assert that the fare is deficient; but judging from islands similarly situated, there can be little doubt that Dominica offers the same kind of deficiency picture observed in St. Kitts-Nevis-Anguilla and St. Lucia. This is confirmed by government health statistics for 1970 which list the most prevalent diseases as "gastroenteritis" and "deficiency diseases."

IV. CONCLUSIONS

Dominica's commercial balance is highly unfavorable. Her exports equal only 32.7 percent of her imports, hence a new source of revenue has to be found if the island is to be placed on a sound economic footing and if British and United Nations assistance is ever to be phased out. At the present time, only tourism is a possible alternative to international dependence.

THE WINDWARD ISLANDS: ST. LUCIA

I. BACKGROUND INFORMATION

A. PHYSICAL SETTING [4] [52] [11]

St. Lucia lies just 25 nautical miles south of Martinique and 20 nautical miles north of St. Vincent, covering 616 square kilometers (see map on page 422). It is an uneven, mountainous volcanic island with peaks rising to 1,050 meters (Mt. Gimie), including an active volcano (Mt. Soufrière). The landscape is cut by deep valleys.

B. CLIMATE [4] [52] [11]

A dry season lasts from January to April and a rainy season from May to August with further rains at the end of the year. Average annual rainfall varies with altitude from 1,500 to over 3,500 millimeters (see map on page 422). The mean annual temperature is 27°C, tempered by the almost constant northeast trade winds.

C. POPULATION [40] [4] [11] [23]

The island's estimated population in 1971 was 123,000 with an annual growth rate of 2.7 percent and a density of 179 per square kilometer. The infant mortality rate is 42.4 per 1,000 live births and life expectancy for men is 55 years, for women 58 years. The population is 60 percent rural. The largest town is Castries, the capital, with 40,000 inhabitants. The relatively large urban population is one factor necessitating a large volume of food imports.

The average monthly income for an urban family is $44, of which 61 percent is spent on food. This is a very high percentage, considering the relative prosperity of the island, but a good indication of the dependence on imported foods.

393

Most of the population is of African or mixed origin, descended from slaves imported to the island in the 17th and 18th centuries. English is the official language, but a French patois is spoken in the countryside. Roman Catholicism is the primary religion, although there are also Anglican and Methodist followings.

D. HISTORY AND GOVERNMENT [11] [36]

St. Lucia is said to have been discovered by Columbus on St. Lucia's Day in 1502, hence its name. The first known attmept to settle the island was made by a group of Englishmen in 1605, but they were driven out by the Carib Indian inhabitants. Another unsuccessful attempt was made from 1638 to 1640. France claimed the island in 1642 and French colonists were finally able to come to terms with the Caribs in 1660. For the next century and a half the island was fought over by Britain and France because of its strategic location, and it changed hands no less than 14 times. It was finally ceded to Great Britain by the Treaty of Paris in 1814. Since 1965 St. Lucia has been one of the West Indies Associated States (see page 348).

E. AGRICULTURAL POLICIES [14]

The Government's agricultural policy aims primarily at increasing the production of food crops for domestic consumption and arresting erosion. To these ends, agricultural credit has been made available and market infrastructure is being developed. An Agricultural Marketing Board has been created to regulate imports and exports, prices, production, processing, grading and transportation. Coconut palm production is being encouraged by providing farmers with seedlings at a subsidized price. Diversification is officially encouraged but difficult to implement because of the banana crop's profitability.

The Agriculture Department operates an experimental station outside Castries and another near Vieux Fort. These stations are concerned with developing ways to increase the production of local crops, demonstrating the use of improved farming methods, selling seedlings (cocoa, coconut, mango, citrus and tomato plants) to farmers for a nominal price, and providing artificial insemination and stud services to livestock raisers.

F. FOREIGN AID

1. Bilateral Aid [11] [4]

St. Lucia receives assistance from Great Britain's Colonial Development and Welfare funds. From 1965 to 1968 this assistance totaled $1,980,000 and from 1968 to 1970 a further $1,320,000 were allocated. The island also receives aid from Canada and the United States.

2. Multilateral Aid [41]

United Nations assistance to St. Lucia has included aid for the Government's integrated health services project and for teacher training. UNICEF has furnished equipment, supplies and transport and WHO workshops and fellowships for the health services program which is aimed at providing better maternal and child care (including nutrition education), communicable disease control, health education, medical and dental care, laboratory services and environmental sanitation. UNICEF has provided teaching and demonstration materials, a bus, and trainee stipends for the Government's teacher training program while UNESCO has provided consultants.

II. FOOD RESOURCES

A. GENERAL [14]

Because of its French heritage, the land tenure in St. Lucia is somewhat different from that in other former British colonies. The land is more fragmented and the holdings are smaller. The total farmland is estimated at 35,000 hectares, representing less than 33 percent of the area. About 21,000 hectares are considered suitable for crops and 3,000 for stock-raising.

B. MEANS OF PRODUCTION

1. Agricultural Labor Force [26]

In 1960 the labor force was estimated at 31,372 and may by now have reached 40,000. Reportedly, 51.7 percent of this force consists of salary earners, 35.4 percent are employers or self-employed individuals, 3.9 percent are unpaid family workers and 9.0 percent cannot be placed in any category.

2. Farms [14]

There are about 13,000 farms on St. Lucia averaging less than 2 hectares each. Over three-fourths of all farms are smaller than 2.5 hectares. Mutliple ownership, a serious handicap to agricultural development, is a frequent occurrence.

3. Fertilizers and Mechanical Equipment [18]

Four hundred tons of nitrogenous fertilizer, an equal amount of phosphatic type, and 600 tons of potassic fertilizer are spread on large farms and estates every year. About 46 tractors are in use on the island.

C. PRODUCTION

1. Crops [18] [23]

Except for bananas, other fresh fruits and edible oil, the food crops, including commercial production of 2,000 tons of corn, are not sufficient to feed the populace. Sweet potatoes and yams are produced at the rate of 1,000 tons per year.

For a long time the most important cash crop was the banana. This preeminence has recently been threatened by adverse weather conditions which have prevented St. Lucia from meeting her banana quota for the United Kingdom. This, in turn, has led the U.K. to grant a quota to "dollar area" banana producers. At 51,034 tons, the 1970 crop on St. Lucia was the lowest in 7 years. Efforts to diversify are being made. Copra is the second largest export crop yielding 2,760 tons and 1,500 hectoliters of oil. Other cash crops include spices and honey. Vegetables and fruits are sold to neighboring islands when there is a surplus.

2. Animal Husbandry [18] [23]

The total cattle herd of 12,000 head is twice the size it was 20 years ago. Still, this is not enough to meet local demand. There are also 19,000 pigs, 8,000 sheep and 5,000 goats, all contributing to the local meat supply, but not in adequate amounts. In 1962 there were two dairies providing milk to the town of Castries. Individual small producers peddle their milk and ladle it out on demand. Two thousand tons of milk are available every year from the area near Vieux Fort where communal pastures are supported by the Government. Eggs are supplied by individual farmers and by two estates which have substantial aviaries. These estates provide broilers as well as eggs to the urban market. Green sea turtles are caught on the island 180 nautical miles away, then brought to St. Lucia and held in a pond for slaughtering. Only one or two turtles are slaughtered each day, but they provide a fairly steady supply of meat for the local market. Turtle eggs are also sold locally.

3. Fisheries [23]

Fish production is expanding. Every coastal village has a small fleet of fishing vessels, mainly 15-18-foot open boats powered by sail, oars or outboard motors. Most of the catch is eaten locally but some is exported. Saint Lucia maintains a fisheries school where 12-15 students are trained each year, using prototype fishing boats which the Government is promoting. The catch of fish is likely to increase as the Government encourages the industry. Some Tilapia for fish ponds are being raised on an experimental basis.

D. FOOD INDUSTRIES [23]

A number of food industries are developing: coconut oil extraction, carbonated beverage production, ice cream manufacturing (one plant), lime juice extraction (12 small factories), sugar refining (one factory) and turtle meat processing (one plant). Although the turtle meat and eggs are sold on the local market, the gelatinous material lining the carapace is removed, processed and exported to Europe for making turtle soup. Each large town has a livestock slaughterhouse. There are two or three dairies supplying small quantities of milk to urban customers.

E. TRADE

1. Domestic Trade [23] [11]

The Government provides large marketplaces in all towns where fruit, vegetables, meat and fish are delivered via a circular road connecting all the major settlements. Buses transport both goods and people and are commandeered by the banana growers when a banana boat is expected. In smaller communities, local general stores provide the people with food staples grown locally or imported.

2. Foreign Trade [11] [4]

The trade balance is constantly negative with a yearly deficit of $10 million which is covered by tourist income, remittances from expatriates and aid from the United Kingdom. The leading imports are fertilizers, flour, cereals (including rice and cornmeal), meat and meat preparations, livestock feed, eggs, milk and milk products, and fish in the form of salted cod, dried fish, or smoked and pickled eel.

III. DIETS

A. GENERAL [23]

A 1961 nutrition survey of several West Indies islands* made by the U.S. Interdepartmental Committee on Nutrition for National Defense (ICNND) covered 99 families (638 individuals on St. Lucia). The results give a fairly accurate idea of the nutritional situation on the island at that time. There is no reason to believe that the relatively favorable picture this survey revealed has changed. On the whole, the diets were found to be good—much better than in most other

---

*Trinidad and Tobago, St. Lucia, St. Christopher, Nevis and Anguilla.

small islands of the area. Local surveys were made in Castries, Choiseul and Dennery (all sizable towns), Gros Islets, Canaries and Anse la Raye (all semirural). The findings shown in the following table are slightly optimistic because the samples tended to lean toward the better-off people. As usual, the worst-fed do not show up in proportion to their social importance.

Average Per Capita Daily Food Consumption – St. Lucia, 1961
(in grams)

	Castries	Gros Islets	Anse La Raye	Canaries	Dennery	Choiseul
Average Monthly Family Income	$58	$48	$22	$38	$74	$26
Food Item						
Cereals	191	130	137	89	281	118
Dried legumes	17	4	4	2	9	3
Greens	23	19	4	5	24	7
Other vegetables	22	36	13	16	29	14
Tubers	40	–	2	–	–	8
Mangoes	180	640	320	240	460	260
Breadfruit	214	1,230	900	1,140	940	1,368
Other fruits	80	77	247	342	469	134
Fish	70	150	80	62	117	121
Meat	100	17	8	6	21	2
Milk and products	151	134	21	58	180	43
Eggs	16	3	–	–	5	2
Fats	24	32	25	19	26	10
Sugar	41	34	35	27	31	21
Miscellaneous	3	3	2	2	3	2

Source: Interdepartmental Committee on Nutrition for National Defense, *West Indies Nutrition Survey.*

Fish was the most important source of animal protein at all locations except Castries, where imported meat was within the means of many families with incomes above the city average of $58 per month. At Castries, the consumption of meat balanced the relatively lower consumption of fish. At Choiseul, Anse La Raye and Canaries, the consumption of meat was practically nil, but was compensated by a relatively good intake of fish. Gros Islets had very modest meat consumption but, being a fishing town, enjoyed the highest level of fish intake. At Dennery the consumption of fish was relatively high, but that of meat only modest. Anse La Raye, the poorest of all locations with an income of only $22 per family per month, not only had poor consumption of meat, but of milk and eggs as well. The basis of the diet in that community was cereals and breadfruit, a mediocre combination. At Choiseul, the consumption of breadfruit was enormous. Breadfruit must have a filling effect which limits the ingestion of most of the valuable foods, such as legumes, greens, milk, meat and eggs.

Dennery is the banana center of the island and the levels of income, education and nutrition are better than elsewhere. Milk and cereals are consumed in higher quantities than in any other location.

Two aspects of the St. Lucia diet are remarkable: the large consumption of mangoes and other fruit, providing generous supplies of vitamin A; and the quantities of breadfruit *(Artocarpus altilis)* eaten, which is unfortunate because this dietary staple is a very poor food, providing only 81 calories and 1.3 grams of protein per 100 grams of edible portion.

B. LEVELS OF NUTRITION [23]

At 2,253 calories, the average St. Lucian daily caloric intake was generally adequate for the places surveyed, yet, as shown on the following table, the families seen at Canaries were eating only 1,854 calories per capita per day, which is slightly under par. Little meat was eaten there and the family income was even lower than it seemed because the households are large.

Per Capita Daily Nutrient Intake – St. Lucia, 1961

Nutrient	Castries	Gros Islets	Dennery	Canaries	Anse La Raye	Choiseul
Calories	2,287	2,582	2,570	1,854	2,187	2,040
Proteins (g)	82	85	86	40	64	61
Percent of animal protein	59	63	23	42	53	57
Carbohydrates (g)	321	460	487	345	369	331
Fats (g)	74	56	59	35	43	21
Calcium (mg)	431	560	553	590	405	431
Iron (mg)	7.7	17.0	16.0	15.6	15.1	12.4
Vitamin A (IU)	4,740	10,000	8,790	11,070	4,320	6,050
Thiamine (mg)	.96	1.4	1.4	1.0	1.0	.96
Riboflavin (mg)	1.4	.96	1.05	.92	.66	1.14
Niacin (mg)	10.6	13.2	18.7	12.3	12.1	13.4
Ascorbic acid (mg)	47	223	186	124	136	250

Source: Interdepartmental Committee on Nutrition for National Defense, *West Indies Nutrition Survey.*

Protein consumption was good in all locations except Canaries, where the intake represented only 84 percent of the requirement. At Dennery the protein intake was good, but the proportion of animal protein was not quite high enough. While protein nutrition was, in general, adequate for adult males, no child among those surveyed met the recommended allowance for his age, sex and weight. Thirty-five percent of the 2-year-olds and 58 percent of the 3-year-olds were consuming less than 50 percent of the recommended protein allowance. Riboflavin intakes were considered to be low everywhere except at Castries where riboflavin was adequate.

All the communities surveyed showed an encouraging use of mangoes and other fruit, which is rather unusual since many people is semideveloped areas have a tendency to forego this convenient resource and like to spend their scarce money on commercial products low in nutrient values. The result of the high consumption of mangoes was that vitamin A and vitamin C intakes were equal to requirements at all locations. The mean carotene levels, however, which were expected to be uniformly high, given the amount of vitamin A apparently consumed, were disappointing. While 42 micrograms of carotene per 100 milliliters of plasma is considered normal in children, 2.1 percent of those surveyed had values below 10 micrograms per 100 milliliters and 37 percent had values below 19 micrograms per 100 milliliters. Vitamin C nutrition was generally good in St. Lucia, rising above 1 milligram per 100 milliliters for all children under 15 years tested. The ICNND investigators found the excretion values of riboflavin on St. Lucia to be the highest among all the islands surveyed; yet analysis of the data seemed to indicate that about 50 percent of each age group was in the "low" category, which was consistent with the findings of consumption of this nutrient. Thiamine excretion was also higher than on the other islands. From these and other data, the conclusion seems to be that St. Lucia is probably one of the better-fed Caribbean islands, although a number of subproblems remain, as shown by the clinical symptoms of nutritional diseases.

IV. NUTRITIONAL DISEASE PATTERNS [23] [29]

The ICNND investigators conducted a clinical and biochemical as well as a dietary survey in 1961. Given the relatively good diet outlined in the previous section, one would not anticipate many incidences of symptoms suggesting nutritional deficiencies. However, findings of the clinical survey were to some extent less favorable than what could have been expected. Many signs of riboflavin deficiency were observed which, of course, reflected the shortage of this vitamin reported in the dietary investigation. In addition, there was a high prevalence of enlarged thyroids, indicative of iodine deficiency which had not been revealed by the dietary survey. Some evidence of other shortages was also noticeable, as shown in the table opposite. The clinical survey also revealed a high prevalence of parasitic diseases, streptococcal infections and respiratory diseases which usually either are correlated with, or are the consequence of, malnutrition.

Dental disease is very common. Sixty-six percent of the people examined in Saint Lucia revealed at least poor oral hygiene, probably coming atop nutritional deficiencies.

Anemia is highly prevalent in St. Lucia. Particularly low hemoglobin levels

Percent Prevalence of Clinical Signs of Nutritional Deficiencies
St. Lucia, 1961
(males and nonpregnant, nonlactating females)

Symptom	Deficiency Presumed to Cause Symptom	Percent Prevalence
Nasolabial seborrhea	Riboflavin	9.2
Angular lesions of the lips	Riboflavin	3.8
Angular scars of the lips	Riboflavin	4.4
Swelling of the gums	Ascorbic acid	1.0
Papillary atrophy of tongue	Riboflavin and/or niacin	13.0
Enlarged thyroid	Iodine	13.0
Follicular hyperkeratosis	Vitamin A and/or vitamin C	1.0
Bilateral edema	Thiamine	1.0
Loss of ankle jerk	Thiamine	1.5
Depigmentation of hair	Protein	6.6
Other		13.0

Source: Interdepartmental Committee on Nutrition for National Defense, *West Indies Nutrition Survey.*

were encountered among children: 85.7 percent of all male children and 75 percent of all females between 2 and 4 years had values inferior to 12 grams of hemoglobin per 100 milliliters of plasma. In addition, 39.1 percent of women aged 15-44 had levels below 12 grams and only 8.7 percent showed hemoglobin values between 14 and 14.9 grams per 100 milliliters.

In 1962 Lees reported that 189 cases of infant malnutrition were identified from January to October. Most cases were in the 10-15 month age range and 163 children were between 4 and 24 months of age. Distribution of dried milk was initiated in December 1962, contributing to a decline in deaths from malnutrition to 115 for the year 1963, compared to 200 in 1962. In 1966 the same investigator reported the results of a survey conducted to discover if social and economic factors were responsible for the persistence of the few residual cases of infant death due to malnutrition. Forty-two families were investigated, both in urban and rural areas, all of whom belonged to the lowest social group. Lees found that income did not play as important a role as could have been expected. Although 88 percent of the children lived with their mothers, 70 percent of the mothers worked outside the home and left their children in the care of some other person. Hence lack of education, ignorance and indifference were probably the reasons that these families still suffered from some level of undernutrition.

V. CONCLUSIONS

Like many other islands of the Caribbean, St. Lucia relies on attracting tourists to meet its deficits and to pay for the imports of food essential to the population's survival. It can only be hoped that the Government's enlightened efforts towards increasing food production will succeed soon enough to ward off the dangers inherent in an economy which is overdependent upon uncontrollable factors such as foreign aid, remittances from abroad and tourism.

THE WINDWARD ISLANDS: ST. VINCENT

I. BACKGROUND INFORMATION

A. PHYSICAL SETTING [52] [12]

The island of St. Vincent lies about 100 nautical miles west of Barbados and 21 nautical miles south of St. Lucia (see map on page 00). It covers 344 square kilometers, extending 29 kilometers from north to south and 18 kilometers from east to west at its broadest point. St. Vincent is of volcanic origin with a mountain ridge running like a north-south dorsal spine. The highest point is at the now dormant volcano Soufrière which in 1902 erupted violently, killing 2,000 people. The crater is located in the north and rises to 1,234 meters. The eastern slope of the mountain range is rugged and deeply dissected, but the western slope is gently rolling. Each side is typified by a number of valleys formed by transverse spurs. Level land is scarce but the northeastern region between Soufrière and the sea is a relatively flat area called "Carib country." Many small streams water the island. Farming is the major occupation with bananas, some sugarcane, coconuts, arrowroot and Sea Island cotton as the major crops.

B. CLIMATE [52] [12]

A dry season occurs from January to May when the climate is mild and northeast trade winds prevail. Throughout the rest of the year, daytime temperatures rise as high as 32°C but the nights remain cool. Average annual rainfall varies from 1,500-2,000 millimeters along the coast to 2,500-3,700 millimeters in the mountains (see map on page 422).

C. POPULATION [12] [40] [52]

In 1970 the population of St. Vincent totaled 89,125 inhabitants, more than half of whom were under 15 years of age. There is an annual rate of increase of

2.0 percent. Overall density is about 245 persons per square kilometer, but actual densities in settled areas are higher due to the fact that much of the island is mountainous and sparsely inhabited. The infant mortality rate is high at about 73.7 per 1,000 live births and life expectancy is only 58.5 years for men and 59.7 years for women. The largest town is Kingstown, the capital (23,482).

The inhabitants of St. Vincent are mostly of African and mixed descent although there are small numbers of Asians, Europeans and Caribs. English is the only language spoken on the island and Christianity is the dominant religion with Methodists, Anglicans and Roman Catholics in the majority.

D. HISTORY AND GOVERNMENT [52] [12] [36]

The island was discovered by Columbus in 1498 on St. Vincent's Day, hence its name. The fierce Carib Indians who inhabited it successfully repulsed all would-be settlers, but nevertheless, the island's possession was a bone of contention between Britain and France until the Treaty of Versailles in 1783 when St. Vincent became an undisputed British colony.

Negro settlers first came to the island in the 17th century when a slave ship was shipwrecked off the coast. The blacks were received hospitably by the same Carib Indians who so furiously fought against any European invasion. Intermarriage began and soon the resulting "Black Caribs" outnumbered the original inhabitants.

The British successfully pacified the island in 1796 and began to settle. In 1846 Portuguese immigrants who came to work on the plantations added to the racial mixture and in 1861 East Indians were brought in as indentured laborers. Although most of the latter eventually returned to India, some remained behind to form the core of a small Asian community which has persisted until the present.

In 1969 St. Vincent became one of the West Indies Associated States with administrative machinery similar to that described for St. Christopher-Nevis-Anguilla (see page 348).

E. AGRICULTURAL POLICIES [14]

The Government's agricultural policy is aimed at stimulating production of domestic foodstuffs and eliminating trade deficits. A law passed early in this century made it compulsory to grow food crops on a certain percentage of the land awarded under a land settlement scheme. The Government provides extension services, agricultural credit and research, and through its Marketing Board guarantees purchase of agricultural products of acceptable quality. The Government also sponsors a soil erosion control program. There is a Banana Growers Association which furnishes credit for the purchase of insecticides, plants and fertilizers and which encourages better cultivation methods. The St. Vincent

Arrowroot Association is a statutory body providing marketing services for its members.

F. FOREIGN AID

1. Bilateral Aid [12]

As of 1968, Great Britain had committed $7.2 million for social and economic development programs in St. Vincent, mainly in the form of grants from the Colonial Development and Welfare funds. Under the 1966-1970 Development Plan for the island, a capital expenditure of $20.6 million was planned for light industry, crop diversification and tourism.

2. Multilateral Aid [41]

United Nations agencies have assisted the Government of St. Vincent with its health services and child feeding programs. UNICEF has provided supplies and equipment and transport and WHO the services of consultants as well as fellowships. Under the program, integrated health services are being established in order to strengthen communicable disease control, health and nutrition education, environmental health, dental and medical care and laboratory services. A network of five health centers and 24 subcenters is being organized to serve the island.

UNICEF is covering freight costs for skim milk powder and corn-soy-milk blend (CSM) donated to the Government's child feeding program. About 5,000 mothers and preschool children and an equal number of schoolchildren receive free rations under this program.

II. FOOD RESOURCES

A. GENERAL [18] [52]

It is difficult to assess the basis for the food resources of the island of St. Vincent because the surface sown is not accurately known. Interspersed sowing, double cropping and unrecorded growing of some crops add to the difficulty. This uncertainty regarding the amount of arable land in use is not, of course, peculiar to the island of St. Vincent; it is a problem in many other parts of the world. It has been said that most estimates of land used for crops in developing countries are understated by 25 percent. Be that as it may, the total land area of St. Vincent is certainly 344 square kilometers. Arable land is officially reckoned to be 18,000 hectares, and prairies and pastures 1,000 hectares. The soil, which in places is highly fertile, has been ruined by erosion in certain areas due to the fact that more than half of the land is on slopes of 30 degrees or more.

B. MEANS OF PRODUCTION

1. Agricultural Labor Force [12] [4]

The labor force numbered 24,856 in 1960 and must have reached 30,000 by 1970. Two-thirds of the force is employed in agriculture, with about 4,000 individuals engaged in commerce in urban areas, 3,000 in industry and the rest in manufacturing. There is considerable seasonal unemployment.

2. Farms [14] [52]

There are about 12,000 farm units of various sizes on St. Vincent, two-thirds of which are very small, not exceeding 2 hectares. There are approximately 30 large estates exceeding 2100 hectares each.

3. Fertilizers and Mechanical Equipment [18]

Five hundred tons each of nitrogenous and potassic fertilizers are used annually by the commercial farm enterprises of St. Vincent. Fewer than 100 tractors are recorded as being in use on the island.

C. PRODUCTION

1. Food Crops [18] [14] [52] [16]

Food crops (whose production is compulsory) are limited to sweet potatoes, yams, manioc, groundnuts, corn (of which 8,000 tons are produced) and vegetables. According to a nutrition survey made in 1967 by the Caribbean Food and Nutrition Institute (CFNI), 78 percent of the families interviewed had gardens where they grew some food. Forty-one percent grew legumes, 43 percent kept chickens, 32 percent had pigs, 1.3 percent raised cattle and 18 percent caught fish. Thus a significant portion of the population had at least a partial subsistence diet but most, if not all, had to enter the money economy to obtain a substantial portion of their food. Unfortunately, they had only cheap products to sell and expensive imports to buy. The table on page 408 shows what portion of the diet was imported.

2. Cash Crops [14] [18] [12] [4]

The St. Vincent Marketing Board is in charge of all exports. Cash crops consist essentially of bananas (averaging 30,000 tons a year and representing about 54 percent of the value of all exports), arrowroot (averaging 2,200 tons and representing 40 percent of total exports), cotton, coconuts, nutmeg and mace. The last two are crops with a future while cotton will probably be abandoned since it is uneconomical under present circumstances.

3. Animal Husbandry [18] [12]

There are about 10,000 head of cattle on the island, providing meat and milk for both local use and export; yet much milk is also imported. Pigs number 19,000, sheep 8,000 and goats 5,000.

4. Fisheries

Fishing is important and remains the best source of animal protein on the island.

D. AGRICULTURAL AND FOOD INDUSTRIES [12] [4]

An arrowroot factory and two cotton gins are operated by the Government. Copra and cottonseed are processed by two privately owned factories. There is a rum distillery and several carbonated beverage factories.

E. TRADE [12] [14] [19]

St. Vincent's principal export by value is the banana crop. Arrowroot is the second most important foreign exchange earner, but world demand is lessening to the point where this plant was grown on only 500 hectares in 1968. However, St. Vincent is still the world's major source of arrowroot. Coconut is next in line, followed by copra, cotton, sugar, fruits and vegetables. The total value of exports in 1967 was $3.4 million while the total value of imports, 33 percent of which were agricultural products, was $9.3 million. The food imported into St. Vincent includes meat and meat products, poultry, salted and smoked fish, dairy products, cereal, flour, fruit and vegetables, tea, coffee, sugar and sugar preparations, animal feeds, oils, vegetable fats and beverages.

F. FOOD SUPPLY [16]

The 1967 CFNI nutrition survey report gives the relationship between locally-produced and imported calories and proteins (see table on page 408). These figures are not absolute. Other foods were probably eaten which corrected to a certain extent the 25 percent shortage of calories and proteins that appears to exist. Notwithstanding the nutritional significance of these values, the economic and social significance of importing 75.6 percent of the calories and protein consumed cannot be overlooked.

III. DIETS

A. GENERAL [16] [52]

Some information is available on the diets in St. Vincent and on the social condition of the population, thanks to the CFNI survey, for which preliminary

Daily Per Capita Supply of Calories and Proteins
St. Vincent, 1966
(proteins in grams)

Food Item	Local Production		Imports		Total Available	
	Calories	Proteins	Calories	Proteins	Calories	Proteins
Cereals	5.0	0.1	660.0	17.0	665	17.1
Roots and tubers	191.0	2.8	–	–	191	2.8
Sugars	–	–	334.0	–	344	–
Pulses and seeds	20.0	1.3	7.0	0.5	27	1.8
Fresh vegetables	21.0	1.2	–	–	21	1.2
Fruits	44.0	1.0	–	–	44	1.0
Meats and products	31.9	2.0	20.1	1.3	52	3.3
Fish	15.1	3.0	17.5	3.4	33	6.4
Eggs	2.7	0.2	4.5	0.4	7	.6
Milk and products	4.4	2.1	67.0	4.8	71	6.9
Fats and oils	–	–	156.0	–	156	–
Miscellaneous	–	–	8.0	0.2	8	0.2
Total	335.1	13.7	1,274.1	27.6	1,619	41.3

Source: Caribbean Food and Nutrition Institute, *A Rapid P.C.M. Survey in St. Vincent.*

results are available. The picture emerging is very similar to that encountered in Jamaica and in Barbados where scientific surveys have also been carried out. Hence it is not stretching the point to surmise that conditions on St. Vincent are by and large representative of conditions in other small Caribbean islands where surveys have not been made.

Most people live in small houses of only one or two rooms. Cooking is done outside, next to or under the house which is often built on stilts or stone pillars. Water is usually brought from a river at a distance. The households are quite crowded: 67 percent include at least seven people, almost half of whom are dependent upon the other half for subsistence because they are too young or too old to provide for themselves. The investigators report that the most reliable source of income is the mother's earnings. The father, if present, may contribute some food for the baby, usually in the form of highly advertised manufactured preparations (usually rich in sugar but poor in nutrients), rather than the nutritious diet needed. The average expenditure for food varies between $2.10 per capita per week in rural areas to $5.30 per capita in urban settlements. In rural areas the staple is homegrown either right around the house or at some distance on a plot known as the "yam piece." Animal protein is purchased and consists of imported salted fish, some fresh fish, some beef, pork or poultry, rice and cooking oil. The housewife usually visits the village store once every other week in order to procure this food. The urban diet is better and more diversified. Food is bought every other day and includes rice, bread, butter and/or marga-rine, meat and fish. It seems that the urban household buys its food in standarized packages which include 1 or 2 pounds of rice, 1 or 2 pounds of sugar and 1 liter of cooking oil.

Two meals a day are usually taken, but there may be snacks in between, expecially for children. Breakfast consists of tea or chocolate and the main meal is a soup with rice and pieces of chicken in it or an African-style stew with fish and yams. Fruits are eaten for dessert. In addition to the main meal, children have snacks of arrowroot and sips of a variety of bush teas.

According to the CFNI investigators, the cheapest 1,000 calories available in the St. Vincent markets in November 1967 were in the form of breadfruit (3¢) or green bananas (3½¢) and the most expensive 1,000 were chicken baby food ($3.25) or strained cream peas ($2.25). The cheapest 20 grams of protein were in the form of dry skim milk (2½¢), while the most expensive were custard powder ($4.00) or arrowroot ($3.00).

The diets themselves, which are based on a variety of foods such as those listed in the table on page 408, do not seem to provide an adequate supply of energy and proteins for the average rural dweller. The CFNI investigators point out that the dairy and poultry industries are working largely for Kingstown and its suburbs, which represent only about 25 percent of the whole population. Fifty percent of the slaughtering is done at Kingstown and the meat is sold locally. The protein-rich imports of frozen or chilled meat are consumed where they are landed, at Kingstown. About 90 tons of nonfat dry milk are imported every year, half through commercial channels, and half through the World Food Program (donations). This, of course, should be reserved for children, but probably is not. The home-raised meat resources listed in the table on page 408 are almost always sold for cash by the livestock owners and hence do not contribute much to the protein rations of these families.

No data have yet been published regarding vitamin and mineral intakes. The consumption of fruit may supply some, but probably not all, of these requirements. Thus the general diet of the adult population is inadequate and as long as it relies on imported foods will probably remain so.

B. SPECIAL DIETS [16]

Infants are usually breast-fed until the age of 9 months. The CFNI investigators found that 33 percent of all infants are off the breast at 6 months and 75 percent at 12 months. The two most common reasons given for weaning (in about the same number of answers) are that the mother is working or that the mother is pregnant again. These are followed by a variety of other reasons, among which illness of the mother is the most common. Supplemental foods are sometimes given as early as 1 month of age. twenty-three percent of these supplements consist of fresh cow's milk, 12 percent of whole dried milk and a variety of other popular imported preparations, 53 percent of dried skim milk and 12 percent of cereal foods, CSM and other products. Peas and beans are used as supplementary foods by 52 percent of the mothers.

After weaning, the children's feeding patterns consist of a portion of whatever is cooked for the family, bush tea with or without milk, snacks of biscuits or bread and porridge based on arrowroot. This diet contains little or no protein except when milk is included, but a worse feature is the reduction of feedings to one or two meals a day which, given the small capacity of the child's stomach, does not allow him to take what he needs for the day at one time. The investigators list as follows the faults of children's diets in St. Vincent: early weaning; excessively diluted and contaminated bottle feeding; early introduction of unwisely chosen supplements; lack of recognition of the special needs of the child; attitudes which prevent a better choice of inexpensive, more nutritious foods; and detrimental meal patterns. These shortcomings are most certainly those of all the islands in the Lesser Antilles.

IV. NUTRITIONAL DISEASE PATTERNS [16]

Obviously, the dietary limitations of the St. Vincent population result in a considerable number of pathological conditions. The CFNI investigators have so far used anthropometric measurements to assess the damage done to child development by the defective diets consumed. Ample evidence of malnutrition has been collected based on weight levels which undoubtedly has application beyond the island of St. Vincent. The following table gives the prevalence of protein-calorie malnutrition among St. Vincent infants and children from 0 to 59 months of age.

Malnutrition Among 2,490 Children of Both Sexes
St. Vincent, 1967

Age (months)	Moderately Severe PCM[a] (percent)	Very Severe PCM[b] (percent)
0–11	21.5	2.5
12–23	31.5	2.0
24–35	23.3	1.2
36–47	24.1	0.6
48–59	28.5	0.5
0–59	25.7	1.5

[a]Weight 61–80 percent of standard.
[b]Weight below 60 percent of standard.
Source: Caribbean Food and Nutrition Institute, *A Rapid P.C.M. Survey in St. Vincent.*

Seventy-six percent of these cases were between 0 and 36 months of age. Marasmus was found to be more common than kwashiorkor (present in 84 percent versus 16 percent of the children examined). These findings undoubtedly could be duplicated in other islands of the area.

The evidence provided by anthropometry, mortality statistics and hospital admissions indicates that protein-calorie malnutrition is common in early childhood, especially in the latter part of infancy and in the second year of life. This is usually moderately severe, although very severe cases are not rare. The PCM seen is mostly of marasmic form, hence more related to calorie deficiency than to protein lack.

V. CONCLUSIONS

The problem for St. Vincent is no different from that for other Caribbean islands. A situation where food imports are essential to survival is acceptable whenever an internationally salable resource exists, such as oil, copper or any other desired commodity. When no such marketable asset exists, future health is, to say the least, vulnerable. St. Vincent is in the same predicament as other islands of the Caribbean whose futures depend on mutual assistance and regional commercial association.

THE WINDWARD ISLANDS: GRENADA

I. BACKGROUND INFORMATION

A. PHYSICAL SETTING [9] [52] [17]

Grenada is the smallest and most southerly of the Windward Islands, lying about 90 nautical miles north of Trinidad and 68 nautical miles southwest of St. Vincent (see map on page 422). Between Grenada and St. Vincent are the Grenadines, a group of islets, some of which belong to St. Vincent, some to Grenada. Carriacou (33 square kilometers) is the largest of the latter. Grenada is about 33 kilometers long and 19 kilometers wide at its broadest point, encompassing 344 square kilometers. The landscape is characterized by volcanic mountains, steep-sided valleys, thick forests and short, swift streams, all encircled by fine, sandy beaches. The mountains run down the center of the island with peaks rising to 820 meters (Fedon's Camp) and 900 meters (Mt. St. Catherine). Agriculture is the island's basic activity although tourism is gaining importance in the economy. Cocoa, bananas, nutmeg, cotton, sugar and food crops are produced.

B. CLIMATE [9] [52]

Grenada experiences a definite dry season from January to May during which the climate is mild, largely due to the prevelance of northeast trade winds. At that time of year, night temperatures fall as low as 18°C while during the rest of the year temperatures may rise to 32°C with little variation between night and day. Humidity is high and rainfall varies from an average of 1,500 millimeters along the coast to upwards of 3,000 millimeters in the mountains (see map on page 422).

413

C. POPULATION [40] [36] [9] [52]

In 1970 the estimated population of Grenada was 97,000, including 6,000 inhabitants of Carriacou. The rate of natural increase is about 2.9 percent per year. The infant mortality rate is 34.1 per 1,000 live births and life expectancy at birth is 60 years for males and 65.6 years for females. The island is densely populated with 305 people per square kilometre. Due to the mountainous interior, the density in areas of settlement is even greater than the overall figure indicates. The population is mostly rural. The largest town is the capital city and principal port, St. George's (8,644 inhabitants).

The inhabitants of Grenada are mostly of African and mixed origin, the descendants of slaves brought to the island in the 18th century. There are some Carib Indians whose ancestors survived the massacres of the 17th century, and some Europeans who are either descendants of early settlers or more recent immigrants. Most of the population is Roman Catholic but a sizable minority adheres to Anglicanism. English is the universal language but a French patois is still spoken among older people of some villages.

D. HISTORY AND GOVERNMENT [9] [36] [52]

Grenada was discovered by Columbus in 1498 but no attempt was made at colonization until 1609 when the British tried to establish a settlement and were repelled by the Carib inhabitants. In 1650 the French purchased the island from the Carib chieftain but the Indians soon wanted their birthright back and bloody hostilities ensued which led to the decimation of the Carib population. For the next century, the French and the British fought over the island and it was finally ceded to Great Britain by the Treaty of Versailles in 1783.

Since 1966 Grenada has been one of the six West Indies Associated States with complete control over its internal affairs. Administration of the island follows the pattern described for St. Christopher-Nevis-Anguilla (see page 348). Grenada is divided into the municipal borough of St. George's and five districts. There is a local authority for Carriacou.

E. AGRICULTURAL POLICIES [14] [9]

The Government of Grenada's first 5-year development plan covered the period 1967-1971 and involved a budget of $22.8 million, 35 percent of which was devoted to modernizing agriculture. Farmers are being encouraged to make greater use of fertilizer, insecticides and improved planting stock and to adopt modern cultural techniques. Agricultural marketing and credit facilities are being established. The Government furnishes cocoa growers with seedlings at subsidized prices and reimburses farmers for 50 percent of the cost of erosion control projects. Two marketing depots are operated by the Grenada Farmers Cooperative Council with assistance from the Government which provides the physical facilities and pays the manager's salary.

F. FOREIGN AID

1. Bilateral Aid [9]

The British Government, through its Colonial Development and Welfare funds, has allocated over $4.2 million in grants and loans to Grenada. The Government of Canada has provided a team of teacher-training advisors.

2. Multilateral Aid [41]

United Nations agencies have provided assistance to the Government's health services program, its child feeding program and a teacher-training project. Under the health services program, an integrated health service is being set up, including maternal and child health, communicable disease control, health statistics, health education, laboratory services and medical care. UNICEF provides equipment and transport, WHO technical advice and fellowships. Through the child feeding program, which began in 1954, approximately 5,000 mothers and preschool children and 5,000 schoolchildren are being reached. Skim milk powder or corn-soy-milk blend (CSM) are supplied by UNICEF while the Government provides cocoa, sugar, yeast and cookies. Under the teacher training program UNICEF makes available supplies, equipment and training grants.

II. FOOD RESOURCES

A. GENERAL [18] [52] [14]

As on most small Caribbean islands, the food resources of Grenada are either grown on uneconomic holdings or imported. The land area of Grenada is 34,000 hectares (344 square kilometers) of which 31,000 are on Grenada and 3,000 on Carriacou. Only half of this land is arable and capable of supporting permanent crops. One thousand hectares are devoted to grazing.

B. MEANS OF PRODUCTION

1. Agricultural Labor Force [9] [14]

The labor force was estimated at 27,314 people in 1960 and must be nearing 30,000 now. Half of the force is employed in agriculture, some as employers or self-employed, some as wage earners or unpaid family workers.

2. Farms [14]

The number of farms is estimated at 15,000, including estates, and they occupy no more than 16,000 hectares. Estates cover about 5,100 hectares, leaving less than 10,000 hectares to be shared by smallholders owning between 1/2 and 1 hectare each.

C. PRODUCTION

1. Crops [18] [14] [9]

As indicated above, the Government is actively engaged in improving agriculture, both to increase the development of cash crops and to stimulate food crops. The latter are the same as in other islands: breadfruit, vegetables, plantains, sweet potatoes, yams and peas. The cash crops include bananas, which exceeded 23,000 tons in 1969 with 25 percent grown on estates, and nutmeg, which amounted to 2,588 tons in 1969, half of it grown on estates. The 1969 output of mace came to 201 tons, that of copra to 635 tons and that of sugar to 1,400 tons. The last two were produced only for domestic use. A small amount of cotton is grown on Carriacou. The rise of bananas as the major crop on the island was the result of the hurricane destruction of cocoa plantations in 1955. But the latter crop is scheduled to be revitalized, probably at the expense of land now planted in bananas.

2. Animal Husbandry [18]

Grenada has a small herd of cattle comprising 7,000 head. There are also 12,000 pigs, 9,000 sheep, 5,000 goats and 150,000 poultry on the island. There is no information on meat, milk and egg production.

D. TRADE [14]

Grenada, like the other Windward Islands, has to import most of its food. These imports represent 22 percent of all foreign purchases and include cereals, feed grains, meats, dairy products, and various food preparations. All imports amounted to $13.2 million in 1968 while exports brought in only $5.1 million.

III. DIETS

No specific data on food intake and nutrition are available for Grenada. The St. Vincent survey should give the reader an idea of the food pattern, which is very similar throughout the Windward Islands and is basically characterized by its high price (due to its being imported) and low vitamin and mineral content.

IV. CONCLUSIONS

The outlook for Grenada seems more favorable than in many places. There is a possibility of increasing local food production and of introducing some light industry to absorb part of the unemployment.

OVERALL CONCLUSIONS

The islands of the Caribbean region in general and those of the Lesser Antilles in particular have been confronted throughout their nearly 500 years of civilized history with similar destinies conditioned by geographical and climatic patterns and by the influence of the European great powers. Although the Lesser Antilles were discovered by Columbus, Spanish influence was never established in the area due to the fierce resistance of the original Arawak and Carib inhabitants. It was not until the 17th century, when France, Britain, and to some extent the Netherlands, began competing for possession of these islands, that the Indians were finally subdued (and even annhilated in places) and permanent European settlements established. Little of the original Indian culture remains today. The islands were important to the French and British both because of their strategic location and because of their potential as foci of sugar production.

Economically, most of the islands have always been dependent upon sugar. The first canes were brought to Hispaniola from the Canaries by Columbus on his second voyage in 1493. From Hispaniola, the cane was spread throughout the Caribbean until almost all of the islands were involved in producing sugar. Very soon this led to the famous—or infamous—triangular trade: home goods from the metropolises were sent to Africa; slaves procured with the home goods were sent to the Caribbean islands; sugar and rum produced by the slaves were sent back to the metropolises. The benefits were enormous. One-third of Great Britain's trade was dominated by sugar by the end of the 18th century. It has been said that during that century, sugar occupied the place which steel held in the 19th century and oil holds in the 20th. These were the days when Guadeloupe was deemed to be more valuable than Canada.

From the beginning, the hypnosis of sugar left little room for growing food crops and in some British islands it took the Second World War for Parliament to pass legislation requiring planters to reserve 12 percent of their land for production of food crops. The shortage of food resulted in the need for imports. In the 17th century, the salted codfish of New England was the least perishable source of animal protein that could be moved over what were then long distances in terms of time. It was and still is also the cheapest. This dependence upon food imports prevented the establishment of a food-oriented agricultural tradition or a farm way of life such as that which supported Europe and North America until the arrival of the industrial age. This situation resulted in an acceptance of high food expenditures as unavoidable which, in turn, necessitated keeping wages high enough to permit the purchase of a minimum diet, yet low enough to keep sugar competitive on the world market. Maintaining such a balance was relatively easy when all sources of sugar were in the sugarcane area, but when at the beginning of the 19th century Napoleon established the continental blockade and European farmers began producing sugar beets, the cane sugar market received a sharp blow. In more recent years the industry has suffered from oversupply and a declining price on the world market.

One of the main problems confronting the Caribbean sugar industry, in addition to hurricanes and other natural catastrophes, has always been the labor force. Three major labor crises have occurred: the first in the early 17th century when the extinction of the Indians through war and disease led the conquering governments to import African slave laborers; the second in the mid-19th century when the slaves were emancipated, requiring the plantation owners to begin paying wages; the third in the mid-20th century after independence when cane cutting ceased to be an attractive occupation because of low wages and social factors affecting the younger generation. This last crisis may be solved if machines can be developed to do the work of cane cutters, but since unemployment is already a problem on most of these islands, automation of the sugar industry is a questionable goal.

The solution to the economic and food problems of the sugar islands has not yet been found, except where some valuable natural resource has been discovered, such as bauxite in Jamaica and oil in Trinidad. Unfortunately, no such discoveries have been made in the islands covered in this chapter where the alternative to an economic fiasco seems to be development of tourism, an uncertain resource at best, but one which will have to serve until a better one can be found.

BIBLIOGRAPHY

1. Ashcroft, M.T., Buchanan, I.C., Lovell, H.G. and Welsh, D. "Growth of Infants and Preschool Children in St. Christopher-Nevis-Anguilla, West Indies." *American Journal of Clinical Nutrition,* 1966, 19, 37-45.

2. Barclay's Bank D.C.O. *Barbados—An Economic Survey.* London, Barclay's Bank, 1967.

3. _____. *The Leeward Islands—An Economic Survey.* London, Barclay's Bank, 1970.

4. _____. *The Windward Islands—An Economic Survey.* London, Barclay's Bank, 1971.

5. *Barclay's Caribbean Bulletin,* June 1971.

6. *Barclay's Overseas Review,* May 1971, 51.

7. British Information Services. "British Virgin Islands." *Fact Sheets on the Commonwealth.* London, BIS, 1966.

8. _____. "Dominica." *Fact Sheets on the Commonwealth.* New York, BIS, 1967.

9. _____. "Grenada." *Fact Sheets on the Commonwealth.* New York, BIS, 1967.

10. _____. "St. Christopher-Nevis-Anguilla." *Fact Sheets on the Commonwealth.* London, BIS, 1968.

11. _____. "Saint Lucia." *Fact Sheets on the Common-wealth.* New York, BIS, 1967.

12. _____. "St. Vincent." *Fact Sheets on the Common-wealth.* New York, BIS, 1969.

13. Brownell, W.N. "Fisheries of the Virgin Islands." *Commercial Fisheries Review.* 1971, 33 (11-12), 23-30.

14. Buck, W.F. *Agriculture and Trade of the Caribbean Region.* ERS-Foreign 309. Washington, D.C., U.S. Government Printing Office, 1971.

15. Caribbean Food and Nutrition Institute. *Barbados Nutrition Survey.* Preliminary Report. Kingston, CFNI, 1969.

16. _____. *A Rapid P.C.M. Survey in St. Vincent.* Preliminary Report. Kingston, CFNI, 1968.

17. *Encyclopedia Britannica.* Chicago, William Benton, Publisher, 1970.

18. Food and Agriculture Organization of the United Nations. *Production Yearbook 1969.* Volume 23. Rome, FAO, 1970.

19. _____. *Trade Yearbook 1969.* Volume 23. Rome, FAO, 1970.

20. *Foreign Agriculture,* 1968. VI (31), 12-13.

21. Gooding, E.G.B. "Diversification of Agriculture in Barbados." *Protein Foods for the Caribbean.* Kingston, Caribbean Food and Nutrition Institute, 1968.

21a. Haidar, W. "Basic Data on the British Leeward Islands." *Overseas Business Reports.* OBR 70-37. Washington, D.C., U.S. Government Printing Office, 1970.

21b. _____. "Basic Data on the Economy of Guadeloupe." *Overseas Business Reports.* OBR 69-50. Washington, D.C., U.S. Government Printing Office, 1969.

22. Hawkins, J. "Barbados Needing Capital Injection." *West Indies,* 1971, LXXXVI (1479), 147-150.

23. Interdepartmental Committee on Nutrition for National Defense. *The West Indies Nutrition Survey.* Washington, D.C., U.S. Government Printing Office, 1962.

24. James, P.E. *Latin America.* Fourth Edition. New York, The Odyssey Press, 1969.

25. Klaidman, S. "Indies' Sugar Blues." *The Washington Post,* July 11, 1971.

26. *Labor Developments Abroad,* 1968, 13 (9), 20.

27. _____, 1970, 15 (11), 19.

28. _____, 1971, 16 (2),

29. Lees, R.E.M. "Malnutrition: The Infant at Risk." *West Indian Medical Journal,* 1966, 15, 221-216.

30. _____. "Malnutrition: The Pattern and Prevention in St. Lucia." *West Indian Medical Journal,* 1964, 13, 97-102.

31. Leung, W-T. Wu. *INCAP-ICNND Food Composition Table for Use in Latin America.* Washington, D.C., U.S. Government Printing Office, 1961.

32. Lowenthal, D. "The Population of Barbados." *Social and Economic Studies.* VI. Jamaica, University College, 1957.

33. McKigney, J.I. "Food Economics in Nutrition Policy and Planning." *Nutrition Newsletter,* 1969, 7 (4), 16-24.

34. *New York Herald Tribune,* December 13, 1959.

35. *New York Times,* February 7, 1971.

36. Paxton, J., Ed. *The Statesman's Yearbook 1970/1971.* New York, St. Martin's Press, 1970.

37. Peronnette, H. "The Community Weight-Profile of Children in Rural Martinique." *Journal of Tropical Pediatrics,* 1968, 14, 43-46.

38. Phillipsen, W.L. "CARIFTA and the Caribbean Market." *Foreign Agriculture,* 1969, VII (21), 10-11.

39. Standard, K.L., Lovell, H.G. and Harney, L. "Heights and Weights of Barbadian School Children." *British Journal of Preventive and Social Medicine,* 1966, 20, 135-140.

40. United Nations (Department of Economic and Social Affairs). *Demographic Yearbook 1969.* New York, UN, 1970.

41. United Nations Children's Fund. *Digest of Projects Aided by UNICEF in the Americas.* New York, UNICEF, 1969.

42. U.S. Department of Agriculture (Economic Research Service). *Agricultural Policies in the Western Hemisphere.* ERS-Foreign No. 36. Washington, D.C., U.S. Government Printing Office, 1967.

43. _____ . *French West Indies: Agricultural Production and Trade.* ERS-Foreign 80. Washington, D.C., USDA, 1964.

44. _____ . *Indices of Agricultural Production for the Western Hemisphere Excluding the United States and Cuba—Revised 1961 through 1969, Preliminary 1970.* ERS-Foreign 264. Washington, D.C., U.S. Government Printing Office, 1971.

45. _____ . *Jamaica, Trinidad and Tobago, Leeward Islands, Windward Islands, Barbados, and British Guiana—Projected Levels of Demand, Supply, and Imports of Agricultural Products to 1975.* ERS-Foreign 94. Jerusalem, Israel Program for Scientific Translations, 1963.

46. _____ /I,. *Prospects for Agriculture in the Caribbean.* FAER No. 58. Washington, D.C., U.S. Government Printing Office, 1970.

47. _____ . *Summary and Evaluation of Jamaica, Trinidad and Tobago, Leeward Islands, Windward Islands, Barbados, and British Guiana—Projected Levels of Demand, Supply, and Imports of Agricultural Products to 1975.* ERS-Foreign 148. Washington, D.C., U.S. Government Printing Office, 1966.

47a. U.S. Department of Commerce (Bureau of International Commerce). "Martinique, Guadeloupe, and French Guiana." *Foreign Economic Trends.* ET 71-056. Washington, D.C., U.S. Government Printing Office, 1971.

48. U.S. Department of Labor (Bureau of Labor Statistics). "Labor Conditions in the British Caribbean Territories." *Labor Digest.* No. 61. Washington, D.C., USDL, 1964.

49. _____ (Bureau of Labor Statistics). "Labor Conditions in the French Caribbean Departments." *Labor Digest.* No. 62. Washington, D.C., USDL, 1964.

50. Uttley, K.H. "The Incidence and Mortality of Disease in Antigua, West Indies, in Recent Years." *West Indian Medical Journal,* 1966, 15, 97-107.

51. *Washington Post,* November 27, 1955.

52. West, R.C. and Augelli, J.P. *Middle America: Its Land and Its Peoples.* New Jersey, Prentice-Hall, Inc., 1966.

53. Williams, E. *From Columbus to Castro: The History of the Caribbean 1492-1969.* New York, Harper & Row, Publishers, 1970.

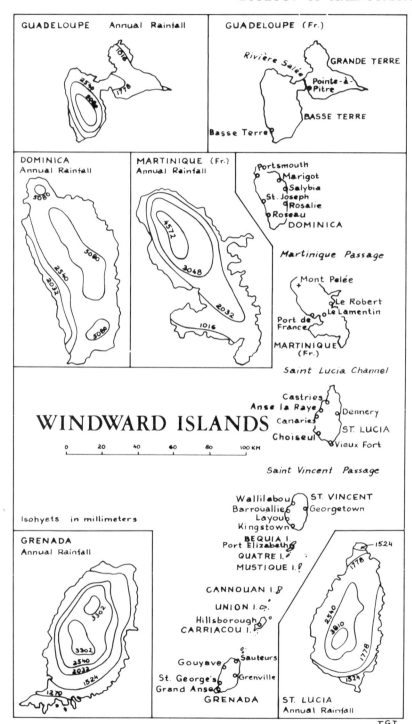

GUADELOUPE   Annual Rainfall

GUADELOUPE (Fr.)

Rivière Salée

GRANDE TERRE

Pointe-à-Pitre

BASSE TERRE

Basse Terre

DOMINICA
Annual Rainfall

MARTINIQUE (Fr.)
Annual Rainfall

Portsmouth
Marigot
Salybia
St. Joseph
Rosalie
Roseau
DOMINICA

Martinique Passage

Mont Pelée

Le Robert
Le Lamentin
Port de France
MARTINIQUE
(Fr.)

Saint Lucia Channel

WINDWARD ISLANDS

Castries
Anse la Raye
Canaries
Choiseul

Dennery
ST. LUCIA
Vieux Fort

0   20   40   60   80   100 KM

Saint Vincent Passage

Isohyets in millimeters

GRENADA
Annual Rainfall

Wallilabou
Barrouallie
Layou
Kingstown

ST. VINCENT
Georgetown

BEQUIA I.
Port Elizabeth
QUATRE I.
MUSTIQUE I.

CANNOUAN I.

UNION I.

Hillsborough
CARRIACOU I.

Gouyave
St. George's
Grand Anse

Sauteurs
Grenville

GRENADA

1524

ST. LUCIA
Annual Rainfall

TGT

TRINIDAD AND TOBAGO

TABLE OF CONTENTS

TRINIDAD AND TOBAGO

I. BACKGROUND INFORMATION

A. PHYSICAL SETTING [7] [17] [35] [34] [1] [23]

Trinidad and Tobago are the southernmost islands of the West Indies, lying off the northern coast of Venezuela between $10°$ and $11°$ north (see Map No. 1). Geologically, Trinidad belongs to the continent of South America, from which it is separated by a fault depression in the Caribbean Coastal Range. At its nearest point, Trinidad lies only 7 nautical miles (across the Dragon's Mouth Channel) from Venezuela. This contiguity is reflected not only in the similarity of surface topography but in the underlying oil-bearing Tertiary formations of southern Trinidad, lying opposite Venezuela's Orinoco delta. The island is approximately 161 kilometers long and 64 kilometers wide, encompassing a total land area of 4,828 square kilometers. The terrain is mostly flat and undulating, although there are three highland ranges crossing the island: the Northern Range and the Southern Range both run from west to east, while the Central Range traverses Trinidad diagonally. The highest peaks are in the Northern Range but they reach only 925.5 meters. However, this chain rises abruptly from the northern shore and its steep sides form a virtual barrier across the northern part of the island for about 80 kilometers. On its southern side, the range slopes gradually to the Caroni Plain. The other two ranges are much lower than the Northern and slope gently to the plains. There are only a few good ports, concentrated along the western side. Elsewhere barrier mountains, coastal swamps, winds and sea currents inhibit ship landings.

The two major rivers of Trinidad are the Caroni and the Oropuche. The Caroni drains the northwestern part of the island, passing through a large mangrove swamp before reaching the sea just south of Port of Spain. The Oropuche drains the southwestern portion and also ends in a swamp near the coast. Another large marshy area, the Nariva Swamp, has been formed on the east coast by a long sand bar (the Cocal) which holds back the waters fed into

425

the swamp by the streams draining the southern flanks of the Central Range. In this area Japanese experts have been investigating the possibility of creating new agricultural lands for the production of rice in the lower plain and possibly watermelons, tomatoes and dairy farming in the higher areas.

The suitability of Trinidadian soils to agriculture varies with location. In general, the soils of the Northern Range are poor but in the sheltered southern valleys and land is appropriate for cocoa production. The clay soils of the central and eastern parts of the island are particularly well-suited to cocoa. In the south, the soil is sandy, unstable and of lower productivity. Fertile soils based on clays and silts support sugarcane in a western coastal belt between the Caroni and Oropuche swamps, while citrus thrives in the soils and climate of the west and northwest.

Tobago lies 20 nautical miles northeast of Trinidad. It is a small island, only about 41.6 kilometers long, 12 kilometers wide and 300 square kilometers in area. Physically, Tobago shows more similarity to its Windward Island neighbors than to Trinidad. A mountainous central spine called the Main Ridge rises to 567 meters and runs almost the entire length of the island. Cocoa is cultivated in the fertile, moist valleys of the Ridge where the plants are sheltered from the wind. The southern flanks of the Ridge slope toward a narrow but fertile coastal plain. To the southwest, an extensive low-lying area comprises a series of flat coral terraces overlaid with thick mud and clay beds. This region is the site of most of Tobago's coconut groves. Soil erosion is a major problem on the island, especially on the interior slopes where most smallholders are settled.

B. CLIMATE [7] [1] [34] [35]

Trinidad and Tobago experience a tropical climate with generally higher levels of temperature and precipitation than are found in other West Indian islands. The hot, humid climate is uncomfortable for man but good for tropical crops. There is little seasonal variation in mean temperatures. The January mean is the year's lowest at 24°C, and the May average the highest at 27.5°C. There are two seasons: a dry period from January to May and a rainy season from June to December. In Trinidad, heaviest precipitation occurs in the Northern Range and in the eastern part of the island where an average of 2,500 millimeters falls annually. The western sector receives about 1,650 millimeters (see Map No. 3) and the southern part of the island is subject to severe drought during the dry season. In Tobago rainfall is heaviest on the crest of the Main Ridge where yearly precipitation never averages less than 3,750 millimeters. Rainfall decreases rapidly toward the southwest. In the lowlands, precipitation averages only 1,125 millimeters and due to the porous character of the coral base, drought is a serious problem during the dry season.

Trinidad and Tobago lie south of the Caribbean hurricane zone and hence are rarely damaged by tropical windstorms. However, in 1963 the two islands were struck severely by "Hurricane Flora" which destroyed 75 percent of the cocoa crop and caused considerable damage to other tree crops such as coconut and banana plantations.

C. POPULATION [25] [35] [1] [7]

The 1970 population of Trinidad and Tobago was estimated at 1,076,263 (see Table No. 1). The annual rate of increase is about 2.0 percent, or perhaps less due to the growing number of people migrating to the United States, Canada and the United Kingdom. The infant mortality rate is estimated at 35.8 per 1,000 live births, down from 41.8 in 1966. Life expectancy is 66 years for females and 62 years for males. The density is 203 inhabitants per square kilometer. In Trinidad the heaviest concentration of population is found along the west coast and in the southwest, reflecting the job opportunities afforded by the sugar plantations, the manufacturing industries, the ports and the petroleum fields located on the occidental side of the island. The southern and eastern coasts of Trinidad are sparsely inhabited due to the unsuitability of the forests and swamplands for crop cultivation and due to the small labor requirements of the coconut plantations located in these areas. In Tobago the densest settlements are established in the southwestern coral lowlands and in the coastal areas. Due to the overpopulation of the agricultural land, many Tobagonians have migrated to Trinidad where the oil industry and new manufacturing enterprises are attracting workers. For this reason, although the population of both islands is still predominantly rural (60 percent), Trinidad has begun to experience a strong trend toward urbanization, particularly around Port of Spain (which now has over 100,000 inhabitants) and San Fernando (which has a population of 48,000). Scarborough, with 3,700 inhabitants, is the largest settlement in Tobago and the market center of the island.

Ethnically, the population of Trinidad is one of the most variegated in the West Indies. About 43.5 percent of the inhabitants are of African descent, 36.5 percent are of East Indian origin, 2 percent are of European background (British, French, Spanish and Portuguese), 1 percent are Chinese and the remainder (17 percent) are mostly of mixed descent, but include some Syrians and Latin Americans. The Tobago population is predominantly Negro. In Trinidad the Negroes (called "Creoles") are concentrated in the cities while the East Indians tend to live in rural areas.

English is the official language, and Creole English the lingua franca, but the various ethnic groups also speak their own tongues, such as Hindi, Urdu and Spanish. The literacy rate is estimated to have risen from 89 percent in 1960 to 94 percent in 1967. The majority of the inhabitants are Christians (35 percent are Roman Catholics; 25 percent are Anglicans). The non-Christians are mainly Hindus and Moslems.

D. HISTORY AND GOVERNMENT [1] [35] [7] [34]

Trinidad was discovered by Columbus on his third voyage in 1498. He named the island La Trinidad because the three hills in the bay where he anchored seemed to symbolize the Holy Trinity. He made no mention of the island of Tobago in his log. Both islands were occupied by Arawak Indians. It was nearly a century before the first Spanish settlement was established on Trinidad at Port of Spain and almost immediately the colony became the victim of successive raids by the English, the French and the Dutch. As on most West Indies islands, the native Indians were soon annihilated by disease and maltreatment and the Spanish imported African slaves to cultivate the fertile soil for cocoa production. During the 16th and 17th centuries the colony suffered from recurring attacks by other European powers and from a blight on the cocoa crop.

In 1783, in an effort to revitalize the island's economy, Spain began encouraging Catholics of any nationality to settle in Trinidad. The French responded to the invitation in largest numbers, introducing coffee, sugarcane and cotton plants and bringing new varieties of cocoa to the island. Settlers began to disperse to the Caroni Plain and the valleys of the Northern Range. In 1797, when Trinidad was captured by the British during the Napoleonic Wars, there were more French than Spanish inhabitants. Trinidad was ceded to Great Britain in 1802 under the Treaty of Amiens and has remained under British influence ever since. The British, being plantation-minded, began to expand the commercial production of sugar and cocoa, the cash crops which provided the basis for the island's 19th century economy. Discovery of oil in 1910 added another source of income. In recent years manufacturing and tourism have contributed significantly to the gross national product.

Tobago was not settled unitl 1632 when a company of Dutch merchants sent settlers to the island. In 1763 the Treaty of Paris gave Tobago to the British, but the island was captured by the French in 1781, then recaptured by the British in 1793, restored to France in 1802 by the Treaty of Amiens and finally ceded to Britain in 1814 by the Congress of Vienna.

The abolition of slavery in 1834 resulted in a depletion of the plantation labor force on Trinidad and Tobago as the Negro freedmen turned to the cultivation of their own small holdings. The estate owners solved the problem by importing indentured laborers from India and thus laid the foundation for the present ethnic diversity of the island nation.

Trinidad and Tobago joined the Federation of the West Indies in 1958 and remained a member until the Federation's dissolution in 1962 when Trinidad and Tobago became an independent state within the British Commonwealth of Nations. A Governor General is the Queen's representative. Executive authority is vested in a Prime Minister who is also the leader of the majority party in Parliament. The legislature is bicameral, consisting of a 36-member House of Representatives and a 24-member Senate. Representatives are elected by universal suffrage while Senators are appointed by the Governor General: 13 from the majority party on the advice of the Prime Minister, four on the advice of the Leader of the Opposition and seven from various religious, economic and social groups deemed important by the Prime Minister. The judiciary consists of a Supreme Court, which includes a High Court and a Court of Appeal, a system of Courts of Summary Jurisdiction, and Petty Civil Courts, Local government is in the hands of three municipal councils (Port of Spain, San Fernando and Arima) and six county councils (including one for Tobago).

Trinidad and Tobago belongs to the General Agreement on Tariffs and Trade (GATT), the British Commonwealth Tariff System, the United Nations, the Organization of American States and the Caribbean Free Trade Association (CARIFTA). It is also a signatory to the Caribbean Fats and Oils and Rice agreements, the Commonwealth and International Sugar Agreements and the International Coffee Agreement.

E. AGRICULTURAL POLICIES [29] [30] [1]

The Government has recognized that the key to Trinidad and Tobago's agricultural development lies not only in modernizing the production of export commodities (sugar, cocoa, citrus and coffee), but also in rationalizing land utilization and increasing and diversifying domestic food production. In its second 5-year Development Plan (1969-1973), the Government allocated $29 million to agriculture, with an emphasis on programs leading to greater self-sufficiency in food. About 20 percent of the agriculture appropriation is to be used for farm credit programs, about 25 percent for distribution of publicly held lands and consolidation of private holdings, and rest for a farm commodity price guarantee program, marketing improvement and rural infrastructure development. Agricultural programs include land settlement schemes, extension education, production subsidies, guaranteed prices (on such crops as corn, beans, pigeon peas, groundnuts, sweet potatoes and plantains), supervised credit, and improved marketing and processing facilities. In 1966 a Central Marketing Agency (CMA) was established and in 1970 the Agency was strengthened by a technical grant from the Inter-American Development Bank. The CMA operates markets, regulates the flow of commodities from producers to retail distribution centers, maintains 12 distribution and purchase centers where food, feed, fertilizers, pesticides and seeds are stored and operates two cold storage plants and a silo. Restrictions on imports are used to protect the local producers against foreign agricultural competition. Special protection has been given to the poultry and livestock industries.

An Agricultural Development Bank (ADB) has been formed with the assistance of the Inter-American Development Bank. The ADB has initiated a $3.6 million credit program for small-and medium-scale farmers.

Since 1965, the Government has been operating a farm demonstration program on Crown Lands. Various types of economically viable small-and medium-sized production units, such as dairy, pig, citrus, food crop and tobacco farms, have been developed and then distributed to independent farmers on a lease basis. With the aid of a World Bank loan, the Government hoped to establish 1,800 farms on about 4,800 hectares of Crown Land by the end of 1971. By the end of 1968 it was reported that 168 dairy, 60 pig, 423 food crop and 9 tobacco farms had been settled through this program. Heavy emphasis has been laid on production of fruit and root crops.

F. FOREIGN AID

1. Bilateral Aid [28] [27]

Between 1962 and 1968 United States assistance to Trinidad and Tobago totaled $22.7 million in long-term Export-Import Bank loans and $32 million in grants, including $0.5 million under Title II of the P.L. 480 (Food for Freedom) program, $0.2 million for support of a Peace Corps contingent and $31.3 in development grants. The Government of Canada has provided a $250,000 loan to develop Trinidad's fishing industry.

2. Multilateral Aid [27] [26] [13] [16]

United Nations Children's Fund assistance to Trinidad and Tobago in the area of food and nutrition has included a health services training project, an applied nutrition program and a child feeding program. Under the health services training project, UNICEF has given supplies, equipment, transport and training grants while WHO has provided a nursing advisor and fellowships. The program is aimed at creating a corps of over 700 nursing auxiliaries to assist in meeting the requirements of public health and hospital nursing services, including pediatric and maternity care.

Through the applied nutrition program, it is hoped to improve the level of nutrition of the rural population by establishing training centers for local personnel, school gardens, small animal projects, fish culture projects and nutrition education programs in schools and health centers. Supplies, equipment, transport and training grants are provided by UNICEF, technical guidance by WHO, and the services of an agricultural extension expert by FAO.

UNICEF has been assisting the Government's child feeding program since 1954 by meeting the ocean freight costs for donated skim milk powder or corn-soy-milk blend (CSM). About 4,000 preschool children and their mothers and 20,000 schoolchildren benefit yearly from this program. Each schoolchild receives a daily ration of milk or CSM and a portion of fresh yeast (supplied by the Government) either in the milk, in cookies, or in soup.

Other UN-supported projects are financed by the United Nations Development Fund (UNDP) from its Special Fund. These include an agricultural and forestry training program ($695,000) conducted at the Eastern Caribbean Farm Institute in Centeno with the aid of FAO advisors. Trinidad and Tobago has also received assistance from the World Bank and the Inter-American Development Bank (IDB). The World Bank has extended a $5 million loan for agricultural development (Crown lands settlement program) and a $3 million loan for family planning activities. Since 1961, the IDB has approved $8.9 million in loans to Trinidad and Tobago, including $3.6 million extended to the Agricultural Development Bank (ADB) for a farm credit program, $2.9 million for agricultural diversification to meet local food demands, and $700,000 to expand farm output ($132,400 to be used to strengthen the ADB and its credit union activities, $31,600 to be utilized by the Central Marketing Agency for consulting services on the warehousing, marketing and transport of agricultural products, and $87,000 to be earmarked for graduate training courses for specialists in the Ministry of Agriculture, Land and Fisheries).

II. FOOD RESOURCES

A. GENERAL [9] [35] [29] [1]

The food resources of Trinidad and Tobago are derived from 139,000 hectares of arable land, 6,000 hectares of pastures, the sea around the islands and from imports. There are 232,000 hectares of forests, some of which could be converted into farmland.

Trinidad and Tobago exhibit a greater agricultural potential than most islands of the West Indies due to generally adequate rainfall, relative protection from hurricane damage, availability of fertile soil and year-round conditions for cultivation. Yet, there is little agricultural tradition in the islands except insofar as cultivation of sugar and cocoa is concerned. Some food crops are grown, but tree crops cover more than half of the cultivated land. These circumstances place Trinidad and Tobago in the same predicament as other islands in the Caribbean area, namely having to import most of the food supply. There is one major difference, however: because of Trinidad's mineral wealth, the country can afford its food imports. Nevertheless, as stated previously, under its second Five Year Plan (1964-1968) the Government has promoted agricultural diversification to increase domestic food resources, with special emphasis on animal husbandry, dairying and truck gardening. The third Five Year Plan, which began in 1969 and is due to end in 1973, continues the policy of the second and aims at ensuring self-sufficiency in food.

The food resources vary with the ethnic group considered. Since Trinidad has a more heterogeneous population than any other Caribbean island, it is not surprising that a variety of menus prevails. Produced on the island are corn and rice (in inadequate quantities), sweet potatoes, yams, manioc, vegetables, bananas, an assortment of other fruits, some meat and some fish. Moreover, while small quantities of fresh milk from local cows are available, most of the milk drunk on Trinidad and Tobago is imported. Pulses, an important item in both the West and East Indian diets, are grown locally but meet only 47 percent of the demand.

B. MEANS OF PRODUCTION

1. Agricultural Labor Force [34] [19] [1] [33]

The labor force in Trinidad increased by 61.4 percent between 1946 and 1965, mainly because of population growth. However, during the same period the participation rate, that is the number of people actually employed compared to the potential able-bodied labor force, declined. This was due in part to the increase of secondary school attendance and in part to the scarcity of jobs.

By 1965 the total labor force amounted to 350,000 people and in 1971 it must have neared 370,000. About 22 percent of this force is still dependent upon agriculture for work, in spite of the growing importance of the oil industry, which is highly automated. As in other sugar islands, the level of subemployment or unemployment is high, estimated in 1965 at 13.7 percent of the total force. Unemployment was lowest in agriculture (5.5 percent) and highest in construction and utilities (25.8 percent). The following table gives an approximate distribution of the labor force in 1965.

Distribution of the Labor Force by Sector – Trinidad and Tobago, 1965

Sector	Number	Percent of Total	Number Unemployed	Percent Unemployed
Agriculture, forestry, hunting and fishing	71,000	20.4	3,900	5.5
Mining, quarrying, manufacturing	63,900	18.3	5,700	8.9
Construction and utilities	50,700	14.6	13,100	25.8
Commerce	55,000	15.8	4,400	8.0
Transport and communication	24,100	6.9	1,900	7.9
Services	72,600	20.8	7,800	10.7
Others	11,100	3.2	11,000	100.0
Totals and Average	348,400	100.0	47,800	13.8

Source: After U.S. Department of Labor, *Labor Law and Practice in Trinidad and Tobago.*

Of the total indicated above, 56,000 or about 16.1 percent were considered to be self-employed, 9,500 (2.7 percent) were employers, 32,100 (9.2 percent) were unpaid workers presumed to be mostly in agriculture working their own subsistence plots, and 70,600 (20.3 percent) were government employees, reflecting once more the need for the bureaucracy to absorb large numbers of people whose level of education causes them to disdain manual work. The level of unemployment is probably higher than shown because the unpaid workers outside the agricultural sector are really among the unemployed, as are an unknown portion of the so-called self-employed.

The islands claim a shortage of skilled manpower and suffer from considerable seasonal variations in employment levels, especially in agriculture where cane cutting and sugar processing activities do not last the year around. Contrary to the case in other Caribbean islands, migration from Trinidad and Tobago is somewhat limited. Fewer than 400 agricultural workers left the islands in 1969 and none were allowed to enter. The Government, however, wishes to increase the emigration of workers to the United States and Canada. After a first period of optimism following the creation of the now dissolved Federation of the West Indies, which it was believed would stimulate employment, stark reality proved it was necessary to restrict immigration and to encourage emigration to ease the unemployment situation.

Wages are generally higher and incomes better than in most Caribbean countries but remain inadequate to purchase a balanced imported diet. Table No. 2 shows the cost of food as a percentage of monthly income among 236 families surveyed in 18 towns in 1961. Average monthly earnings of agricultural workers in 1965 were around $36.50 for males and $21.75 for women. Field work is often paid by the task under rates which vary with each estate but most farmhands are paid hourly wages. These agricultural rates are the lowest offered in all sectors of employment and contrast with an average per capita income of $50.00 per month for the Trinidad and Tobago population as a whole (rural and urban combined). Keeping in mind that among the employed, agricultural workers represent the highest percentage of the labor force, this discrepancy between their earnings and the monthly average per capita is suggestive of significantly short diets. Fringe benefits are not unknown in the islands and some are assured to seamen, waterfront workers and oilfield workers, but there is no legislation to cover them and no evidence that any of these benefits apply to agricultural laborers.

2. Farms [1] [34] [35] [15]

Half of the island land is owned by the Government which rents certain portions out for 25 years at a time. After emancipation, many freed slaves settled on little holdings which have become the small farms of today. There are about 35,800 farms, the vast majority of which are less than 2 hectares in size. Less than one-third of the total number of farms were estimated to have more than 6 hectares each. Only about 1 percent of the farms are large estates, but these occupy over 40 percent of the farmland. All the farms cover about

215,000 hectares, which must include a sizable amount of undeveloped forest-land since arable land totals only 139,000 hectares.

Half of the agricultural output is grown for local consumption, the other half for export. While most of the farms are merely subsistence enterprises, 9,693 farmers grow sugarcane which they sell to the large companies. The farmhouse *(ajoupa)* is usually poor, often limited to a mud structure with no flooring and a thatched or corrugated iron roof. Better-off farmers have houses of wood and concrete. Thanks to loans provided by the Sugar Industry Labor Welfare Fund, many of these *ajoupas* are now being replaced by better structures. The Government has also started a Better Village Program in the hope of improving village life and slowing down the cityward drift.

3. Fertilizers and Mechanical Equipment [1] [15] [30] [9]

Fertilizers have long been used in Trinidad and Tobago. Truck farmers apply pen manure, supplementing it with appropriate mixtures of phosphatic and potassic fertilizers. Some fertilizer is produced in Trinidad through Federation Chemicals Limited, an affiliate of W.R. Grace and Company. Its plant at Point Lisas produces anhydrous ammonia, ammonium sulphate and urea. Plant capacity reaches 75,000 tons of urea and 90,000 tons of sulphate of ammonia. In addition, 60,000 tons of nitrogenous fertilizer and 7,000 tons of phosphate fertilizer are purchased abroad.

It is believed that at least 500 tractors are in use on the islands. Subsidies are paid by the Government towards the purchase of fertilizer and agricultural equipment.

C. PRODUCTION [29]

Agriculture is of great importance to the islands, perhaps first because it gives employment to over 20 percent of the labor force, second because it produces some food that does not have to be purchased, and finally because it provides cash crops. The area sown and the production of major crops are shown in Table No. 2 (see also Map No. 2).

1. Food Crops [9] [1] [32] [35] [15] [29]

Food crops are produced on the lands of many smallholders who usually are undercapitalized and follow poor farming practices. The result is low yields. Rice, corn, pulses, roots, fruits and vegetables are the mainstay of this subsistence production; any surpluses are sold on the domestic market. The kinds of food grown or purchased (from domestic or imported resources) to provide the daily menu of the average Trinidadian are listed in Table No. 3.

Rice has been grown on the islands for many decades without any changes in technique. It is cultivated mainly by East Indians who plow with the aid of water buffaloes, as in Asia. The growing season for rice is from June to December (the wet season); during the rest of the year vegetables are often planted in the rice fields. Since 1952, the area sown has covered 6,000 hectares, primarily in the Caroni Swamp area of Trinidad. Eighteen thousand tons of paddy were produced in 1948-52, dropping to 10,000 tons thereafter. The yield remained static since 1961 at 1.7 tons per hectare (compared to 5.7 tons in Japan). Apparently, the multiple varieties of rice grown make it difficult to establish proper quality standards. Local production supplies only 15 percent of domestic requirements and this rice is consumed mainly by the farmers themselves. Additional amounts of rice are imported from Guyana according to the provisions of CARIFTA. Guyana, in return, buys petroleum and fertilizers from Trinidad and Tobago. The consumption of rice is on the increase and self-sufficiency is not in sight.

Corn is a minor crop. It does not even figure in Table No. 3 because it did not emerge as a frequent staple at the time of the survey on which the table is based.* The area sown has remained at 2,000 hectares for 20 years with a stable output of 3,000 tons annually and a yield of 1.8 tons per hectare (compared to 4.9 tons in the U.S.). The demand for corn seems to be growing, to some extent because of the population increase, but mostly because of the Government's interest in promoting the livestock industry. Yet, there does not seem to be any indication of a resurgence of this cereal, probably because no crop can really compete with sugar and because U.S. corn is of superior quality and is reasonably priced.

Sweet potatoes, yams, taro and manioc are part of the basic diet of the Trinidad and Tobago people. Since 1964, only 2,000 hectares have been planted in sweet potatoes and yams, yielding 18,000 tons a year. The acreage in manioc is not recorded but it is estimated that a crop of 5,000 tons is produced annually. The trend for the traditional tubers is downward as the popularity of European potatoes increases, indicating a growing preference for imported food items and an increased availability of money. This does not necessarily mean an increased standard of living and better nutrition, however. Pigeon peas and all other pulses are popular and widely cultivated in unrecorded quantities. Pigeon peas are subsidized by the Government under a price support policy and the crop is commercialized. Two private firms collect, process and can pigeon peas. Many vegetables are grown: onions, garlic, cucumbers, cabbages, etc.

---

*1961 nutrition survey sponsored by the Interdepartmental Committee on Nutrition for National Defense.

Oils and fats are derived mainly from coconuts, but due to the continued ravages of the Red Ring disease, the production of this crop has been declining steadily. Between 1952 and 1956 an estimated annual average of 146 million nuts were harvested, but by 1968 the output had dropped to 110 million.

2. Cash Crops [29] [1] [35] [9]

The most important cash crop is sugarcane, followed by cocoa, coffee, citrus fruit and bananas. About 24 percent of the cropland is now in sugarcane, all located in Trinidad because the climate and the soil of Tobago do not lend themselves to this culture. Sugar and related products represent 60 percent of all agricultural output. The area sown in cane has remained between 32,000 and 36,000 hectares during the last 20 years but, thanks to good practices, the yields have increased considerably from 42.5 tons per hectare to 68 tons in 1969. This is remarkable, considering the rapid deterioration and impoverishment of tropical soils under intensive cultivation and the fact that some fields have been under sugar for 150 years. Cane is grown between the Caroni and Oropuche swamps along the west coast. This area is drier than other parts of the island and the drier the climate, the more concentrated the sugar in the cane.

Sixty percent of the sugarcane acreage is in large estates, the rest in smallholdings numbering about 11,000. The former are highly mechanized, although a gradual plan was introduced by the Industrial Court to minimize the unavoidable unemployment which follows mechanization. Individual farmers do not enjoy the benefits of mechanization due to the small size of their holdings. The large companies produce about twice as much sugar as the smallholders and they purchase the farmers' output for processing along with their own. One factory produces the sugar needed for domestic consumption (10 percent of the total crop) and three more manufacture the rest for export. The annual production of cane has varied from an average of 1,441,000 tons per year during the 1948-1952 period to 2.5 million tons in 1968, and that of sugar from 174,000 tons per year from 1952 to 1956 to 243,000 tons in 1968. The yield of sugar per ton of cane is about 10 percent. Trinidad is in the same position as the other Commonwealth sugar islands: her market is protected until January 1, 1975 by the Sugar Agreement with the United Kingdom but the situation will change when Britain becomes a member of the European Economic Community.

By-products of the sugar industry are bagasse (fibers left after the cane has been processed) and rum. The former is used for fuel in local factories and the latter partly consumed at home and partly exported. From 1962 to 1968 an average of 65,400 hectoliters of rum was distilled every year, of which about 30,000 hectoliters or 3 liters per capita were consumed at home.

Cocoa was the leading product of the islands during the first quarter of the 20th century but yielded first place to sugar in the 1930's. The drop in world prices about that time, combined with the damage done by the "witch's broom" disease resulting from a fungus, caused the crop to lose prestige. The main areas of cocoa production are the central and eastern parts of the islands. The best region for the crop is the Central Range where clay soil, rainfall in adequate quantities, and shelter from the winds favor cocoa. It is believed that the area under this crop extends over 28,000 hectares and that 6,000 tons of beans are now harvested yearly between October and March. This is a drop from the yearly average of 7,900 tons between 1948 and 1952. The exact total harvested is not known because farmers have planted hitherto abandoned areas and the Government has subsidized further extension. The entire crop is subsidized through the Cocoa Board which also grades the product, an essential step if the market for Trinidad, and Tobago cocoa is to be kept up.

Coffee is the third cash crop. It is believed that Robusta trees thrive best on Trinidadian soil and some planters concentrate on these, but Arabica trees are also grown. Coffee is in part a subsistence crop, as many farmers grow coffee for their own consumption. The total area under production is not certain because trees are planted on the edge of cocoa groves. The crops harvested have varied from a low of about 1,000 tons per year between 1948 and 1952 to a high of 4,500 tons in 1964 and 1970. Exports have increased in recent years, allegedly reaching 8,700 tons in 1968. This figure would have to include stored reserves from previous years. FAO gives a 1969 export figure of 2,760 tons.

Citrus fruits grow well in Trinidad, especially in the valleys of the Northern Range where soils, temperature and rainfall combine to create a favorable environment. The crop, principally grapefruit, is harvested from October to the following June, with the peak in January. In 1968 about 16,000 tons were produced, the lowest crop on record since 1948. In 1970 production rose somewhat to 18,000 tons. Oranges and tangerines, by contrast, increased from an average of 9,000 tons between 1948 and 1952 to 14,000 tons in 1964 but decreased recently to 11,000 tons. Lemons, limes and other citrus fruit add about 2,000-4,000 tons a year to this bounty. The total area devoted to citrus is believed to be about 8,000 hectares. Because the citrus harvest period is about the same in all the Caribbean islands, the competition on the world market is serious. The Trinidadian Cooperative Citrus Growers Association, founded in 1932, sees that quality grades are kept up. In 1968 about 2,278 tons of citrus of all kinds were exported, indicating that a substantial portion of the crop is eaten at home where an average of about one orange every 5 days should be available to each Trinidadian.

Bananas in small amounts are commercialized through the office of the Central Marketing Agency. Coconuts are cultivated along the coasts of Trinidad and on the leeward side of Tobago. The 1969 harvest totaled 113 million nuts, about three-fourths of which were produced on estates. Most of the crop is dried for copra (13,000 tons in 1970) which is then used in the manufacture of edible oils, soap and cosmetics both for domestic use and for export to other West

Indian islands. The local copra output does not supply the domestic processing industry and must be supplemented by imports.

3. Animal Husbandry [9] [11] [1]

a. *Livestock and Poultry*

Animal husbandry, although established on a small base, has been very successfully developed. Self-sufficiency in pork and poultry seems to have been reached. Yet, much meat and many meat products still have to be imported. Cattle production has risen from about 32,000 head 20 years ago to 63,000 head in 1970. The subsidies and constant support given the industry by the Government, including the importation of breeding stock, the distribution of corn feed and the expansion of veterinary services, have brought about this increase. The country's livestock wealth also includes 50,000 pigs, 6,000 sheep and 35,000 goats. The pork meat industry has been handicapped by storage problems in the past but presently seems to have surmounted them. Eighty pig farms of 2 hectares each are, or soon will be, established. Forty pigs will be raised for slaughter on each farm. A processing plant capable of handling 500 pigs a week and 100 head of cattle is being completed.

There are an estimated 5 million chickens or other poultry. Since 1961, the Government has supported the poultry industry by: 1) encouraging the development of hatcheries; 2) increasing production of feed; 3) controlling infectious diseases; 4) providing financial aid for and abolishing customs duties on medicine and equipment that could be useful to the industry; 5) promoting better marketing practices; and 6) developing local breeders. After 1965 Trinidad practically ceased to import poultry and a drastic reduction in price, from $1.00 to 45¢ per pound, resulted from the expansion of the local industry. The following table illustrates this development.

Poultry – Trinidad, 1961-1967

Year	Local Production (1,000 tons)	Imports (1,000 tons)	Total (1,000 tons)	Consumption Per Capita Per Year (kilos)
1961	3.4	2.8	6.2	7.1
1963	5.1	2.7	7.8	8.6
1965	10.4	.45	10.8	10.4
1967	9.4	–	9.4	9.4

Source: After F.O. Gonzalez, "Programme to Increase Protein Products in Trinidad."

b. *Meat, Milk and Eggs*

At 1,000-2,000 tons a year, the production of meat from local cattle is insufficient to meet demand and considerable amounts have to be imported. The

Government's continuous effort to stimulate pork production, however, has resulted in tripling the output from 1,000 tons in 1966 to 3,000 tons in 1970, making the country self-sufficient in this kind of meat. The amount of available milk is rising slowly and reached 6,000 tons in 1968. This has been greatly encouraged by the prices paid by Nestlé Products of Trinidad, Limited. With Government help, 3,000 Holstein Friesian cattle have been imported. Milk production was expected to reach 12 million liters (12,000 tons) in 1971.

To increase the country's milk resources, the Government plans to develop 8,000 hectares of Crown Land into a number of dairy farms and other food crop holdings (see *Agricultural Policies*). The World Bank will finance the development of 5,000 hectares. Eventually there should be 200 dairy farms of 8 hectares each. These were expected to be operational by the end of 1971. Each farmer will be granted 12 cows, eight of them already lactating. Experimental studies have satisfied the Government that each farmer could make $1,000 a year on this basis. The land chosen was formerly used as an American base. The fertility of the soil is low but it will be seeded with drought-resistant Pangola grasses. It is hoped that by 1973 the dairy farms will have an output of 20 million liters of fresh milk, representing 40 percent of the present level of imports.

Trinidad still imports some hens but claims to be already self-sufficient in egg production, although the demand for eggs does not seem to exceed 104 million units a year or just about two eggs per capita per week. If the cost is brought down, however, the market may increase.

4. Fisheries [6a] [15] [6b]

Until very recently, the fishing industry remained unorganized and the production of fresh fish is still inadequate. Since 1967 a fishing cooperative which has helped in building more ice-making plants and refrigerated storage space, has been in charge of sales. While quite a number of people are fulltime fishermen, it is only now that this food resource is becoming important. In June 1968, Canada announced a $250,000 development loan for fishing projects in Trinidad. The loan will pay for the salary of an advisor on fishing research, for the training of fishing specialists in Canada and for biological station officials. A trawler with skipper and engineer and two refrigerated trucks have already been shipped. The 3 percent loan has a 30-year duration and carries a 7-year grace provision.

The third Five Year Plan (1968-1973) provides for a multimillion dollar fisheries project involving all CARIFTA nations but based on Trinidad and Tobago. The United States will provide $7.1 million for the establishment of a single company responsible for: a) a fleet of seiners and trawlers; b) support vessels with all that is needed from port to fishing grounds and back; c) a special fishing harbor with cold storage and facilities for manufacturing ice and dry ice;

d) a maintenance shop for engines and a small shipyard for the fishing fleet; e) a repair shop for fishing nets; f) a store for spare parts; g) processing facilities for canning, filleting, smoking, salting, and dehydrating fish and for producing fishmeal; h) distribution centers in Trinidad and Tobago and other CARIFTA member countries to market fresh, chilled and frozen fish, etc. The United Nations is helping with this undertaking by providing a grant of $1.5 million (susceptible to increase) for technical assistance. The fishing port will be at Sea Lots, Chaguaramas or Point Lisas. A fishery training school will be established at the University of the West Indies to provide technological training.

D. FOOD INDUSTRIES [1] [15] [30] [8]

The food industries of Trinidad and Tobago which once were the most important have now ceded first rank to petrochemicals, fertilizers and oil. Industry is encouraged by the Trinidad and Tobago Industrial Development Corporation established in 1959 to promote development in the islands. The industrial establishment includes the following food industries: bottling of aerated waters and alcholic drinks, meat processing, vegetable and fruit canning, coffee and cocoa processing, milk and milk products processing, bakeries, macaroni manufacturing, jam and jelly preserving. Canned foods are popular in the islands for those who can afford them. The Citrus Growers Association has a cooperative for canning orange and grapefruit quarters and producing juice. The Association handles both domestic and foreign trade. As in Jamaica, much imported food is repackaged in Trinidad for sale abroad. The processing of cereals into pasta and macaroni seems to be among the most efficient enterprises. Annual production amounts to 1,800 tons of flour and 900 tons of pasta items. The "Pioneer Status Law" allows subsidies to be granted to incipient processing industries. For example, a recently established feed processing plant and flour mill was permitted duty-free imports and a 5-year tax relief on profits. Public slaughterhouses exist in most sizable towns under the supervision of public health authorities. As mentioned previously, a meat processing plant is being built which will be able to handle the meat obtained from 500 pigs and 100 head of cattle per week. Cold storage space is available throughout the islands, which has helped the development of the meat industry. A total of 247,000 square meters of space are supplied by a number of companies, such as Union International, International Foods, Furness, Wethy and Company, and the Electric Ice Company. Two of these plants are at Port of Spain and allow direct discharge of cold storage cargo.

E. TRADE [1] [15]

Like other countries of the area, Trinidad and Tobago has an official food crop organization called the Central Marketing Agency. Its function is to provide the farmer with a sure market and to reduce the cost of foodstuffs for the consumer. Unfortunately, the system does not always fulfill its objective, often because of a lack of competent personnel to issue adequate regulations on time. Some specific items, such as milk and pig products, are assigned to the private sector for marketing. Most towns have markets where fish and foods other than preserved goods can be sold and general retail stores where not only food but also utensils and dry goods are sold.

1. Domestic Trade [1] [8]

All internal marketing comes within the purview of the Government Development Plan, which has assigned the distribution of certain products to private industry or to the Central Marketing Agency of the Government. Milk marketing is undertaken by Nestlé Products, Limited, of Trinidad. In the case of pigs, the agency is a meat processing plant (Trinidad Packers, Limited) which produces all kinds of pork and pork products. The Central Marketing Agency also buys pigs from the pig farmers on a graded basis. Private concerns are encouraged to can peas and beans through the Pioneer Aid Program. Fresh agricultural products are sold directly by the Central Marketing Agency. The marketing channels for processed food items follow the usual chain: producers to wholesalers, wholesalers to retail grocers, and the latter to consumer. Infant foods donated by foreign assistance agencies, both national or international, go directly to the Government, which distributes them through schools or welfare clinics.

2. Foreign Trade [1] [32] [10]

Trinidad is dependent upon imports for much of its food and this represents a serious burden to the economy (see Table No. 5). Hence, a policy was devised to try to make Trinidad and Tobago self-sufficient in as many staples as possible. The policy seems to have succeeded to an encouraging degree. Imports of fresh and frozen meat have dropped almost one-third from $2,979,000 in 1961 to $2,042,000 in 1968. Poultry imports are virtually nonexistent now; imports of fresh milk and milk products have diminished by half. The increased importation of dry and condensed milk certainly includes donated nonfat dry milk, which does not cost the Government anything. Both live animals, probably breeders, and animal feeds have increased substantially, indicating a determined effort to continue the trend towards self-sufficiency in meat other than pork and in milk. There seem to be enough processed foods to permit the export of miscellaneous food preparations. These brought $1.4 million in 1968 against only $313,000 in 1961. Moreover, the balance of payments is favorable, with $465 million coming in and only $428 million going out. The income, of course, is mainly due to oil exports and tourism.

F. FOOD SUPPLY

1. Storage [1] [61]

There is no readily available information on the food storage facilities of Trinidad. Much of the food supply is located in the cold storage plants mentioned previously, in the baskets of the housewives and in the stores of the Central Marketing Agency. The Agency keeps surplus food in its warehouses and sells it to regulate prices.

2. Transportation [15] [35]

Communications within the islands are satisfactory and meet the needs. The railroad was closed down in December 1968 and replaced by bus service. Roads radiate from Port of Spain on Trinidad and reach almost every point on the island. As early as 1961, Trinidad had succeeded in building a road system adequate to support all food and agricultural distribution needs. In Tobago a circular road runs along the coast, connecting all villages and towns.

III. DIETS

A. GENERAL [15] [24]

Our knowledge of diets in Trinidad is provided by two good surveys which were carried out almost 10 years apart in 1961 and 1970. The first was carried out under the auspices of the U.S. Interdepartmental Committee on Nutrition for National Defense (ICNND) and the second under the sponsorship of the Caribbean Food and Nutrition Institute (CFNI).

The ICNND survey covered 266 families which included 1,951 people. The 24-hour recall questionnaire method was used with spot check weighing of the household food to verify the accuracy of replies. The average monthly family income was found to be $70 in Trinidad and $63 in Tobago and the cost of food represented 61 percent of family income in Trinidad, or $6.80 per capita per month.

Table No. 3 shows the different kinds of food available in Trinidad and Tobago and the differences in consumption among the various ethnic groups in 1961. The sources of energy were somewhat diversified. All groups ate rice but the Hindus consumed more than the others. Negroes ate as much bread as the three other groups put together and four times more bread daily than the Hindus who, however, used as much flour for their *chapatties* (pancakes or *roti*) as the Moslems and the Negroes together. Hindus traditionally ate *dal* (legumes) which gave them some good vegetable protein in larger amounts than that consumed by Negroes and Moslems. Hindus ate little meat while Negroes ate as much as they could afford and Moslems ate some beef (which was mostly imported and hence expensive) and some mutton but no pork. As a result of the combined diet restrictions of Hindus and Moslems, pork was in small demand and sufficiently available from domestic sources to satisfy the home market (see *Livestock and Poultry*). Fish was very popular, especially among Hindus and Moslems. Fresh fish mostly entered the diets of people living near the sea, and especially in the Diego-Martin, Mayaro and Fyzabad areas. Dried cod, an inheritance from the days of the triangular trade (see page 417), was eaten mostly by Negroes and by less affluent people who also made use of pigs' feet, pigs' snouts and pigs' tails.

Vegetables, whether green and leafy or yellow, were not consumed in large quantities in 1961, especially by the Negro group, although Moslem farmers ate more of them than urban residents. The local mixed ancestry group was the largest consumer of vegetables of all kinds. It was found that there was a correlation between income and amount of vegetables consumed. Tomatoes were appreciated but costly, a fact which limited their consumption. When income permitted, white potatoes were preferred to sweet potatoes, yams or manioc. This is another important symptom of Westernization. Mangoes were popular, especially with Moslems, and when in season provided a good substitute for oranges whose commercial export value made them scarce on the domestic market even when they were in season. Bananas, citrus fruit and avocados were preferred by the Negro group.

Milk was expensive, and when fresh was drunk in significant amounts only in certain areas. In 1961 the greatest consumers of milk were the East Indians.* Among processed types of milk, condensed was the most popular. This is unfortunate because its sweetness limits the level of intake and hence the amount of protein consumed. This is one of the very weak aspects of the Trinidad and Tobago diet for reasons given on page 446. The school system is, of course, provided with nonfat dry milk through UNICEF donations. This improves the diets of the children 5-7 years of age. Yet, at the time of the 1961 survey, mothers did not generally understand how powdered milk should be reconstituted. The children found it too thick and did not like it, creating an unfavorable bias against milk.

The fat used for cooking was most generally coconut oil.** Butter and margarine were used as a spread; East Indian families also used ghee in their foods. Margarine fortified with vitamin A was available.

Fresh vegetables, fruits and roots were bought on market days but canned food and nonperishable items were bought from the village grocer at any time. Only sugar, flour, rice and condiments were stored in the house. Cooking fuel

---

*The 1970 survey indicates that the Chinese are now the chief consumers of milk.

**Rich in saturated fatty acids.

was frequently kerosene, called "pitch oil" in Trinidad and Tobago. Utensils were iron pots or, in better-off homes, items similar to those used in the United States.

Negroes and Chinese start the day with a continental type breakfast: cocoa, tea or coffee with milk and sugar, bread and butter. East Indians eat *roti* and drink milk. The midday meal is the most important. A local recipe calls for dried codfish cooked in coconut oil, seasoned with tomatoes and onions, followed or accompanied by sweet potatoes, plantains, breadfruit or any other starchy vegetable. Another local dish liked by both East Indians and Africans is rice and beans eaten with eggplant, onions, garlic and pepper. The Chinese eat their usual varied menu, rich in vegetables and pork with large quantities of rice. The evening meal is more spartan with only *roti* for the East Indians, cheese and sardines for the Africans, and tea, coffee, cocoa or fruit juice, and fruit. Snacks are common; their nature varies mostly with income and opportunity. Far too many carbonated beverages—expensive calories—are drunk by all, including children. Rum is a staple of the diet, available at an estimated rate of 5 liters per capita per year (excepting most of the East Indian population).

As shown in Table No. 4, the ICNND investigators found that in 1961 on the average, families in the 18 Trinidadian towns surveyed spent 61 percent of their income on food. In Tunapuna the average rose as high as 85 percent. A study prepared by the Central Statistical Office of Trinidad and Tobago in 1960 estimated the following breakdown of the average family's food budget:

Percent Distribution of Family Food Budget – Trinidad, 1959

Item	Percent
Cereals	23.0
Meat	14.5
Fish	4.7
Oils and fats	3.8
Sugars	3.6
Dairy products	16.6
Fruits and nuts	7.6
Potatoes and vegetables	16.4
Beverages	2.8
Soft drinks	2.1
Other manufactured foods	3.9

Source: Interdepartmental Committee on Nutrition for National Defense, *The West Indies Nutrition Survey.*

The budget confirms what our knowledge of the availability of foods has already told us. Most of the money is spent on cereals and starchy foods, then on dairy products, fruits and nuts, fish, miscellaneous manufactured foods, oils and fats, sugar, beverages and soft drinks.

The 1970 CFNI survey was conducted from February to May and covered 1,050 households—637 rural and 413 urban—which included 5,822 individuals.

The food consumption of each household was inventoried by weight and cost for five consecutive days. The foods were grouped into 12 different categories and weighed. The nonconsumed balance after 5 days was deducted. Taking into consideration the number of people partaking in the meal, the weight and cost of the diet per household and per capita was evaluated.

The 1970 survey found the average family income of its sample to be $149 and the average cost of food to be 50¢ per capita per day or $15 per month. Obviously, the cost of food had more than doubled or the value of the currency had declined more than 50 percent or both since 1961. The cost of feeding a family of 5.5 in 1970 had risen to $82.50 but this represented only 55.3 percent of the income compared to 61 percent in 1961.

The CFNI found that the urban consumption of vegetables, meat, eggs and milk was higher than in the rural areas and that conversely, the villagers ate more cereals and legumes than the urbanites, other items being consumed at the same levels. This confirms that vegetables are now more readily available than they used to be. Perhaps better nutrition education has stimulated increased production. Moreover, Table No. 5 shows that fewer vegetables were exported in 1968 than in 1961, leaving more for domestic consumption. The 1970 survey also revealed less seasonal variation than expected (except for citrus fruit) because more vegetables were grown, more meat available and more food imported.

The 1970 survey confirms that most East Indians are rural and most Negroes urban; the former seem to consume more cereals and the latter more root crops and sugar. Contrary to expectation, milk consumption is higher among Trinidadians of Chinese ancestry and lower among East Indians. If correct, this is a very significant change from ancestral habits.

Comparing the percentages spent on food with those shown on page 444, the 1970 survey revealed 21 percent of the budget to be spend on meat instead of 14.5 percent, 15 percent on cereals instead of 23 percent and, surprisingly (since more vegetables are eaten), 10 percent on vegetables instead of 16.4 percent. Barring error, this could reflect a considerable drop in price due to greater production. However these changes, which could be an indication of some improvement in the food purchases pattern, are not true throughout the islands. In the rural area of Victoria for instance, 25 percent of the food budget is still spent on cereals and only 10 percent is spent on meat compared to 14.5 percent in 1959. In Caroni up to 12 percent of the food budget is spent on soft drinks, chocolate and beer instead of only 4.9 percent in 1961. But higher percentages are spent on vegetables, fruits, milk and meat. In Tobago, the 1970 investigators found food to be more expensive than in Trinidad but the proportion of higher incomes was greater, a factor already noticeable in 1959 when Scarborough, the capital, had an average monthly income of $87 compared to $70 in Trinidad. The 1970 survey stressed an improvement of incomes and diets in the larger cities, reflecting the existence of a larger high income group swollen by the oil industry, but the impact of this improved sector on the diet of the still large lower class is not clear. It was found, however, that in both rural and urban areas the weighted average consumption of vegetables, meat, fish, eggs and milk decreased as the size of the household increased. Since these items are not grown but purchased, the adverse influence of larger families on the quality of diets is once more obvious.

Table No. 6 gives the consumption figures found in 1970 by the CFNI. The figures represent an average of surveys made in nine areas. These are compared to the findings of the 1961 ICNND survey. It is interesting to note that the amount of cereals consumed was very nearly the same, at least when comparing the results for Trinidad in 1961 and the average for both islands 9 years later. The consumption of legumes, vegetables and fruits had increased as a result of considerable increases in production. The consumption of meat seemed to have increased as had the consumption of milk, milk products and eggs. On the whole, the average diet seemed to have improved during the 9 years that elapsed, but as will be shown, significant percentages of populations were still found to be under- and malnourished.

B. SPECIAL DIETS [3] [15] [24]

Chopra and Gist made a study of the infant feeding practices among Trinidadians of both Negro and East Indian extraction. Ten (26.3 percent) of the 38 Negro mothers surveyed were found to breast feed their children exclusively from birth to 1 year; 12 (31.5 percent) breast-fed them at night but used bottles during the day; and 16 (42.1 percent) bottle-fed their babies at all times. Frequent feedings, probably on demand, seemed to be the prevailing attitude. All the totally breast-fed children were also given orange juice, but no supplementary semisolid food. The other children received orange juice at least three times a week and most received arrowroot or another starchy supplement such as potatoes or other roots, and even eggs, peas and beans, carrots and pumpkins. The degree of dilution of the orange juice was always uncertain.

When their infants reach 1 year of age, most Negro mothers stop breast feeding, although some continue for a while beyond that age. All, however, give condensed milk to their infants by the age of 1 because of its many advantages, the most important of which is its easy preservation due to the sugar content. The drawback, of course, is the excessive proportion of sugar to protein. Free donated skim milk is available and distributed at welfare clinics. Seventy-seven percent of the mothers surveyed also gave meat to their weanlings in the amount of 15-30 grams per serving. Some fish and eggs were also offered, but 6.6 percent of the children received nothing but condensed milk. Legumes were also available, and, in certain cases were even served every day. Citrus fruit and mangoes were provided as often as available, but leafy or yellow vegetables only infrequently. Unfortunately, 79 percent of the children were treated to sweet drinks regularly.

In contrast, none of the East Indian mothers fed their babies solely on breast milk and the majority used bottle feeding exclusively. Frequency and amounts remain undetermined. Few of these children received orange juice every day. Some received it twice a week, some never; 20.3 percent of the infants were given semi-solid supplements, most commonly mashed white potato, together with crackers, vegetables, and occasionally rice or macaroni or even split peas, fish and eggs.

The East Indian children 1-5 years of age fared somewhat differently from the Negro youngsters. Most received skim milk from the clinics and mothers resorted to condensed milk only when the former was not available. Breast feeding, where and if started, seemed to last longer among Indians than among Africans. Sixty-eight percent of the children of this group received eggs, meat, poultry and fish at least twice a week, and vegetables (green or yellow) about once a week. Citrus fruits and mangoes were popular and eaten in quantities in season. Sixty-eight percent of the children were not given beef because of religious beliefs but they ate eggs and other meats twice weekly.

In conclusion, there is a short breast feeding spell, followed by a diet relying too heavily on starches and carbohydrates. Condensed milk seems to be a necessary evil because of its good storing qualities but it probably does little to improve the diet.

C. LEVELS OF NUTRITION [15] [21] [24]

The ICNND survey was made at 22 points in Trinidad and at three points in Tobago. These locations were considered representative of the seven regions in which they were distributed. As Table No. 8 shows, the caloric intake of the average population reached 96 percent of the requirements but in places like San Juan, Barataria, Morvant and El Soccoro only 71 percent of the requirements were met. This must have meant very low levels for a significant number of people. A similar situation was observed in 1946 by Platte visiting the same suburbs of Port of Spain. This is a good example of suburban malnutrition which, when present, is usually far worse than its rural counterpart. Other areas, like Sangre Grande, Biche and Rio Claro, were not very much better off in 1961 while isolated examples of very poor families were found in Tobago. The most typical family almost reached the daily requirement.

As indicated on page 442, two types of examinations were conducted by the ICNND investigators, one through the questionnaire method, the other through family visits during which the food intake was weighed. The differences are important, and almost uniformly the data obtained by visits indicated a lower intake than that compiled from questionnaires. While the average caloric intake according to the questionnaires was 1,954, according to the weighed intake it was only 1,502. In one instance, a very destitute family of 10 people was found in a poor suburban area where the average caloric intake was 666 calories (see

Table No. 8). Protein nutrition appear to be almost satisfactory, at least on the basis of recall questionnaires, with an average individual intake of 62 grams. Yet, as expected, this dropped to 45 grams in the vulnerable suburban areas where the caloric intake was low. Protein intakes were also computed on the basis of the nitrogen/creatinine excretion ratio. In no case did the children surveyed meet the protein allowance recommended by the U.S. National Academy of Sciences. Thirty-five percent of the 2-year-olds and 53 percent of the 3-year-olds seemed to consume less than 50 percent of the recommended allowances. The 4-6-year-olds did not do any better. (These allowances were met by children of California in a comparable study made by Morgan in 1959.) However, most of the Trinidadian children met the minimum requirements set by FAO, which of course are lower than recommended allowances. On the basis of visits, three of 19 families had a protein intake below requirements. Yet, total plasma protein values were always above the norm of 6.4 grams per 100 milliliters of plasma. In certain localities, such as Tunapuna, the average protein intake was as low as 43 grams. Obviously there is no hard and fast line concerning optimal allowances of dietary proteins but considerable doubts exist as a result of these observations on the adequacy of protein intakes among children in Trinidad. These doubts are further supported by the common prevalence of protein-calorie malnutrition syndromes in the country (see *Nutritional Disease Patterns*).

Thiamine nutrition offers the same uncertainty. While questionnaire replies could be interpreted as meaning acceptable levels of thiamine intake, weighed food yielded low amounts in four of the 19 families visited. Riboflavin consumption was low in all families seen at .76 milligrams per milliliter and was in agreement with the findings of the questionnaires. The ICNND investigators ascribed this deficiency to the high cost of milk in the islands. Vitamin A consumption was low at all locations but one. This can be explained by the preference for cheap cereals and by the lack of enthusiasm for green and yellow vegetables. Vitamin C values were also low but this was explained by the recent expiration of the mango season at the time of the survey and the fact that the orange season had not yet begun. Iron intakes were low even on the basis of the questionnaires, and of course much lower on the basis of weighed intakes. Calcium consumption varied widely in relation to family income and the ability to buy milk. Many values of plasma vitamin A were low, which surprised the investigators because the plasma values of carotene, the precursor of vitamin A, were almost uniformly high. In Trinidad and Tobago 6 percent of the people less than 15 years of age who were surveyed had vitamin A values of 10-20 micrograms per 100 milliliters. No satisfactory explanation can be given for the discrepancy, except perhaps that carotene levels were sustained by the daily intake of carotene-rich foods but that the stores of vitamin A in the liver had not yet been rebuilt through conversion of carotene into vitamin A. The assumption was that the stores of vitamin A were depleted during the previous season when no carotene or vitamin A had been ingested.

Comparing the level of nutrition of 1,197 individuals belonging to 193 Negro, Hindu and Moslem families (see Table No. 9), the ICNND investigators found the best caloric intake among the Hindus who also enjoyed the highest protein consumption, largely because of their milk, legume and cereal combination. Calcium consumption was low in all groups; iron was acceptable only among the Hindus and vitamin A only among the Moslems. Thiamine and riboflavin levels were low across the board and niacin acceptable in all groups; ascorbic acid consumption was on the low side but this is usually a seasonal shortage which changes with the arrival of the citrus fruit season.

The nutritional levels evidenced by the 1970 survey indicated that 16 percent of all households surveyed received below 2,000 calories per capita per day and 42 percent received more than 3,000 calories. The distribution of sources of calories was found to be as follows:

Sources of Calories in the Diets – Trinidad and Tobago, 1970

Food Categories	Percent	Total (Percent)
Cereals	39.5	
Roots	4.4	
Vegetables	1.4	
Fruits	2.9	
Sugar	11.1	
Total carbohydrates	59.3	59.3
Legumes	5.5	
Milk	10.0	
Eggs	0.9	
Meats	6.6	
Fish	1.3	
Total protein-rich foods	24.3	24.3
Fats	13.5	13.5
Miscellaneous	2.9	2.9
		100.0

Source: Government of Trinidad and Tobago, *Report on National Household Food Consumption Survey in Trinidad and Tobago 1970.*

On the average, 59.3 percent of the calories were provided by carbohydrates (more in the rural than in the urban areas), 24.3 percent came from protein-rich foods and 13.5 percent were derived from fat (also more marked in rural than in urban areas). Cereals were the most important source of protein (35 percent) followed by meats (17 percent) and milk (16.5 percent). However, the quality of the protein seemed low. The limiting amino acids were found to be sulphur-containing methionine and cystine. Although lysine was in highest amounts of all amino acids, it was not adequately provided by the diets. Neither was tryptophane. The protein/calorie ratio was inadequate everywhere and the ratio of animal protein to total protein was low. The main sources of calcium were milk and milk products (56 percent). Fresh vegetables and milk products provided most of the vitamin A. Milk and cereals provided 40 to 44 percent of the riboflavin while meat (26 percent) and cereals (34 percent) contributed the niacin.

These findings underscore the importance—in the overall health picture—of the percentage of households that are deficient in meeting requirements. Averages may not reveal existing malnutrition and even conceal the importance of certain pockets that just do not rise above the mathematical waterline, but nevertheless are of considerable public health importance.

In Nariva, Victoria and St. Patrick, 61 percent of the households did not meet their caloric requirements and 31 percent failed to meet their protein needs; 22 and 25 percent were short in calcium and iron daily allowance; 29 percent were low in vitamin A, 12 percent in vitamin C, 33 percent to 47 percent in thiamine, 51 percent in riboflavin and 44 percent in niacin. These deficiencies were more marked among middle and low income groups. In Tobago under- and malnutrition were evidenced at different income levels.

It is impossible to draw close comparisons both in diets and nutritional levels between the 1961 and the 1970 surveys. The two methods used were too different and both have built-in biases which prevent researchers from comparing results without running into misleading conclusions. Only general impressions can be drawn.

Both surveys indicate that although a wide variety of food is available, the nutritional values of the diets consumed by the different population groups are very uneven. In many cases they do not provide the basic minimum nutrient requirements. While the overall average caloric intake in 1961 was about 83.6 percent of requirements, in suburban areas such as Barataria, Morvant and San Juan there were conglomerations of people whose average intake dropped to 72 percent of requirements (see Table No. 8). In 1970 it was found that in urban areas only 57 percent of all households surveyed met their caloric requirements. This, of course, places some groups, and some individuals among these groups, especially children, far down the ladder. This was true both in 1961 and in 1970. With a population as diversified as that of Trinidad and Tobago, tradition, religious beliefs and, of course, income and opportunities create a wide range of diets, many of which are faulty on one count or another. There seems to be among certain groups an improvement in the quality of the diet between the two dates. But no definite conclusion can be drawn except that whatever improvement has taken place for some, too many people are still suffering from shortages of one nutrient or another. A percentage of the population has moved up on the income scale. On the other hand, this is balanced by the fact that the number of children whose mothers work has increased with a probable consequent rise in infant malnutrition.

IV. ADEQUACY OF FOOD RESOURCES [31] [15]

Table No. 10 gives a food balance sheet for Trinidad and Tobago based on FAO's projected needs for 1970 made in 1964. It was then estimated that the population should reach 1,120,000 by 1970, a figure which closely approximates reality. Wheat continues to be imported as none is grown on the island. Rice and corn also require strong supplements from external sources. Potatoes are the main imported root, and legumes are purchased abroad in increasing amounts in spite of the existence on the domestic market of an abundance of canned peas. Milk, meat and fish are not available in adequate quantities and the shortage is made good by imports. Table No. 9 suggests that 2,700 calories should be available to the average person, as well as 69.3 grams of protein and 74 grams of fat. But this rather high level of caloric intake includes 405 calories provided by sugar, a high level when compared to nonsugar calories. These resources would be satisfactory if equally distributed according to needs, but we know that this is not the case.

The table suggests a serious inadequacy in the indigenous food resources since Trinidad and Tobago imports 61 percent of the population's overall needs and about 50 percent of the calories. Further industrialization will bring about more transfers of the population to the cities and further discrepancies between wages and cost of foods. The solution is obviously to keep people in the rural areas by stimulating food production which, if successfully carried out, will bring wages and cost of living into closer balance. The Government of Trinidad and Tobago seems to be well aware of this situation.

V. NUTRITIONAL DISEASE PATTERNS [15] [24] [6] [5] [4] [2] [12] [20]

The relative status of nutrition in a given community can be measured by comparing heights and weights for a given age and sex with accepted standards corrected for local factors. Such studies were made in 1961 by the ICNND group. It was soon recognized that the mixed racial situation in Trinidad and Tobago influenced the results to a considerable extent. The Africans seemed to be heavier than the mixed individuals who, in turn, appeared to be heavier than the East Indians. On the whole, very few people were found to fall in the less than 70 percent of standard height and weight categories, which is the minimal accepted criterion for "normalcy," but a substantial number of individuals fall in the over 120 percent category, reflecting the unusual number of obese persons, especially among women, found in Trinidad and Tobago. Because significant deviations from standards have been observed, the conclusion can be inferred that important pockets of malnutrition do exist in Trinidad together with the inevitable nutritional diseases which accompany malnutrition.

Table No. 11 shows the percentage and medical significance of certain nutritional diseases in eight locations of Trinidad and Tobago. The data reveal the existence of vitamin B complex deficiencies, inadequate iodine intake and protein-calorie deficiencies which, if diagnosed on the basis of hair depigmentation, should be carefully weighed, given the mixed ethnic character of the population. These clinical findings confirm the biochemical results and are generally what they led us to expect. The most obvious symptoms were found in Port of Spain and revealed riboflavin deficiencies as indicated by nasolabial seborrhea, papillary atrophy of the tongue, and lesions of the lips with scars indicating cured anterior lesions. In certain seasons (particularly that during which the survey was made), the relatively high level of swollen gums in Port of Spain could be due to a shortage of ascorbic acid. This symptom does not seem to exist in other more rural areas where the consumption of citrus fruit and mangoes is probably more extensive and more frequent. Goiter is less prevalent in these islands than it is in other parts of the Caribbean or Central America. The highest level of prevalence seems to be in Tobago where about 19.9 percent of the population is affected.

The investigators made a detailed study of pregnant and lactating women and compared them with nonpregnant and nonlactating females of the same ages. They found higher prevalences of symptoms of riboflavin deficiency and goiter among the pregnant and lactating women, suggesting a shortage of these nutrients in body stores, preventing the women from coping with the additional stresses of their condition. The rate of incidence of diarrhea in children and of streptococcal and respiratory ailments in adults indicates a synergistic action between infection and malnutrition. It is hard to tell whether malnutrition increases the predisposition to infection or whether the frequency of infection, along with intestinal parasitism, causes malnutrition.

Protein-calorie malnutrition is present and has been reported by several investigators. Chopra, Tantiwongse et al., for example, have observed 22 cases of it at the second- and third-degree levels. They have explored the relationship between this condition and anemia. The children of their samples were of Negro, East Indian and mixed (Creole) origin between 1 month and 4 years of age. All showed retarded growth compared to established Boston standards which other Trinidad children do meet. Fifty-nine percent revealed diarrhea and enlargement of the liver, and 72 percent had abnormal pallor, apathy, marasmus and edema. Most of these children came from families with low incomes where 62 percent of the family's resources was spent on food without providing enough for an adequate diet. The majority of families did not grow their own food, and those who did cultivated such poor nutritive resources as manioc and turnips, although some also grew carrots, spinach, and corn, and cultivated fig trees. Milk was the preferred supplemental food. Three of these 22 children had not been breast-fed at all because the mothers thought bottle feeding was the best, the modern way of raising children, an attitude quite common in the developing world. The mixtures were always made of powdered milk and water in overly diluted proportions. At the average age of 4 months, starchy supplements such as arrowroot flour and infant cereals were given. Fruit juices and eggs were offered to some, meat to others. The average daily nutrient intake of these diets revealed an 89 percent caloric deficiency, 74.9 percent protein deficiency, 83.4 percent iron deficiency and 70.3 percent calcium deficiency. Among the vitamins, A seemed to be practically absent, niacin was 96 percent short, riboflavin 50.6 percent and ascorbic acid (vitamin C) 55.1 percent inadequate.

Many investigators find that anemia is usually not severe in kwashiorkor cases. Chopra, Perelta et al. found this to be the case in Trinidad. Yet, average values for hemoglobin showed 8.7 grams (instead of 12 grams) per 100 milliliters in 54.5 percent of the cases; all these anemias were of the macrocytic type. Normocytes were deficient in 31.8 percent and microcytes in 13.7 percent of the cases examined. The prevalence of anemia was low in the age group considered (0-6 months) as long as breast feeding was continued. However, among groups where, for cultural or economic reasons, breast feeding was discontinued early and not adequately replaced, anemia became an important problem. These findings confirmed those of the ICNND investigators who found that there was a high prevalence of anemia in Trinidad and Tobago. The ICNND findings showed that 8 percent of all male adults and nearly 40 percent of all female adults had values of less than 12 grams of hemoglobin per 100 milliliters. Pregnant and lactating women had hemoglobin concentrations in their blood well below those of nonpregnant and nonlactating women of the same age, showing again that their reserves did not support the additional stress created by pregnancy and lactation. Particularly low hemoglobin concentrations were found among children.

Chopra, Noe et al., further investigating the frequency of anemia in pregnant women, found that 34 percent of a sample of 535 women had hemoglobin values below 10 grams per 100 milliliters. These investigators also observed that anemia seems to increase as pregnancy develops, the highest level being reached during the eighth month. There also is a positive correlation between the number of pregnancies and the degree of anemia. Additional analysis by Chopra and Byam showed that more of the East Indians (38 percent) than of the Negroes or Creoles (26 percent) had values of hemoglobin below 10 grams per 100 milliliters and one speculates that the East Indians, being mostly rural, are more subject to contamination by hookworms and perhaps also by the malaria parasite prior to its eradication. The nutritional origin of this anemia may be questionable, although the consumption of iron, at 10.3 milligrams a day in 31.4 percent of the people, was well below standards. Habib, working at Trinidad

General Hospital, recorded 10 cases of megaloblastic anemia between 1959 and 1961, suggesting the possibility of folic acid deficiency somewhere in the metabolic process. All were Hindus, all were found to have low intakes of vitamin B_{12}, and all but one were lactovegetarians.

Several researchers, including the ICNND investigators, found a high prevalence of obesity among women in Trinidad and Tobago. McCarthy made a study in 1963 of 63 obese women and 26 controls. The results indicated low caloric intakes in both groups. No correlations were found between these caloric intakes and energy expenditures. Familial obesity was highly prevalent among the patients, and 66 percent of the subjects indicated that the years between 13 and 19 saw the beginning of their obesity. The investigator found a high level of acceptance of obesity as a normal condition, and noted that the patients all led monotonous existences with lack of intellectual and social contact. Other data revealed a high prevalence of anemia and of parasitic diseases, such as those caused by hookworm, ascarids and others, whose action combines with poor diets to worsen malnutrition.

The occurrence of dental caries is widespread, and the infinitesimal content of fluorine in local waters affords no protection against tooth decay. Periodontal disease is also reported to be highly prevalent, but in Trinidad it seems to be slightly less common in the cities than in the rural areas, perhaps because treatment of dental caries is more readily available at an earlier date.

Trinidad and Tobago is part of that extensive category of countries where malnutrition is preventable. It occurs in specific pockets, where the authorities are aware of its existence and want to eradicate it. The problem, however, it made more complex than elsewhere because of the racial and religious backgrounds of the population. The French, Spanish, Dutch and British have left their mark on the local food habits; Africans, East Indians and Chinese have brought their way of life; and mixtures of all these ingredients have occurred which have created a diversity of traditional patterns of living which, in turn, have influenced the pattern of disease. The various religions practiced in the islands, such as Christianity, Islam and Hinduism, have also shaped the way of life. For example, most East Indian Hindus remain in the countryside near their cattle, leaving the urban jobs open for Negroes. Perhaps more than elsewhere these differences have influenced the pattern of disease.

VI. CONCLUSIONS

Trinidad and Tobago is among the fortunate developing countries. In another chapter we stated that sugar was to the economy of the 18th century what oil has been to the economy of the 20th century. Trinidad and Tobago among all the Caribbean islands has had the benefit of both sugar and oil and a comfortable tourist trade besides. While the sugar industry suffers here as elsewhere from the current crisis, the impact is blunted by the availability of a marketable product, oil. No one need starve. Yet some do, mostly in the suburban shanty-towns. The danger for Trinidad is not of the kind that threatens other developing countries. There is no fear that funds to finance purchases of food abroad will not be available. The danger facing the country is that the number of jobs open in the industrial sector does not rise as fast as urban migration, and simultaneously that the number of jobs in the civil service and commerce, the so-called white collar jobs, do not increase as fast as does the number of young people leaving school. The result is an unavoidable concentration of job seekers in the cities, some of whom, the school leavers, would not soil their hands with earth or oil.

The cityward trend in Trinidad is a fact. Its causes are the same as elsewhere: inadequate size of rural holdings making food production insufficient to support life in the subsistence sector, and unrewarding on farms large enough to produce commercial surpluses; disaffection from village life; attraction to city life—hopes for excitement, wealth, power and comfort, etc. Its consequences are also the same as elsewhere: unreadiness of the towns and cities to absorb more immigrants; inability of the factories to absorb more manpower; unreadiness of the world markets to accept more industrial production; and competition from the more advanced countries. All this and more causes the shantytowns surrounding industrial cities, where many wait in squalor for the development of their country to catch up with their expectations. This is the nutritional danger one can fear for Trinidad and Tobago. The malnutrition in the suburbs of the cities is just as severe as rural malnutrition can be, but permanent, not just seasonal, and money is the most important element in its cure. In the rural areas, a good harvest can suddenly change the whole picture.

The national survey made by ICNND gives us a glimpse of the situation. It is in the areas around Port of Spain, in Barataria, Morvant and San Juan, that the most serious malnutrition is found among people who wait for a salary but have no land on which to grow food in the meantime, among those whose wages have not risen enough to meet the cost of imported foods and whose salaries cannot rise much more without causing the product they help create to price itself out of the world market. These are the nutritional problems Trinidad and Tobago has to face. They are no easier to solve than those arising in other islands where no oil is available.

BIBLIOGRAPHY

1. Barclay's Bank D.C.O. *Trinidad and Tobago*. London, Barclay's Bank, 1969.
2. Chopra, J.G. and Byam, N.T.A. "Anemia Survey in Trinidad and Tobago." *American Journal of Public Health*, 1968, 58, 1922-1936.

3. —————————————— and Gist, C.A. "Food Practices Among Trinidadian Children." *Journal of the American Dietetic Association*, 1966, 49, 497-501.

4. —————————————— , Noe, E., Matthew, J., Dhein, C., Rose, J., Cooperman, J. A. and Luhby, A.L. "Anemia in Pregnancy." American Journal of Public Health, 1967, 57 (5), 857-868.

5. —————————————— , Perelta, F., Villegas, N. and Everette, L. "Anemia in Lactation." *West Indian Medical Journal*, 1964, 13, 252-265.

6. —————————————— , Tantiwongse, P., Everette, L. and Villegas, N. "Anemia in Malnutrition." *The Journal of Tropical Pediatrics and African Child Health*, 1965, 11 (1), 18-24.

6a. *Commercial Fisheries Review*, 1968, 30 (10), 69.

6b. ——————————————, 1969, 31, (3), 50-51.

7. *Encyclopedia Britannica*. Chicago, William Benton, Publisher, 1970.

8. Food and Agriculture Organizations of the United Nations. *Report to the Governments of Guyana, Jamaica and Trinidad and Tobago. Industrial Production of Protein Foods for Infants and Young Children in the Caribbean—A Feasibility Study*. Nutrition Consultants Reports Series 15. Rome, FAO, 1970.

9. —————————————— . *Production Yearbook 1970*. Volume 24. Rome, FAO, 1971.

10. —————————————— . Trade Yearbook 1969. Volume 23. Rome, FAO, 1970.

11. Gonzalez, O. "Programme to Increase Protein Production in Trinidad." *Protein Foods for the Caribbean*. Kingston, Caribbean Food and Nutrition Institute, 1968.

12. Habib, G.G. "Nutritional Vitamin B_{12} Deficiency Among Hindus." *Tropical and Geographical Medicine*, 1964, 16, 206-215.

13. Inter-American Development Bank. *Eleventh Annual Report 1970*. Washington, D.C., IDB, 1971.

14. —————————————— . *Socio-Economic Progress in Latin America*. Washington, D.C., IDB, 1970.

15. Interdepartmental Committee on Nutrition for National Defense. *The West Indies Nutrition Survey*. Washington, D.C., U.S. Government Printing Office, 1962.

16. International Bank for Reconstruction and Development. *Statement of Loans June 30, 1971*. Washington, D.C., IBRD, 1971.

17. James, P.E. *Latin America*. Fourth Edition. New York, The Odyssey Press, 1969.

18. *Labor Developments Abroad*, 1968, 13 (9), 16-25.

19. —————————————— , 1971 16 (4 and 5), 79.

20. McCarthy, M.C. "A Study of the Nutritional and Other Environmental Factors Associated with Obesity Among Women in Trinidad." Cambridge, Massachusetts Institute of Technology, Mimeographed, 1963.

21. Morgan, A.F. *Nutritional Status, U.S.A.* Bulletin No. 769. California, Agricultural Experiment Station, 1959.

22. National Academy of Sciences (National Research Council). *Recommended Dietary Allowances.* Seventh Revised Edition, 1968. Washington, D.C., NAS, 1968.

23. Paxton, J. (ed.). *The Statesman's Yearbook 1970-1971.* New York, St. Martin's Press, 1970.

24. Trinidad and Tobago, Government of and Caribbean Food and Nutrition Institute. *Report on National Household Food Consumption Survey in Trinidad and Tobago, 1970.* St. Augustine (Trinidad), CFNI, 1971.

25. United Nations (Department of Economic and Social Affairs). *Demographic Yearbook 1969.* New York, UN, 1970.

26. United Nations Development Program. *Projects in the Special Fund Component As of 30 June 1971.* DP/SF/Reports Series B, No. 12. New York, UNDP, 1971.

27. United Nations Children's Fund. *Digest of Projects Aided by UNICEF in the Americas.* New York, UNICEF, 1969.

28. U.S. Agency for International Development. *A.I.D. Economic Data Book – Latin America.* Revised February 1970. Washington, D.C., AID, 1970.

29. U.S. Department of Agriculture (Economic Research Service). *Agriculture and Trade of the Caribbean Region.* ERS-Foreign 309. Washington, D.C., 1971.

30. _____ . *Agricultural Policies in the Western Hemisphere.* ERS-Foreign 36. Washington, D.C., U.S. Government Printing Office, 1967.

31. _____ . *Food Balances for 24 Countries of the Western Hemisphere Projected 1970.* Supplement 1 to *The World Food Budget, 1970.* Washington, D.C., USDA, 1964.

32. _____ (Foreign Agricultural Service). "Trinidad Agriculture." Port of Spain (American Embassy), Mimeographed, 1964.

33. U.S. Department of Labor (Bureau of Labor Statistics). *Labor Conditions in Trinidad and Tobago.* Labor Digest No. 57. Washington, D.C., 1964.

34. _____ . *Labor Law and Practice in Trinidad and Tobago.* BLS Report No. 319. Washington, D.C., U.S. Government Printing Office, 1967.

35. West, R.C. and Augelli, J.P. *Middle America: Its Lands and Peoples.* Englewood Cliffs (New Jersey), Prentice-Hall, Inc., 1966.

36. Williams, E. *From Columbus to Castro: The History of the Caribbean 1492-1969.* New York, Harper & Row, Publishers, 1970.

LIST OF TABLES

LIST OF MAPS

TABLE NO. 1

Population by Principal Cities and Counties –
Trinidad and Tobago, 1960-1970

Cities	1960	1970 (estimate)
Port of Spain	93,954	122,139
San Fernando	39,830	51,779
Arima	10,982	14,276
Counties		
St. George	256,478	333,419
Caroni	90,513	117,666
Nariva	17,226	22,392
Mayaro	6,080	7,904
St. Andrew	32,590	42,367
St. David	6,032	7,871
Victoria (without San Fernando)	132,721	172,437
St. Patrick	108,218	140,681
Tobago	33,333	43,332
	827,957	1,076,263

Source: After U.S. Department of Labor, *Labor Law and Practice in Trinidad and Tobago.*

TABLE NO. 2

Area and Production of Major Crops – Trinidad and Tobago, 1948-1970
(area in 1,000 hectares, production in 1,000 tons)

Crop	Annual Average 1948-52		1964		1966		1967		1968		1969		1970	
	A	P	A	P	A	P	A	P	A	P	A	P	A	P
Rice	7	18	6	11	6	10	6	10	6	10	6	10	6	10
Corn	2	4	2	3	2	3	2	3	2	3	2	3	2	3
Sweet potatoes and yams	3	18	2	15	2	15	2	18	2	18	2	18	2	18
Manioc	—	5	—	5	—	5	—	5	—	5	—	5	—	5
Sugarcane	34	1,441	33	2,570	33	2,330	32	2,185	36	2,468	36	2,485	35	2,254
Sugar (raw value)	—	151	—	229	—	204	—	247	—	244	—	221	—	256
Cocoa	—	7.9	—	5.3	—	4.2	—	6.1	—	4.7	—	6.0	—	6.0
Coffee	—	1.0	—	4.5	—	3.2	—	4.3	—	3.1	—	2.0	—	4.5
Grapefruit	—	26	—	36	—	24	—	18	—	16	—	16	—	18
Oranges and tangerines	—	9	—	14	—	14	—	9	—	11	—	11	—	11
Lemons, limes and others	—	4	—	2	—	2	—	2	—	2	—	2	—	2
Coconuts (million nuts)	—	129	—	113	—	110	—	110	—	110	—	113	—	—
Copra	—	15.9	—	13.2	—	13.0	—	13.0	—	13.0	—	13.0	—	13.0
Bananas	1	10	2	27	2	27	2	27	2	30	2	30	—	—

A=area
P=production

Source: Food and Agriculture Organization of the United Nations, *Production Yearbook 1970*.

TABLE NO. 3

Average Daily Food Consumption by Ethnic and Religious Groups
Trinidad and Tobago, 1961
(Grams per Person per Day)

Ethnic Group / Food Item	Negroes	East Indians			Trinidad	Tobago
		Hindus	Moslems	Others	Avg.*	Avg.**
No. of Persons	561	429	207	135	1,725	226
Food Item						
Cereals						
Bread	90.4	21.0	20.4	49.8	60.4	71.1
Rice	115.4	138.0	124.1	116.3	118.7	74.6
Flour	71.2	272.6	179.3	129.6	142.9	100.0
Legumes						
Peas, dry	11.0	35.3	17.5	24.4	19.6	2.6
Beans, dry	0.5	3.4	7.7	–	2.1	2.7
Lentils	1.2	–	–	–	1.1	2.2
Green and Yellow Vegetables						
Spinach and leafy greens	13.8	17.9	21.9	16.7	18.2	8.2
Beans, green	3.4	8.4	–	13.5	4.6	–
Carrots	0.2	0.1	2.2	1.7	0.3	0.6
Miscellaneous (cabbage, peppers, pumpkin, ochroes (okra), lettuce)	3.0	0.8	0.7	5.4	2.7	4.6
Other Vegetables						
Cucumbers	4.3	7.2	7.6	1.7	5.3	2.1
Eggplant	8.5	12.1	13.3	6.7	9.7	4.4
Onions	8.1	10.2	8.5	7.8	8.9	8.5
Tomatoes	16.2	19.4	13.6	21.9	18.3	4.2
Tubers and Roots						
Manioc	0.1	3.1	–	5.0	0.9	6.2
Potatoes	11.4	27.4	21.0	30.7	22.7	12.2

TABLE NO. 3 (continued)

Average Daily Food Consumption by Ethnic and Religious Groups
Trinidad and Tobago, 1961
(Grams per Person per Day)

| Ethnic Group | Negroes | East Indians | | | Trinidad | Tobago |
| | | Hindus | Moslems | Others | Avg.* | Avg.** |
No. of Persons	561	429	207	135	1,725	226
Potatoes, sweet	2.1	–	–	–	0.7	21.1
Taro (dasheen, eddoes, tannia)	1.6	5.3	–	0.3	2.3	16.2
Yams	8.5	–	–	–	1.8	4.6
Fruits						
Avocados	12.8	8.0	9.8	6.2	8.7	14.6
Bananas (green figs)	14.7	22.7	3.3	11.9	15.2	94.0
Bananas, ripe	5.4	3.7	–	–	3.6	8.0
Breadfruit	9.4	2.1	–	35.8	9.0	8.8
Citrus	1.0	3.8	–	0.8	1.9	2.3
Citrus, sweet, canned	25.7	9.0	14.0	7.4	18.2	23.4
Mangoes	11.4	9.1	18.1	0.8	8.6	12.4
Plantain	18.9	1.1	8.7	9.3	8.5	15.0
Miscellaneous fruit (plums, sweetsop, etc.)	0.8	0.5	–	10.0	1.0	–
Sugar	48.4	48.7	44.8	44.1	46.0	62.7
Meats						
Beef	16.5	4.2	13.1	3.4	10.5	25.4
Crabs	–	9.0	8.7	7.6	4.0	–
Fish, fresh	48.1	40.5	61.3	44.8	49.5	54.0
Fish, dried, salted	12.2	10.2	7.2	3.9	7.2	8.1
Fish, sardines, can	–	2.5	2.0	–	–	–
Goat, lamb	1.2	2.9	–	–	1.0	–
Liver	–	–	–	3.4	2.0	–
Pork, pigs feet, tails, etc.	7.6	–	–	3.4	–	2.3
Poultry	22.4	4.7	15.2	38.2	20.1	16.7
Miscellaneous (salami, bacon, manicou, etc.)	3.3	1.1	–	4.2	2.0	1.5

Milk Products						
Milk, condensed	14.9	9.7	7.1	18.4	13.1	24.9
Milk, evaporated	9.0	–	0.3	6.1	5.3	–
Milk, dried, whole	14.0	6.2	3.3	4.1	9.2	9.9
Milk, fresh	1.5	46.2	25.5	20.6	18.8	20.7
Milk, skim, dried	0.8	0.2	0.3	–	1.0	–
Cheese	5.5	0.7	0.5	4.6	3.6	6.4
	6.4	2.7	7.3	5.8	5.6	8.8
Eggs						
Fats and Oils						
Butter (and ghee)	11.3	3.6	6.9	7.2	8.6	11.3
Oil (coconut)	12.3	16.7	13.3	11.2	14.1	14.0
Other fats (margarine, etc.)	5.6	0.3	3.3	2.8	3.9	4.3
Miscellaneous						
Cocoa	2.5	1.6	2.6	3.4	2.4	2.3
Coconut	4.3	2.1	–	–	1.4	6.5
Chocolate	0.6	0.1	0.3	0.2	0.4	1.5
Coffee	0.2	0.1	0.3	–	0.2	–
Total	719.6	856.2	715.0	751.0	745.8	805.9

*Includes all ethnic groups and is average (unweighted) for 18 survey areas in Trinidad.

**Average for 2 survey areas in Tobago. No ethnic study as respondents were 95 percent Negro.

Source: Interdepartmental Committee on Nutrition for National Defense, *The West Indies Nutrition Survey.*

TABLE NO. 4

Monthly Income and Food Expense of Families Questioned in Nutrition Survey –
Trinidad and Tobago, 1961

Location	No. of Families	Average Monthly Family Income $	Monthly Food Cost per Person $	Food Cost as Percent of Income
Trinidad				
Port of Spain	34	109	10.5	51
Diego-Martin	16	80	6.5	59
San Juan	16	92	7.6	55
Barataria	8	57	5.8	57
St. Joseph	12	64	6.7	53
St. Augustine	10	74	7.5	68
Tunapuna	10	67	7.7	85
Arima	10	74	6.5	58
Sangre Grande	9	40	4.2	75
Couva	13	55	6.6	70
San Fernando	17	115	8.9	50
Princes Town	16	72	6.8	60
Moruga	6	45	5.0	60
Mayaro	11	35	6.1	82
Rio Claro	13	48	4.6	60
Siparia	15	73	5.8	58
Fyzabad	9	76	6.1	54
Point Fortin	11	82	10.3	46
Average of 18 Towns	236	70	6.9	61
Tobago				
Scarborough	15	67	8.5	57
Speyside-Charlotteville	15	40	5.3	70

Source: Interdepartmental Committee on Nutrition for National Defense, *The West Indies Nutrition Survey.*

TABLE NO. 5

Food and Agricultural Trade – Trinidad, 1961-1968

Item	Exports (in $1,000) 1961	Exports (in $1,000) 1968	Item	Imports (in $1,000) 1961	Imports (in $1,000) 1968
Cereal preparations	1,093	257	Live animals	155	540
Fresh fruit and nuts	951	421	Meat, fresh and frozen	2,979	2,042
Fruit and nuts, prepared	1,715	2,354	Poultry	1,787	39
Vegetables, fresh and dried	447	177	Other meat preparations	2,367	2,159
Sugar, raw and refined	24,644	22,758	Milk and milk products	2,797	1,312
Molasses	1,642	1,450	Milk, condensed and dry	3,150	3,735
Coffee	848	2,737	Butter	1,244	1,564
Cocoa	3,847	4,084	Cheese and curd	747	932
Spices	85	48	Eggs	253	640
Animal feed	157	549	Rice	4,085	4,286
Miscellaneous food preparations	313	1,413	Corn	623	2,356
Beverages	1,919	1,207	Wheat and flour	6,426	5,270
Animal and vegetable fats	389	417	Cereal preparations	884	904
Other agricultural exports	548	701	Fruits and vegetables	5,014	5,073
Total agricultural exports	38,598	38,573	Sugar, candy and honey	452	554
Total exports	346,162	465,071	Coffee, tea, spices	1,561	1,503
Agricultural export percentage	11	8	Animal feed	2,467	4,173
			Miscellaneous	1,993	1,976
			Beverages	2,708	1,295
			Animal and vegetable fats	1,677	1,948
			Other agricultural imports	3,626	5,162
			Total agricultural imports	46,995	47,463
			Total imports	340,634	428,237
			Agricultural import percentage	14	11

Source: U.S. Department of Agriculture (Economic Research Service), *Agriculture and Trade of the Caribbean Region.*

TABLE NO. 6

Average Daily Food Consumption by Food Groups –
Trinidad and Tobago, 1961 and 1970
(in grams per person per day)

	1961		1970
Item	Trinidad	Tobago	Trinidad and Tobago
Cereals	322.0	245.7	325
Legumes	22.8	7.5	43
Vegetables	68.0	32.6	171
Roots and tubers	28.4	60.3	161
Fruits	74.7	178.5	173
Sugar	46.0	62.7	86
Meats	35.6	45.9	103
Fish	96.3	62.1	40
Milk and products	50.9	61.9	115
Eggs	5.6	8.8	18
Fats and oils	26.6	29.6	50
Miscellaneous	4.4	10.3	67

Sources: Interdepartmental Committee on Nutrition for National Defense, *The West Indies Nutrition Survey.*

Government of Trinidad and Tobago, *Report on National Household Food Consumption Survey in Trinidad and Tobago 1970.*

TABLE NO. 7

Average Calculated Daily Nutrient Intake Per Person – Trinidad and Tobago, 1961
(Questionnaire Method)

Location	Port-of-Spain / Diego Martin	Barataria / El Socorro / Morvant / San Juan	St. Joseph / St. Augustine / Curepe / Tunapuna / Arima	Sangre Grande / Biche / Rio Claro	San Fernando / Princes Town / Couva	Mayaro / Moruga	Siparia / Fyzabad / Point Fortin	Speyside / Scarborough / Charlotteville	Average Nutrient Intake per Individual Trinidad and Tobago
	Trinidad							Tobago	
No. of Families	56	29	51	27	50	21	42	40	316
No. of Individuals	331	200	347	183	313	102	249	226	1,951
Calories	1,812	1,458	2,080	1,895	2,152	2,054	2,138	1,933	1,954
Calorie intake as percent of requirement	87	72	100	94	106	106	106	94	96
Percent of Calories from fats	26	23	21	13	18	24	18	25	21
Protein, g	63	49	64	57	66	65	72	58	62
Percent of protein as animal	53	48	36	28	31	49	41	52	42
Protein intake as percent of requirement	150	123	154	144	165	176	182	140	154
Carbohydrate, g	270	233	345	346	371	321	342	309	319
Fat, g	53	37	49	27	43	54	45	54	46
Calcium, mg	411	378	350	188	256	313	272	322	318
Iron, mg	9.6	5.5	7.7	7.3	8.7	6.7	12.2	6.4	8.3
Vitamin A, IU	4,343	3,583	2,949	2,791	2,684	2,172	6,400	2,460	3,536
Thiamine, mg*	0.86	0.54	0.79	0.76	0.83	0.72	0.83	0.60	0.76
Thiamine, mg/1,000 Calories*	0.47	0.37	0.38	0.40	0.39	0.35	0.39	0.31	0.39
Riboflavin, mg*	1.00	0.75	0.69	0.57	0.72	0.66	0.88	0.75	0.77
Niacin, mg*	12.2	7.2	10.6	10.0	10.7	10.9	12.4	8.6	10.5
Vitamin C, mg*	36	26	27	31	23	34	46	45	33

*Corrected for cooking losses.

Source: Interdepartmental Committee on Nutrition for National Defense, *West Indies Nutrition Survey.*

TABLE NO. 8

*Average Nutrient Intakes Calculated from Chemical Analyses of Family Diets,
Compared with Data Obtained Through Questionnaire Method – Trinidad and Tobago, 1961*

								Averages		
								For 19 Family Visits		Questionnaire
Location	Port-of-Spain / Diego Martin	Barataria / San Juan	St. Joseph / Tunapuna / Arima	Biche*	San Fernando / Couva	Siparia / Fyzabad*	Scarborough / Charlotteville	Chemical Composites	Calculated Intakes**	Ave. of 20 Areas
No. of Families	6	2	4	1	2	2	2	19	19	316
No. of Individuals	46	22	30	10	16	10	16	150	150	1,951
Calories	1,613	1,487	1,173	666	1,403	1,009	1,712	1,382	1,502	1,954
Calorie intake as percent of requirement								66	73	96
Protein, g	63	52	43	31	55	31	39	49	45	62
Protein intake as percent of requirement								111	102	154
Carbohydrate, g	212	236	208	124	243	166	175	204	240	319
Fat, g	55	36	14	5	12	25	35	32	41	46
Calcium, mg	558	324	294	149	584	195	338	398	360	318
Iron, mg	14.1	13.0	9.8	5.7	12.7	8.3	5.8	11.0	6.6	8.3
Vitamin A, IU	1,512	4,600	1,300	300	450	460	450	1,394	2,648	3,536
Thiamine, mg	0.55	0.87	0.46	0.46	0.53	0.36	0.50	0.53	0.63	0.76
Thiamine, mg/1,000 Calories								0.38	0.42	0.39
Riboflavin, mg	1.07	0.52	0.42	0.18	0.73	0.20	0.57	0.65	0.76	0.77
Niacin, mg	11.1	8.3	6.9	5.2	8.7	4.2	5.8	8.1	7.9	10.5
Vitamin C, mg	34	15	18	12	18	8	13	21	32	33

*Severe poverty cases included.

**"Recipe method."

Source: Interdepartmental Committee on Nutrition for National Defense, *The West Indies Nutrition Survey.*

TABLE NO. 9

*Average Per Capita Calculated Nutrient Intake for Negroes and
East Indians (Hindus and Moslems) — Trinidad, 1961
(Questionnaire Method)*

| | Negroes | East Indians | |
		Hindus	Moslems
No. of Families	111	56	26
No. of Individuals	561	429	207
Calories	1,912	2,325	1,979
Protein, g	62	79	66
Carbohydrate, g	286	427	325
Fat, g	57	41	43
Calcium, mg	350	264	213
Iron, mg	6.6	9.5	7.8
Vitamin A, IU	2,660	2,711	3,962
Thiamine, mg*	0.68	0.90	0.73
Riboflavin, mg*	0.83	0.81	0.73
Niacin, mg*	12.6	13.9	13.9
Vitamin C, mg*	33	32	32

*Corrected for cooking losses.

Source: Interdepartmental Committee on Nutrition for National Defense, *The West Indies Nutrition Survey.*

TABLE NO. 10

Adequacy of Food Resources – Trinidad and Tobago, Projected, 1970
Population: 1,120,000 (estimate)

Product	Supply					Nonfood use				Utilization			Supply for food Net				
						Seed					Ex-trac-		Per	Per capita			
						and		Indus-		Total	tion		year	Per day			
	Pro-duction	Im-ports	Ex-ports	Chan-ges in stocks	Total supply	waste	Feed	trial	Total	gross	rate	Total	Kilo-grams	Calo-ries	pro-tein	Grams fat
	1,000 tons	1,000 tons	1,000 tons	1,000 tons	1,000 tons	1,000 tons	1,000 tons	1,000 tons	1,000 tons	1,000 tons	Per-cent	1,000 tons	Kilo-grams	Calo-ries	Grams tein	Grams fat
Wheat	–	55	–	–	55	–	–	–	–	55	72	40	35.7	356	12.4	1.1
Flour	–	40	–	–	40	–	–	–	–	40	–	40	35.7	356	12.4	1.1
Corn	8	30	–	–	38	–	36	–	36	2	90	2	1.3	13	.3	.1
Rice	20	53	–	–	73	3	2	–	5	68	63	43	38.0	375	6.9	.7
Other cereal prod.	–	3	–	–	3	–	–	–	–	3	–	3	2.8	28	.6	.1
Total cereals													113.5	1,128	32.6	3.1
Sugar: centrifugal	318	–	272	–	46	–	–	–	–	46	93.5	43	38.2	405	–	–
Potatoes	–	17	–	–	17	–	–	–	–	17	–	17	15.0	29	.7	–
Sweetpotatoes	20	5	–	–	25	2	–	–	2	23	–	23	20.5	53	.8	.1
Cassava	6	–	–	–	6	–	–	–	–	6	–	6	5.2	16	.2	–
Pulses	7	9	–	–	16	–	–	–	–	16	–	16	14.2	136	8.2	1.6
Other vegetables	52	9	–	–	61	3	–	–	3	58	–	58	51.8	65	1.9	.3
Bananas	38	2	3	–	37	5	–	–	5	32	–	32	28.6	56	.6	.2
Other fruit	73	9	35	–	47	8	–	–	8	39	–	39	34.8	42	.5	.5
Cacao	11	–	9	–	2	–	–	–	–	2	88.5	2	1.5	14	.3	1.0

Beef	3	6	—	—	—	—	—	9	9	8.0	48	3.3	3.7
Other meat	10	10	—	—	—	—	—	20	20	17.9	126	5.6	11.2
Total meat										25.9	174	8.9	14.9
Fish	6	9	—	—	—	—	—	15	15	13.5	23	3.2	1.0
Vegetable oils	9	6	—	—	—	—	—	15	15	13.7	332	—	37.5
Butter	—	4	—	—	—	—	—	4	4	3.3	65	.1	7.3
Total fats										27.0	397	.1	44.8
Whole milk	25	—	—	—	—	—	—	25	25	22.3	38	2.1	2.0
Dried milk	—	6	—	—	—	—	—	6	6	5.3	52	5.2	.1
Canned milk	—	12	—	—	—	—	—	12	12	10.7	41	2.1	2.3
Cheese	—	2	—	—	—	—	—	2	2	1.5	12	.7	1.0
Total milk and cheese											143	10.1	5.4
Eggs	4	—	—	—	—	—	—	4	4	4.0	16	1.2	1.1
Total consumption											2,700	69.3	74.0

Source: U.S. Department of Agriculture (Economic Research Service), *Food Balances for 25 Countries of the Western Hemisphere Projected 1970.*

TABLE NO. 11

Clinical Findings – Trinidad and Tobago, 1961

Symptoms	Port of Spain	San Juan	St. Joseph	Sangre Grande	Couva	Moruga	Siparia	Tobago Scarborough	Total or Average
No. of cases examined	437	471	963	358	643	273	527	447	4,119
					Percent of Prevalence				
Nasolabial seborrhea	8.2	3.4	7.6	3.6	3.9	4.8	7.6	11.8	6.4
Lip lesions	.9	1.3	1.0	.8	1.9	.7	.2	.4	.8
Lip scars	3.4	3.8	10.8	2.5	8.7	1.8	4.0	6.0	6.5
Swollen gums	6.0	1.1	.8	—	.8	.7	1.1	—	1.3
Slight papillary atrophy of the tongue	12.8	.8	.9	—	.3	—	.4	—	1.8
Moderate to severe papillary atrophy of the tongue	.2	.2	—	.6	—	—	.2	—	.1
Goiter	3.9	6.6	5.1	3.9	7.3	3.3	13.7	19.9	8.0
Follicular hyperkeratosis	.8	1.8	.3	.6	—	—	—	—	.4
Bilateral edema	2.1	.4	.2	.6	.2	.4	.2	2.0	.5
Bilateral loss of ankle jerks	2.5	.6	1.3	1.4	1.4	3.7	.9	.2	1.5
Depigmentation of hair	2.1	1.2	1.1	—	—	.4	—	.4	.6

Source: Interdepartmental Committee on Nutrition for National Defense, *The West Indies Nutrition Survey.*

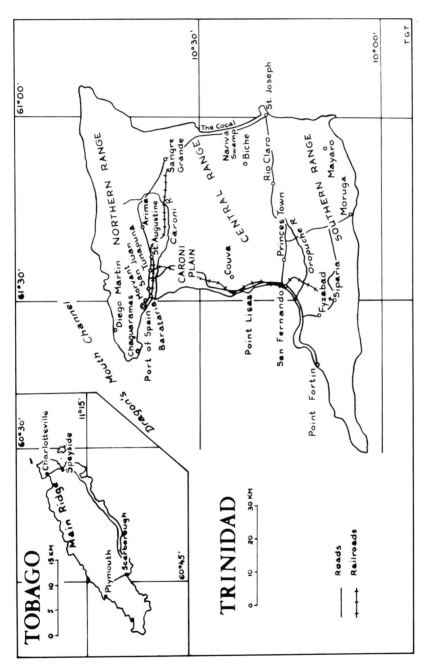

MAP NO. 1.

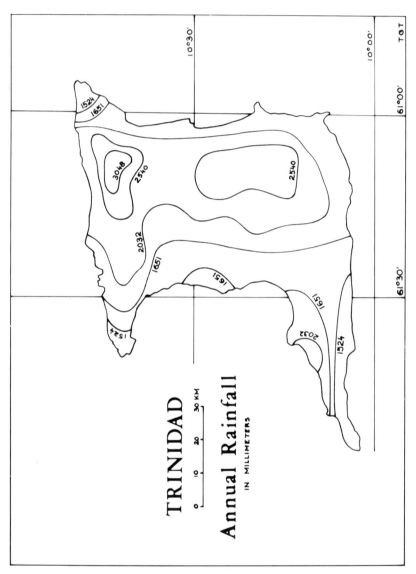

TRINIDAD

Annual Rainfall
IN MILLIMETERS

MAP NO. 2.

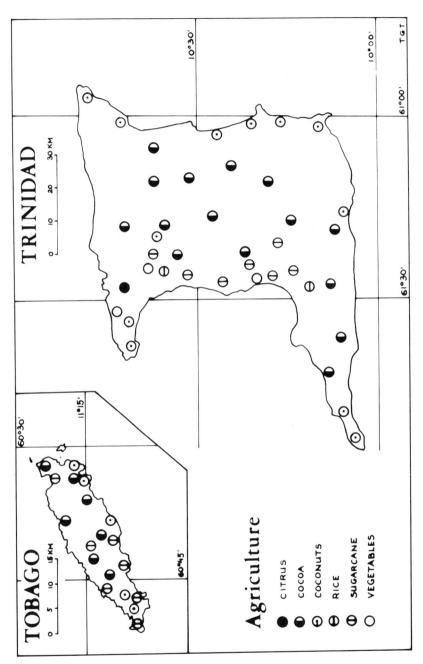

MAP NO. 3.

INDEX

477

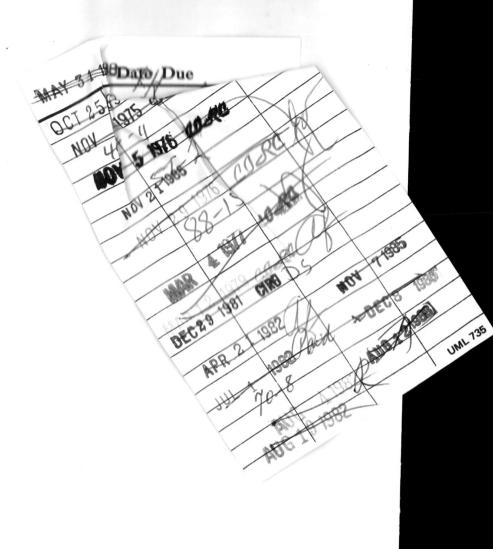